Rhetoric of a Global Epidemic

Rhetoric of a Global Epidemic

Transcultural Communication about **SARS**

Huiling Ding

Southern Illinois University Press / Carbondale

Library of Congress Cataloging-in-Publication Data
Ding, Huiling.
Rhetoric of a global epidemic : transcultural communication about
SARS / Huiling Ding.
    pages cm
Includes bibliographical references and index.
ISBN-13: 978-0-8093-3319-6 (pbk.)
ISBN-10: 0-8093-3319-8 (paperback)
ISBN-13: 978-0-8093-3320-2 (ebook)
1. SARS (Disease) 2. Communication in public health. 3. World
health—Forecasting. 4. Epidemics—Prevention. I. Title.
RA644.S17D56 2014
362.1962—dc23   2013032383

Contents

Acknowledgments

A book is never written alone. I am fortunate to have mentors all along the way when working on this book. I thank first and foremost Patricia Sullivan for guiding me to think seriously about research methodologies and for inspiring me to undertake challenging work. Michael Salvo, Thomas Rickert, and David Blakesley helped me tremendously in the development of this project. In addition, Steven Katz and Blake Scott read my manuscript and offered extremely insightful criticisms for the book. My dear friends Jingfang Ren, Amy Ferdinandt Stolley, Tarez Samra Graban, Nicole Livengood, and Xiaoye You helped me to sharpen my arguments in initial drafts by raising difficult questions.

I also benefited greatly from scholarly conversations with my colleagues at Clemson University. A number of colleagues read parts of the manuscript: Lee Morrissey, Michelle Martin, Joe Sample, Teddi Fishman, Cameron Bushnell, Brian McGrath, Kimberly Manganelli, and Shannon Walter, among others. My research assistants Ali Ferguson, Carly Finseth, Elizabeth Pitts, and Beth Wilkerson copyedited the manuscript at different stages.

Part of the research for this book has been generously supported by a yearlong Purdue Research Fund in 2006–7 and a summer fellowship and a travel grant from Clemson University in 2008.

I especially thank Karl Kageff, editor-in-chief, Southern Illinois University Press, for his patient guidance, good humor, and encouragement. My reviewers, one of whom was Blake Scott, offered invaluable feedback. Blake's work on both HIV testing and transnational pharmaceutical responses to bioterrorism inspired my work throughout the revisions.

Finally, I thank my family members for their boundless love. My parents, Peican Ding and Jinlan Xiao, collected numerous materials in China about SARS for me. My in-laws, Hongxiao Zhang and Shennian Jiang, supported my work with encouragement and confidence. My husband, Xun Zhang, always cheers me up with his humor and support. My daughter, Vivian, patiently waits for mommy to "return from work at home" through my long writing hours before lighting up my days with her smiles and delightful talk.

Portions of this book were previously published. I am grateful to the following publisher and journals for allowing me to reprint them here: Taylor & Francis Ltd., http://www.informaworld.com, "Rhetorics of Alternative Media in an Emerging Epidemic: SARS, Censorship, and Participatory Risk Communication," *Technical Communication Quarterly* 18.4 (2009): 327–50; "New Directions in Intercultural Professional Communication," *Technical Communication Quarterly* 22.1 (2013): 1–9; and "Transcultural Risk Communication and Viral Discourses: Grassroots Movements to Manage Global Risks of H1N1 Flu Pandemic," *Technical Communication Quarterly* 22.2 (2013): 126–49.

Rhetoric of a Global Epidemic

Introduction: Transcultural Flows, Communication, and Rhetorics during a Global Epidemic

Somewhere in the world the wrong pig met up with the wrong bat.
—A memorable line from *Contagion*

Imagine that you go to bed early after a long day at work. After midnight, you are awakened by a phone call from a friend who lives far away. He sounds frantic: "People are dying. The epidemic is spreading. There are no masks left here, and online orders won't arrive for at least two weeks."

You're tired and immediately think he must be overreacting. Rumors have been flying on the Internet. But for the sake of politeness, you promise to buy him some masks the next morning. Calmer now, he warns you to stay away from crowds. His suggestions seem trivial: washing your hands often, taking herbal medicines to boost immunity, and avoiding travel.

You head to the drugstore the next day after a few early-morning meetings. Panicked early-bird shoppers have cleared the shelves of masks. Soon you find out from various cashiers that local TV stations have reported more suspected and confirmed cases. You try to order online, but masks are out of stock. Realizing the severity of the situation, you call friends in other parts of the country to warn them. You urge them to buy masks, to send you some, and to get prepared for the quickly spreading epidemic. Then you send text messages or mass e-mails to alert other contacts to the situation.

You may or may not receive any masks during the entire outbreak.

Sound familiar? If you happened to be in or near the epicenters in the first two global epidemics of the new millennium, you may, like me, have been both the panic shopper and the friend who tries but fails to find masks.

During the global epidemics of severe acute respiratory syndrome (SARS) in 2003, I frantically sought masks in a small college town in Illinois after China officially admitted to having underreported the spread of disease. Like hundreds of other Asian students, I wanted to send much-wanted supplies to

1

friends and relatives back in China. During the H1N1 flu pandemic in 2009, I went through the same experience again, now in another college town in South Carolina. The only difference is that with a spouse working at a medical institution and a newborn child at home, I was now worried about my own household. Friends around the country reported the same experience: they drove to the local CVS or Walgreens but failed to find any masks.

Widespread panic buying accompanied both emerging epidemics, but fatality rates and treatment differed widely: unlike SARS, H1N1 was soon found to be curable with Tamiflu.[1] So whereas mass panic continued for months in SARS-affected countries and regions, the panic that H1N1 inspired was short-lived; by the end of 2009, it received no more media coverage than other types of seasonal flu.

After the first human case of H1N1 flu was diagnosed on April 13, 2009, the epidemic quickly spread across North America and Europe along heavily treaded routes of international travel. Reports of a possible pandemic flooded the global media within a couple of weeks. Many discussed global emergency-response systems, travel advice, public health preparedness, and global risk management. Comparisons with SARS were frequently made in the hopes that lessons learned from one epidemic would help to manage the risks associated with another. Reports were often highly emotional, using terms such as "anxiety," "disruption," "havoc," "scare," "scar," "panic," "shame," "haunting ghosts," "looming biological nightmare," and "deadly killer." Journalists used military metaphors, that is, "combat," "battle," "contain," "quarantine," and "closure," to stress the need for an immediate, calculated response. Global media also paid attention to the viral nature not only of both epidemics but also of the discourses surrounding them. A *Toronto Star* editorial claims

> media coverage of swine flu [. . .] went viral quicker than the flu itself. As one US pundit put it: "if as many people had swine flu as those that [were] covering it, then it would be a pandemic to reckon with." ("When Coverage Goes Viral" IN06)

Contagion, a 2011 Steven Soderbergh thriller, dramatizes the horrors of emerging global epidemics at a scale rivaling that of the 1918 Spanish flu. Many of its scenes bear disturbing resemblance to the first two epidemics of the twenty-first century: a mysterious start in the world's largest metropolis; rapid spread through familiar routines, such as handshakes and money exchanges; heightened confusion, helplessness, outrage, mass panic, and social distancing; long lines for antibiotics and vaccinations; vicious rumor-mongering via guerrilla media; and the heroic efforts of those fighting the epidemic, from both within and outside the Centers for Disease Control and Prevention (CDC). Other scenes show viruses jumping species, overcrowded quarantine shelters, the disproportionate toll taken on Third World poor, the epidemic's exponential spread, and its capacity not only to kill millions but also to dissolve civil society (Denby; Jones). To some extent, *Contagion* tells a story of a pandemic yet to come, a pandemic worse than SARS.

As the first global epidemic in this millennium, SARS taught the world invaluable lessons. Numerous studies have been published about the economic, medical, historical, public health, and communication aspects of the crisis, which will certainly help to improve our ability to better cope with future pandemics (see Kleinman and Watson; Duffin and Sweetman; Powers and Xiao; and *SARS Investigation*). SARS also brought about profound changes in public health legislation and infrastructure in many affected countries, particularly those in Asia. Overall, SARS occupies a key position in our understanding about transcultural risk management of global epidemics.

This book adds to existing conversations by focusing on the intersections among economic, cultural, and grassroots globalization, risk politics, digital media, and transcultural rhetoric. Its central questions are, How did forces of globalization transform these two limited, regional outbreaks into global epidemics affecting over thirty countries and regions, and how did the world communicate about such quickly spreading novel epidemics, as in the case of SARS? Taking SARS as a historical case, the current volume explores how various cultures and transcultural communities make sense of and communicate about emerging global epidemics. It also investigates the way knowledge production and legitimation operate in global epidemics, the roles that professionals and professional communicators play in the communication processes, points of contention within these processes, and possible entry points for ethical and civic intervention.

Patient Zero and Medicalized Globalization

On February 21, 2003, sixty-four-year-old nephrologist Dr. Liu Jianlun checked into a room on the ninth floor of the Metropole Hotel in Hong Kong to attend a family wedding. The next day he became ill and walked five minutes from the hotel to the Kwong Wah Hospital. During his stay at the hospital, he did not respond to antiviral treatments commonly used for pneumonia, and his situation quickly deteriorated. He told a group of physicians, who were appalled and dumbfounded about his mysterious pneumonia, about the local outbreaks of a so-called atypical pneumonia in the neighboring Guangdong Province and advised them, "Lock me up. Don't touch me. I have contracted a very virulent disease" (C. Taylor, "China"). In addition, he recommended that his medical care workers wear protective gloves, masks, and gowns. He died on March 4, 2003. Within a month of his arrival, seventy medical staff and seventeen medical students at the hospital were infected.

Much later, after SARS had spread to various parts of the world, Liu was epidemiologically identified as the "Patient Zero" at the center of a global health emergency. Even though he was not the first SARS patient in mainland China or Hong Kong, Liu attracted a lot of epidemiological attention because he was constructed not only as the "face and human form" of the then-unknown virus (Wald 226) but also as the embodiment of the crucial linkage between him and those who got infected and carried the deadly virus to other parts of the world. In scientific and popular accounts, the contact he made with other guests staying on the same floor was seen as the tipping point in which a previously regionally confined epidemic quickly developed into a massive global outbreak. In addition, he came to represent one of the largest, most at risk, and most stigmatized populations of the SARS epidemic: the medical care workers.

Before his deadly trip to Hong Kong, Liu worked as a physician and professor of nephrology at Sun Yet-sen Memorial Hospital in Guangzhou, about seventy-five miles northwest of Hong Kong. Liu's occupations put him in contact with over 200 atypical pneumonia patients (Chen and Jia). A SARS superspreading event took place in the same hospital in late January, with a seafood salesman causing 130 primary and secondary infections, of which 106 were hospital-acquired cases (Bloom 701). The salesman became known as "Du Wang," or the "Poison King," whose coughs worked like "biological bombs," infecting and killing many hospital staff (C. Taylor, "China"). It is highly likely that Liu was among these infected staff.

Reincarnated as Patient Zero in later accounts of the epidemic, Liu metamorphosed into the familiar human-virus hybrid who unknowingly yet carelessly transmitted the mysterious virus to international travelers staying in the same Hong Kong hotel and later to the medical care workers who tried to treat his conditions. He becomes a key figure in the analysis of the cultural logic of the SARS outbreak and its accompanying narratives. Particular emphasis was put on the medicalized globalization as demonstrated in the rapid and global spread of SARS during Liu's one-night stay at the hotel. Constructed as a viral protagonist, Liu embodied "the apocalyptic scenarios of infections emerging elsewhere, increasingly in Asia" (Wald 217). A later study claims that over half of the SARS infections all over the world can be directly traced to Liu through chains of transmission, which offers a "dramatic illustration of the impact of modern air travel on the spread of an emerging human infection" (Poon, Guan, Nicholls, Yuen, and Peiris 663).

The March 28 update on SARS in the CDC *Morbidity and Mortality Weekly Report* (*MMWR*) contains a figure that visually illustrates how Liu as the index patient triggered a global outbreak (see fig. i.1). Placed near the center of the figure and identified as A in Hotel M Hong Kong, Liu is portrayed as the index patient who traveled from Guangdong (note the use of solid black for both A and Guangdong) to Hong Kong and stayed at Hotel M for one night on February 21 before he got "admitted to hospital on February 22 and died the next day" (Centers, "Update" 242). Via the air, Liu infected at least sixteen guests, tourists, and visitors staying in the same hotel. These infected people traveled back to Toronto, Singapore, and Hanoi or checked into hospitals in Hong Kong, carrying the fatal virus with them. Within a couple of weeks, outbreaks with different degrees of severity were seen in Hong Kong, Canada, Singapore, and Vietnam. According to the *MMWR* report,

> epidemiologic investigations have identified patients from this cluster as index patients in subsequent clusters in Hong Kong and other areas. Patient B is the index patient for the outbreak in Hanoi involving 59 HCWs and close contacts and also is linked to one case in Thailand. Patients C, D, and E are associated with 70 cases in Singapore and three cases in Germany. Patient F is linked with a cluster of 16 other cases in Toronto. (Centers, "Update" 242)

The report brings "the variable of person, place, and time into focus" by incarnating Liu as the epidemiological index as well as the "archetypal carrier" of SARS (Wald 229). He treated atypical pneumonia patients in Guangzhou in early February and began demonstrating symptoms on February 15. Figure i.1 emphasizes this geographical designation by coding both him and Guangdong, where he had traveled from, in solid black. Circles depict contaminated locations, such as hotel and hospitals in Hong Kong, and infected travelers are represented by squares on the circumference of the hotel circle.

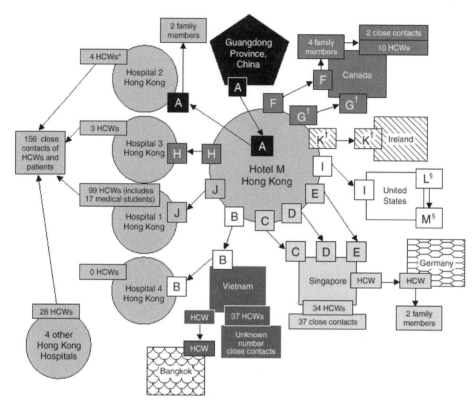

Figure i.1. Chain of transmission among guests at Hotel M–Hong Kong, 2003. * *HCWs*, Health-care workers. † All guests except G and K stayed on the ninth floor of the hotel. Guest G stayed on the fourteenth floor, and guest K stayed on the eleventh floor. § Guests L and M (spouses) were not at Hotel M during the same time as index guest A but were at the hotel during the same time as guests G, H, and I, who were ill during this period. From Centers for Disease Control and Prevention, "Update: Outbreak of Severe Acute Respiratory Syndrome—Worldwide, 2003," *MMWR* 52.12 (2003): 241–48

Juxtaposing a spatial dimension with the temporal dimension of the event, figure i.1 groups those contracting SARS according to their subsequent movement, that is, visiting various hospitals in Hong Kong where they initiated superspreading events and traveling to other destinations in Vietnam, Singapore, Canada, the United States, Germany, or Ireland. Fiona Fleck, news editor for *Bulletin of the World Health Organization*, laments the rapid speed by which "those travelers fanned out across the world, triggering [explosive] outbreaks in Singapore, Toronto in Canada, and Hanoi in Viet Nam as well as in Hong Kong itself."

Excluded from this figure are earlier SARS cases and the temporal and spatial dimensions of outbreaks in various countries. This strategic exclusion helps to metamorphose Patient Zero from "an epidemiological index case" to the "index case and source of" SARS outbreaks in multiple countries (Wald 229). As Priscilla Wald points out, the scientific and popular construction of Gaetan Dugas as Patient Zero of "North American AIDS" lacks scientific validity because the construction fails to distinguish between "the epidemiological index and the index case of an epidemic" (230). The same can be said about depictions of Liu: even without the superspreading event in Hotel M, SARS would still have circulated to numerous countries because many other international travelers were infected. As Panem says, "anyone knowledgeable knows that to pin a global epidemic on the action of a single individual is absurd" (1040).

Globalization of SARS?

The pieces of the mysterious pneumonia puzzle were put together in late March and early April 2003 when the World Health Organization (WHO) figured out that the epidemic had begun in November 2002 in Guangdong Province. China sent WHO a report in February 2003 that offered an update about the outbreak and claimed that it was "under control." In mid-February, a false alarm of an avian flu outbreak was issued when a Hong Kong resident died of pneumonia and his son was hospitalized because of pneumonia. H5N1 virus was identified in the tissues gathered from both cases. WHO issued a pandemic-flu alert soon afterward, which diverted media attention but was later found unnecessary.

While SARS silently spread to Beijing, Hong Kong, Toronto, and other parts of the world in March 2003, China underwent a top-level power transition. The new fourth generation of leaders, Hu Jintao, the president of China and secretary of the Communist Party (CPC), and Wen Jiabao, China's premier, succeeded President Jiang Zemin and Premier Zhu Rongji after the convention of the National People's Congress (NPC) in Beijing around the same time. The transition was not smooth—which was unsurprising given that since the foundation of the People's Republic of China, the party has "repeatedly failed to execute orderly successions" (Kahn, "Hu Takes Over" 1). Jiang retained his position as chief of the military while Hu commanded only the state and the party, a direct contradiction of Mao Zedong's famous preaching "The party directs the gun." With the new president coexisting with his predecessor, China's disjointed power distribution left the country open to confusion. In addition, Jiang "retained his enormous political muscle" not only by keeping "allies in key positions" in the politburo but also by using his allies to restrict coverage of sensitive topics, including SARS and corruption scandals, in the government-controlled press (Kahn, "Analysts See Tension" A1). Jiang would not give up his position as China's military chief until nineteen months later, on September 19, 2004, when the party completed the first orderly transfer of power in its history.

Beijing witnessed its first SARS outbreak when a businesswoman who had contracted SARS during a trip to Guangdong infected her family and medical workers in the Shanxi Province and was then transferred to a Beijing military hospital in early March. On March 10, 2003, the Ministry of Health (MOH) in China asked WHO for technical support to investigate the cause of the atypical pneumonia outbreak in Guangdong. Also in March 2003, WHO received numerous alarming reports about a mysterious and highly contagious pneumonia in Vietnam, Hong Kong, and Guangdong. For the first time in its fifty-five-year history, WHO issued an unusual global alert on March 12, warning national health departments of the new threat. On March 15, WHO issued another travel alert recommending screening measures to control the spread of the epidemic. On March 18, in response to the widespread suspicion of China as the origin of the new epidemic, WHO announced that it remained "undetermined whether an outbreak of atypical pneumonia in southern China [was] related to the current outbreaks" ("Update 3").

In its March 18 SARS update, WHO announced that SARS was transmitted via direct and close contact ("Update 3"). This theory, however, could not explain a massive outbreak that took place in the Amoy Gardens apartment blocks in Hong Kong. Later research told a story reminiscent of Typhoid Mary: many SARS patients excreted coronavirus in their stool (Peiris, Lai, Poon, et al.). The dangerous yet unsuspected bodily discharge could result in the dissolution of the border between the healthy and the sick and in the "careless" ingestion of others' bodily waste due to a faulty sewage system in the building (Wald 73). Environmental contamination, in this case, a faulty sewage system, caused the infection of 321 people in that one building by April 15 (Parry). Further investigation found that "the index patient in this outbreak was a 33-year-old" visitor who developed SARS symptoms on March 14. He had "diarrhea and used the toilet there" on March 19 (Hung 374). Later, "as many as two-thirds of the patients in the Amoy Gardens outbreak had diarrhea," which caused the discharge of "a very substantial virus load" into the faulty sewerage and resulted in the massive outbreak there (Hung 375). This incident caused immense uncertainty and fear about the little-known epidemic, and local media and grassroots forces started to employ different tools to intervene in the risk management processes. One instance widely reported in transnational media was the civilian website of sosick.org, which provided location-specific information about infected SARS buildings after Hong Kong's Department of Health repeatedly rejected public requests for such risk information.

China started its belated, full-scale anti-SARS campaign after WHO issued a travel advisory on April 2, 2003, recommending the postponement of nonessential travel to Hong Kong and Guangdong Province. Jiang's protégé Zhang Wenkang, the health minister, insisted "SARS was under control" from March to mid-April. He and Meng Xuenong, the Beijing mayor, were fired on April 20 because of their failure to effectively contain SARS and communicate about SARS in Beijing. This unusual firing of high officials symbolized Hu's and Wen's dramatic breaks from Jiang's cover-up policies and media control. It also served as the turning point at which both the party-oriented and market-oriented newspapers started to cover not only SARS but also WHO's inspection trips in a transparent manner (Huang and Hao).

As many studies point out, SARS posed the first major challenge for China's new generation of leaders, threatening national stability as well as economic development and the legitimacy of Hu and Wen (Eisenman; Kahn, "Analysts See Tension"; Lin; X. Lu, "Construction of Nationalism"). Suffering from corruption and tight restrictions of political freedom, Beijing relies on economic development and party-centric nationalism to maintain social stability. Unfortunately, SARS "hit both the investment and production side of the economy" (Eisenman). The "politics of silence" in play until April not only produced mass panic and mounting international criticism for China but also the medicalized globalization of SARS (C. Taylor, "China"). Hu and Wen took rigorous measures to ensure transparent case reporting and sufficient material support for SARS-related research and medical facilities. With full media coverage, the country launched a people's war against SARS. Hero narratives were constructed about patriotic medical care workers risking their lives to save patients; governmental institutions' full engagement in anti-SARS campaigns were highlighted; and community participation and personal sacrifices were enlisted. With national commitment and mass mobilization in place, Beijing was removed on June 24 from both WHO's travel advisory and the list of areas with recent, local transmission. On July 5, 2003, WHO declared that SARS had been contained throughout the world.

As the first deadly global epidemic in the twenty-first century, SARS had spread to twenty-nine countries and three regions by August 2003, with a cumulative total of 8,422 cases and 916 deaths. According to the WHO cumulative SARS case report issued on August 15, the total numbers of SARS cases were 5,327 for mainland China, 1,755 for Hong Kong, and 251 for Canada. A heavy economic toll follows the trace of global epidemics. SARS caused "a total loss of US$25.3 billion to China's economy" (Hai, Zhao, Wang, and Hou 57) and "cost the Canadian economy $519 million in 2003 alone and $722 million between 2003 and 2006" ("Economic Impact"). As WHO's "World Health Report for 2003" points out,

> SARS caused widespread social disruption and economic losses. Schools, hospitals, and some borders were closed and thousands of people were placed in quarantine. International travel to affected areas fell sharply by 50%–70%. Hotel occupancy dropped by more than 60%. (78)

A *Lancet* editorial considers SARS as a "model" emerging epidemic for the twenty-first century that "demonstrates how changes in society, the environment, and our increasing global interconnectedness converge to enhance the likelihood of disease emergence" ("Reflections on SARS" 651). The 2004 avian flu outbreak and the 2009 H1N1 flu pandemic further demonstrate the rapid speed with which any regional epidemic may develop into a global public health crisis. Factors contributing to such quick dissemination of novel viruses include the heavy intercontinental traffic of people and goods, the unpredictability of such epidemics, and the need for cross-boundary collaboration to deal with epidemics defying any national boundaries. As Ulrich Beck, a German sociologist, points out, in the current world-risk society, undesirable events can no longer be geographically contained. Instead, they unfold on a planetary scale. We have "*globalization of disease as a consequence of economic globalization*" (Stein A11; emphasis added).

The Need to Study

Transcultural communication/rhetorics studies the exchange of information and cultural flows not only among individual nation-states but also among diverse cultures as represented by communities of different geopolitical, ethnic, class, and gender compositions.[2] Focusing on the circulation and transformation of global flows of people, ideas, and discourses across localities (both national and regional), transcultural rhetorics examines the interactions and negotiations between localities and larger global processes, flows, and structures. Three central reasons dictate the need for scholarly attention to the transcultural communication about global epidemics and to the rhetorical constructions of the stories we tell about global epidemics. First, given the constant threat of pandemics, such as the avian flu or bioterrorist attacks and the rapid spread of infectious viruses via routes of intercontinental travel, the study of transcultural rhetorics about global epidemics becomes a necessity for us to better understand and evaluate the narratives different cultures tell about such epidemics. Second, global epidemics offer a perfect opportunity to examine the way transcultural communication operates in such epidemics, the problems existing in such communication processes, and the complicated networks made up of cultural narratives, ideological/political values, historical contexts, science, and media. Third, global epidemics are understudied in the fields of professional communication and rhetoric. Focusing mostly on individual affected countries or regions, the existing scholarship on epidemics (Barnes; Epstein; Erni; Iezzoni; Rosenberg; Scott, *Risky Rhetoric*; Ziporyn) has yet to produce compelling transcultural analyses of the competing forces operating in outbreak narratives.

As a global epidemic, SARS has received little attention from rhetoricians and professional communicators because of its short outbreak, quick containment, and sudden disappearance. Yet, despite its short lifespan, SARS functioned as a site of competing ideologies and knowledges and, more important, can serve as an important opportunity to study transcultural communication in global epidemics. In her brief analysis of American media coverage of SARS, Wald explores the connections among emerging epidemics, preexisting biases and values, poverty, and global economy. John H. Powers and Xiao Xiaosui's edited collection examines how SARS was socially constructed by national media, public health experts, and interest groups in East Asia. With most chapters focusing on one particular country or region, their collection works well to provide cross-cultural perspectives about the way media, institutions, cultural values, and local communities worked together to make sense of SARS. In addition, many popular and scientific discourses on H1N1 flu return to SARS in their discussions of lessons learned about global epidemics, such as appropriate communicative practices in such events, risk management tools and approaches, and global collaboration and sharing of resources and information (Chen, "Statement"; Derfel; Ding and Zhang; Fang; "Japan"; Jordans and Cheng; Trifonov, Khiabanian, and Rabadan). But how do institutions, media, and communities from different cultures communicate about an emerging and quickly spreading global epidemic? What challenges and problems do they encounter in such processes? What issues should be taken into consideration? Why? How?

Issues in the Study

Before WHO's intervention in mid-March 2003, mainstream media in China remained silent about the emerging epidemic (Brookes and Khan). My examination of the SARS media coverage from February to March, however, shows that a wide range of cultural sites were seething with rumors, speculations, and contradictory risk messages. Indeed, such speculations came not only from mainstream, commercial, and alternative media but also from various regions, nation-states, and international organizations (e.g., the Guangdong Province, Hong Kong, Chinatowns in Europe and North America, transnational pharmaceutical corporations, and WHO). The mysterious pneumonia was described as anthrax, a bioterrorist attack from the United States, bird flu, *Pestis*, Legionnaires' disease, and the bubonic plague. Hoax e-mails and text messages claimed that that the invasion of Iraq would cause food shortage in China; that Guangzhou "banned the export and import of commodities," such as rice, salt, and cooking oil (M. Lee, "Hunan in Panic"); that those who got infected would die within twenty-four hours from lung puncture; and that the outbreak had turned Guangzhou into a ghost city ("Pestis in Guangzhou"). Another rumor widely circulated in the Internet claimed that "200 people became sick and 30 died after being exposed at Guangzhou's World Trade Centre building alone" (Ying and Lee).

Chinatowns all over the world witnessed rumormongering, which often targeted individual businesses. Such rumors often falsely announced that employees returning from Hong Kong or mainland China had died from the mysterious pneumonia. They created panic and discrimination by urging people to "stay away from Chinatown and other predominantly Asian neighborhood[s]" to avoid contracting the killer disease ("SARS Virus Infects"). WHO exacerbated the confusion by issuing an avian flu alert in mid-February, indicating a possible avian flu outbreak in Hong Kong. In addition, Roche, a transnational pharmaceutical company, exploited the avian flu incident in Hong Kong and held a press conference in Guangzhou on February 9, announcing that "the flu resembled Hong Kong's deadly bird flu outbreak in 1997" (Ying, "Roche Denies" 1). The company then claimed that its drug Tamiflu was the only cure for avian flu. The claim was widely disseminated via text messages and Internet reports, which resulted both in radically increased sales of fifteen thousand boxes of Tamiflu over the Lunar New Year and charges of profiteering from local newspapers in Guangdong Province (Ying, "Roche Denies" 1). Meanwhile, the Chinese Center for Disease Control and Prevention (China CDC) announced on February 18 that its research team had identified the Chlamydia pneumonia bacteria as the cause of the outbreak. This claim was quickly challenged and rejected by leading clinicians treating atypical pneumonia patients in Guangdong. Medical experts, including Zhong Nanshan, a senior academician of the Chinese Academy of Engineering, provided clinical evidence of hundreds of atypical pneumonia patients who did not respond to antibiotic treatments for Chlamydia pneumonia. In early May, at the height of the SARS epidemic, several versions of underground, superstitious rumors traveled quickly in poor rural areas in at least fourteen provinces in central China. These rumors typically announced that in local towns, "a newborn baby talked" or "a lifelong deaf-dumb person spoke," both to deliver SARS prevention tips. Such tips were quick, simple, and inexpensive: "Play with fire crackers; hang ai leaves, a popular bug-repelling herb, over your door; drink green bean soup. These measures will protect you from SARS" (Hua). From late January to early June, most regions in mainland China witnessed rumormongering, mass panic, and rushes for and the subsequent price hikes of commodities, such as antibiotics, flu medication, masks, vinegar, rice, salt, and edible oil.

Further complicating an already hectic scene, "flexible citizens"—immigrants, international travelers, and overseas Chinese holding multiple passports in many countries across the world—began using the Internet both to pass on risk messages they learned from personal networks and to seek more risk information for their families in China (Ong, *Flexible Citizenship*). Moreover, despite China's official control of the Internet, many technology-savvy users circumvented official censorship and posted inside stories in major overseas Chinese websites to send out risk messages.

Complex global communication scenarios such as this one pose great challenges for intercultural communication theories. They raise multiple layers of issues including transcultural connectivities through online and interpersonal networks; competing transcultural narratives and rhetorical networks surrounding global events and the vastly different conditions that help to shape such narratives; power apparatuses and disciplinary technologies employed by nation-states, institutions, and local communities; impacts of local media structures on communicative practices; and local resistances taking place as extra-institutional risk communication and information leakages.

To help address the multifaceted issues raised by global communication about emerging epidemics, I propose a new theoretical framework of transcultural communication that makes use of and, in some cases, revises concepts such as transnational connectivities (Grewal), flexible citizenship (Ong, *Flexible Citizenship*), and global cultural flows (Appadurai). Before discussion of the proposed theoretical framework of transcultural communication is a review of existing theories of intercultural communication and intercultural professional communication and an examination of these theories' limited explanatory power when applied to the study of global epidemics.

Limitations of Rhetorical Inquiries in Cross-Cultural Contexts

Three main areas of inquiry investigate rhetorical interactions and communicative practices in cross-cultural and international contexts: intercultural communication, contrastive rhetoric, and comparative rhetoric. However, their focus on nation-states as the unit of analysis seriously restricts their analytical capacity to engage with rhetorical and communicative practices in a transcultural context.

Intercultural Communication

Courses of professional communication and rhetoric and composition often have intercultural or multicultural components in their curricula. Their approaches are limited, however, because of their reliance on oversimplified notions of cultural variables and cultural dimensions. Such theories focus on intergroup or face-to-face communication across individual nation-states and teach principles of intercultural communication as something transferable to various intercultural settings (Gudykunst, Lee, Nishida, and Ogawa; Hall; Hoftstede; Kim; Martin and Nakayama; Ting-Toomey). By emphasizing face-to-face communication and objectivist research approaches, the field of intercultural communication relinquishes the larger and more influential arena of governmental and nongovernmental intercultural communication, while offering an inadequate framework to consider the impacts of communication technologies or the intercultural communication processes concerning science, trade, technologies, and media that take place outside of typical face-to-face settings. In addition, studies of localization, globalization, and translation in intercultural professional communication suffer from their preoccupation with industrial needs and have limited explanatory power when transferred to the study of global events.

Intercultural Professional Communication

The study of intercultural professional communication has gained increasing importance in the field of professional communication. Numerous studies have focused on cross-cultural events and methodological approaches. Both Libby Miles and Dànielle Devoss, Julia Jasken, and Dawn Hayden employ textbook analysis to examine discussions about intercultural communication and offer suggestions to better address intercultural communication in professional communication pedagogy. Barry L. Thatcher examines ways to design more valid and ethical empirical studies in intercultural professional communication research. Huatong Sun and Beth Kolko and Carolyn Y. Wei explore possible ways to integrate cultural and social contexts in empirical research methodologies to study the use of technologies, such as mobile phones and the Internet, in different cultures. Timothy Weiss proposes the understanding of intercultural professional communication as translation to cultivate a sensibility to better deal with "absence, indirection, and plurality of meanings" (323). Many studies also offer suggestions about possible ways to internationalize professional communication classrooms and to teach global literacies (Alred; Andrews; Maylath; St. Amant; Starke-Meyerring).

However, little attention has been paid to the study of professional communication practices in cross-cultural events in its full complexity. At first glance, the absence of a systematic methodology to study professional communication in cross-cultural events does not seem particularly problematic because of the possibility of transferring existing methodologies, such as rhetorical analysis, textual analysis, and empirical methods, from monocultural to cross-cultural contexts. Yet, this transfer of existing methodologies becomes far more problematic than it initially appears when one considers confounding factors, such as the involvement of cultural, institutional, and regional players; the impact of cultural differences and power relations; and the wide geographical distribution and temporal duration of such events. Furthermore, as Thatcher eloquently points out, existing methods "seem derived from and designed for predominantly U.S. cultural and rhetorical values" and need to be "critically adapted for intercultural studies" (459). To answer Thatcher's call for critical adaptation of existing methodologies and methods for studies of intercultural communication, chapter 1 proposes a critical contextualized methodology that draws strength from institutional critique, Foucauldian genealogy, complexity theory, critical and cultural rhetorical theories, and transnational research. Engaging with these diverse approaches enables the invention of a robust heuristic tool to tackle the complex task of studying intercultural communication practices of global events.

Contrastive and Comparative Rhetoric

The field of contrastive rhetoric, later renamed intercultural rhetoric, compares writing styles in different countries to enable better teaching of writing to English as a Second or Foreign Language (ESL or EFL) learners. This field suffers from a limited definition of "culture" as monolithic nation-states and from its focus on textual analysis to identify essential features of rhetorics and writing practices (Kaplan; Connor). To cope with the severe constraints imposed by these oversimplified concepts of culture, Dwight Atkinson and Ulla Connor argue that scholars should move away from conflating culture with national entities. They also suggest a need to examine culture at various levels, in various locations, while incorporating historical contexts and power relations.

Comparative rhetoric, according to George Kennedy, is "the cross-cultural study of rhetorical traditions as they exist or have existed in different societies around the world" (1). Using Greco-Roman rhetorical theory as the foundation of his work, Kennedy applies its concepts to non-Western traditions to test the universal applicability of these concepts and to better understand rhetoric as a general phenomenon of human life (5–6, 217). Studying rhetorical theories and practices in different cultures (e.g., Egypt, Ireland, China, and India), comparative rhetoric focuses on nation-states as the unit of analysis and examines various schools of dominant rhetorical theories—for instance, Confucian rhetoric in China (Ding, "Confucius;" Mao; You, "*Way*"). The field has suffered from a deficit model in which individual non-Western cultures are examined in search for rhetorical theories, which are then often compared with the Western model to demonstrate the non-Western cultures' inadequacy and incompleteness.

Efforts have been made to better explore the numerous schools of rhetorical theories within individual cultures (X. Lu, *Rhetoric in Ancient China*; Yameng Liu). Scholars have argued for the need to study such rhetorical theories in their own contexts and on their own terms instead of imposing Western concepts on non-Western cultures with vastly different historical, social, and political contexts (Mao). Despite its increasing attention to local contexts and its methodological complications, comparative rhetoric "may not sufficiently analyze the interrelations and interconnections between and across nations" because of its nation-centric mindset (Hesford and Schell 465–66).

Transnational Approaches to Rhetoric

Innovative scholarship is moving beyond the existing ethnocentric focus on North American and European rhetors, texts, and contexts to examine discourses produced in non-Western cultures and globally circulated afterward. Such theoretical efforts not only surpass past preoccupations with nation-states but also expand the focus of mainstream rhetorical studies beyond Western rhetoric to examine the way transnational discourses are mediated by technologies, media, and imagination. In a *College English* special issue on transnational feminist rhetorics, Wendy Hesford and Eileen E. Schell delineate possible approaches to study transcultural rhetorical practices. They stress the need to consider the "complex histories of capital, power, nationalist discourses, and global interconnectivities" as well as "networks and relations across cultural groups" (465). They also call for the establishment of reciprocity between rhetorical studies and postcolonial and transnational studies by shifting the field's emphasis to "the study of transnational *interarticulations* and [by] mobiliz[ing] and revis[ing] theoretical constructs to accommodate this new knowledge" (466; emphasis original). Similar arguments have been made elsewhere. For instance, A. Suresh Canagarajah and Xiaoye You criticize the field of rhetoric and composition for its isolationist tendency and its nationalist paradigm because the field fails to respond effectively to the globalization of English composition courses, the global politics surrounding language resources and language use, and the rise of world Englishes. Such rhetorical studies help to better address the challenges posed by ever-increasing globalization processes and transnational movements of goods, capital, technology, and people.

The problem posed by transnational connectivities is not unique for rhetoric and composition. The field of professional communication faces similar challenges to move beyond its current focus on service to industry in North American contexts and its oversimplified nation-state–centered ideology. Several worthwhile efforts have been made to explore possible approaches to study transcultural professional communication among transnational groups and communities. Distinguishing culture from cultural identity, R. Peter Hunsinger stresses the "intertextual connections" between cultural identities and extracultural factors, such as economic, political, historical, or technological contexts as well as the dynamism of globalization (36). Highlighting the need to "address the specifically dynamic problems that stem from cultural conflict or confusion," Hunsinger suggests that "researchers study the ways cultural issues reflect many of the underlying antagonisms of the globalizing world" (42).

J. Blake Scott explores how the pharmaceutical industry employs transnational rhetorical discourses to manage and respond to the global risk of bioterrorism ("Kairos"). Investigating the constantly shifting power networks and the contradictory processes of intervention and mediation, his historical case examines the flow of risk discourses across institutional and extra-institutional boundaries at local and global levels. Navigating the rhetorical networks employed by multiple players, it clearly illustrates possible ways to explore the global cultural flows and the intertextual connections surrounding the global risks of bioterrorism.

The current volume shares the emphases of many theorists on global and local contexts, transcultural connectivities, and global power dynamics. It builds on existing theoretical discussions about intercultural professional communication by offering (1) a new conceptual framework of transcultural professional communication as a robust way to examine intercultural communication practices; (2) operational theoretical tools for the study of transcultural communication; and (3) a critical contextualized methodology to study transcultural communication. It also demonstrates ways to move beyond current preoccupations with nation-states and institutions in the study of intercultural communication practices. I argue that one entire yet essential research dimension is missing: to be specific, the undercurrents of everyday practices of and power struggles made by individuals, communities, and other extra-institutional players. Indeed, these powerful and omnipresent undercurrents *go undetected* by our current theoretical engines on intercultural communication. We are doing a huge disservice to both our profession and the public if we continue to ignore these tactical transcultural communication practices instead of engaging them and perhaps suggesting ways to boost their rhetorical and practical impacts.

Transnational Connectivities and Flexible Citizens

Inderpal Grewal defines the myriad connections that characterize the transnational arena as transnational connectivities "within which subjects, technologies, and ethical practices [are] created through transnational networks and connections of many different types" (3). Connectivities refer to information technologies, such as networks; the economics of information technologies as demonstrated in issues of access, transportation, delivery, and costs; and "discourses that travel through these networks" and become circulated, translated, transcoded, articulated, connected, or neglected (23). For Grewal, connectivities serve as a metaphor both for "the links and routes within which cosmopolitan discourses of power constitute the 'global'" and for the study of immigrants, diasporic citizenship, nationalism, and consumer culture.

When applied to the case of China, the concept of transnational connectivities takes on a unique new meaning: the cultural and ethnic interconnectedness between mainland China and overseas Chinese, particularly those in Hong Kong, Taiwan, Singapore, Macao, Southeast Asia, Europe, and North America. Although overseas Chinese live in various countries and regions, they share the same language and culture and have numerous informal personal networks of relatives and friends in China. Such connectivities bring not only cultural affinities but also capital inflow to China. For instance, the foreign direct investment (FDI) inflow from Hong Kong, Macao, Taiwan, and Singapore accounted for 61.9 percent of the total amount of FDI from 1983 to 2000 (State Statistical Bureau).

It should be stressed that global cultural flows take place not only among long-term immigrants and refugees but also among short-term "sojourners," including diplomats, students, researchers, teachers, journalists stationed overseas, employees of multinational corporations, and volunteers for organizations, such as the Peace Corps (Jackson). Aihwa Ong calls those two groups of people "flexible citizens," who shuttle across national borders in constant pursuit of capital and social prestige. Her concept of "flexible citizenship" can help us understand the various types of "condition[s] of cultural interconnectedness and mobility across space," or transnationality (*Flexible Citizenship* 7). Flexible citizenship refers to "the cultural logics of capitalist accumulation, travel, and displacement that induce subjects to respond fluidly and opportunistically to changing political-economic conditions" (Ong, *Flexible Citizenship* 7).

Ong's definition only includes people who enjoy sufficient economic and cultural capital to travel across national borders; it is problematic and limited in terms of class and income levels because of her exclusion of disadvantaged groups. For instance, seasonal, lower-class migrant farmworkers travel from Mexico to Texas or California to pick cotton or fruit for better pay, and illegal Hispanic immigrants from Mexico or Cuba travel to the United States to escape political control and to pursue a better life. Furthermore, developing countries with huge regional economic disparity, such as China, India, and Mexico, have been experiencing unprecedented scales and frequencies of human migration. In China, every year hundreds of millions of migrant workers leave their hometowns in the countryside to look for employment and better income in manufacturing or service industries. Even though they do not enjoy as much privilege or flexibility as transnational business travelers, these two types of migrating groups still have a lot in common in terms of motivations, goals, and patterns of behaviors. Finally, medical tourists represent another type of flexible citizens in emerging epidemics. Sick people travel across national and regional borders in search of better medical treatment, as illustrated by the first death of H1N1 flu in the United States and the numerous superspreading incidents in Beijing that took place because affluent people from the Shanxi Province sought the best hospitals in the capital city. Medical tourists may unknowingly introduce new and little-understood viruses to neighboring countries and areas.

The issue of flexible citizens poses difficulty for existing theories of intercultural professional communication, which assume discrete, coherent topics, such as national values and communicative practices, as their subjects of research. With transnational flows becoming the dominant scene of global capitalism, the increasing number of communities of flexible citizens calls for a more powerful theoretical framework to study cultural hybridity, contact zones, and multiculturalism. Flexible citizens often live in long-existing ethnic communities, such as Chinatown and Little Italy, big cities in the United States and Canada, and high-tech zones like the Silicon Valley. They can also be found in newly emerging communities, such as Korean villages in Beijing, luxurious house complexes provided for foreign managers and their families in cosmopolitan cities like Guangzhou and Seoul, and designated residential areas for foreign workers and students in big cities in many countries. Such communities develop hybrid cultures through constant exchanges with their host countries and with translocal business networks.

New Framework: Transcultural Professional Communication

Dwight Atkinson reviews various conceptualizations of culture and stresses the need to apply different ways of thinking about culture to "do justice to the ways cultural phenomena currently impact people's lives" (287). In his study of the cultural dimensions of globalization, Appadurai criticizes the noun form of culture for its implication of culture as a substance and advocates a shift to the adjective form of the word, *cultural*; for him, the adjective sense of culture stresses the "idea of situated difference" and the "contextual, heuristic, and comparative dimension" of individual cultures (13). Appadurai also redefines culturalism as "the conscious mobilization of cultural differences in the service of a larger national or transnational politics," which is "frequently associated with extraterritorial histories and memories" (13). As a form of cultural differences, cultural movements require the "deliberate, strategic, and popularist mobilization of cultural materials" in the era of "mass mediation, migration, and globalization" (14).

Cuban anthropologist Fernando Ortiz coined the term *transculturation* in 1947 to describe the convergences of various cultures and various phases of transition from one culture to another. These phases include the acquisition of another culture (acculturation), the loss or uprooting of a previous culture (deculturation), and the consequent creation of new cultural phenomena (neoculturation) (102–3). Transculturation can be used to describe a wide variety of global phenomena, including exile, immigration, multicultural contact, ethnic conflicts, interracial marriages, overseas sojourns, and transnational tourism.

To meet the challenges posed by global cultural flows, I propose the theoretical framework of transcultural professional communication. The proposed theory shifts the focus from the study of culture as substances to that of cultural as differences. It enables us to ask new, pressing questions and to acquire new insight through in-depth investigation of interactions between localities at various levels and the larger cultural and economic global flows.

Appadurai characterizes five global flows of textuality as ethnoscape, mediascape, technoscape, financescape, and ideoscape, which function as useful heuristic tools to explore global cultural flows, or landscapes of people, media, technologies, capital, and ideologies (see more detailed definitions and examples in chapter 1).[3] He employs the suffix "scape" to describe "the fluid, irregular shapes of these landscapes" that function as "building blocks of imagined world" (33). As deeply perspectival constructs, these scapes "are inflected by the historical, linguistic, and political situatedness of different sorts of actors: nation-states, multinationals, diasporic communities, as well as subnational groupings and movements" (33). My analysis of the transcultural rhetorics of SARS demonstrates the highly interactive and interconnected relationship among the five scapes. For instance, the global mediascape and ideoscape were full of competition, contestation, and contradiction in their constructions of SARS. Deeply inflected by ideological, political, and cultural values, the media at different cultural sites told drastically different stories about SARS. Meanwhile, when it came to the international, national, and institutional responses to SARS, the seemingly distinct concepts of ethnoscape, technoscape, and financescape became highly blurred and indistinguishable because of the impact of epidemics on the constant flows of people, of industrial and biopolitical technologies,[4] and of global capital in pursuit of profit. Chapter 1 examines in more depth the ways the five scapes unfolded and functioned in transcultural communication about SARS.

Complexities of Transcultural Communication

This book conducts a critical and rhetorical study of the transnational construction of SARS as a medical, social, and cultural epidemic and as a global risk. To meet the challenge of studying transcultural communication about global epidemics, I propose a new methodology, *critical contextualized methodology*, which can be readily adapted and transferred to the study of transcultural professional communication about global events (see chapter 1 for more detail). To develop a rhetoric of global epidemics, this book examines the way various institutional and extra-institutional players communicated and negotiated about the emerging risks of SARS and, less systematically, about the risks of H1N1 flu, within and across cultures at different stages.

Using the *extreme case sampling method* (Goubil-Gambrell),[5] this study focuses on China, Canada, and the United States for two reasons: (1) to include examples from the wide spectrum of countries most and least influenced by SARS and (2) to investigate the responses from countries that took a reactive or proactive approach to SARS. Because of the prominent role that WHO plays in global health issues, also explored is the way WHO negotiated about SARS with its member states to offer a fuller picture.

In addition to these four national and international key players, this study considers various transnational and transcultural forces—for instance, transnational media, different localities affected by SARS, overseas Chinese communities inside and outside Chinatowns, and flexible citizens (such as foreign students and workers), whistle-blowers, virtual communities, and international travelers in SARS-affected countries. This book examines the ways deterritorialized and reterritorialized communities were influenced by SARS and the rhetorical strategies that they employed to resist the stigmatization and exclusion they encountered in their host and home cultures.

Besides the focus on transcultural rhetorics, this book also explores how the two major institutional players (mass media and public health) and competing extra-institutional players interacted with and influenced one another in the construction of SARS narratives. Michel Foucault sees epidemics as being caught in a double system of observation: a social/political gaze "re-absorb[ing] it into all the other social ills to be eliminated" and a medical gaze isolating it "to circumscribe its natural truth" (*Birth of the Clinic* 43). SARS is converted into an object of knowledge by the complex network of public health procedures and by the "representing codes, statements, narratives, and images" appearing in scientific and popular discourses (Erni xii). SARS discourses across institutions and cultures are characterized by confusion, tension, and contradiction as well as conjoinment and reinforcement. This project sheds light on the discursive representations of SARS as an invading epidemic, which includes the construction of the entire event and its legitimation processes; the network of technologies, apparatuses, and actions operating in the event; the cultural narratives and fantasies that represented and sustained it; and the wider historical contexts from which it emerged and evolved. Rhetorical and critical analysis of the construction of SARS as a social/cultural disease, in addition to being a medical one, can help shed light on the interplay among medicine, politics, culture, ideology, and power in various genres of SARS discourses. It also provides an arena to explore the medical-cultural-rhetorical construction of the epidemic, thus the power-knowledge relationship in the transcultural discourse networks about SARS.

Toward a Rhetoric of Global Epidemics

This book draws some inspiration from existing studies on AIDS as a social/cultural disease (Epstein; Erni; Murphy and Poirier; Scott, *Risky Rhetoric*; Singer; Sontag; Treichler, *How to Have Theory*; Wald; Waldby) that pay particular attention to underlying ideological and cultural values, sociopolitical impacts of scientific discourses, practices of social stigmatization, and the way biopolitical technologies change the lives of carriers and high-risk populations. Given that SARS as a global epidemic originated in a communist country, China, and transmitted via large air droplets, this book involves a very different set of preexisting values, assumptions, and networks of communications. The ultimate goals of this volume are to construct an international rhetoric of global epidemics that emphasizes transnational connectivities and cultural flow, to create a conceptual mapping for transcultural communication about global epidemics, and to highlight the interplay among complicated ideological, cultural, and political values in such rhetorical constructions. This examination of the transcultural rhetorics about SARS can also serve as a historical case study on the way discourses work to interpret emerging, foreign, and urgent health menaces; to negotiate the sociocultural understanding of such events; and to package them as coherent, dramatic stories. Thus, the research questions are as follows:

- What conditions shape the coverage and construction of a global epidemic within and across cultures?
- What transformations do such constructions undergo as they circulate across national borders and are disputed, distributed, accepted, and put to use?
- How does rhetoric interact with other cultural, ideological, and political forces to shape the constructions of global epidemics and health crises within and across cultures?
- Where do the networks of public health and the media extend within and outside individual cultures? How are these networks interlinked and interacting with one another?

- How can we study both emergency health risk communication and transcultural communication about global epidemics to better facilitate the transcultural negotiation and collaboration to contain the epidemic?[6]
- What kinds of entry points can professional and health communicators employ to actively participate in and to help shape ongoing transcultural conversations about global epidemics?
- What literacy practices should be incorporated into communication classrooms to better prepare future professional and health communicators for challenges they may encounter in such difficult communicative events?

Given the constant threat of avian flu outbreaks and bioterrorist attacks, this study is both historically significant and highly relevant. This research contributes to the theoretical study of the interaction among transnational connectivities, medicine, culture, ideology, and mass media in global health crises. The investigation of the transcultural rhetorics about SARS enables a comprehensive, diachronic, and multidimensional study about SARS from different perspectives and at different developmental stages. This approach allows identification of important problems in the transcultural construction of SARS and points of departure in the transcultural negotiations about SARS. Further, this research highlights issues, challenges, and possible approaches for affected countries with different ideologies and economic interests to cope with disagreements that may arise in future pandemics. In other words, the current volume offers vocabulary and heuristic tools that professional communicators and health workers in outbreak areas can use to invent approaches of research, negotiation, and intervention.

This study makes two major theoretical contributions. First, chapter 1 develops a critical contextualized methodology as an analytical framework to investigate transcultural communication about SARS and H1N1 flu that can be readily applied to the study of global medical, scientific, and environmental events. Second, a vocabulary and language begin to be developed to discuss transcultural communication about global epidemics and to build an international rhetoric of global epidemics. To illustrate the methodological and theoretical potential of these proposed tools, a discussion for each of chapters 2, 3, 4, and 5 explains how both critical contextualized methodology and transcultural communication theory are employed (see appendix).

Doing so helps to outline the ways in which these tools operate in my studies and the ways that they can be employed to navigate overwhelmingly complicated and widely distributed transcultural narratives to better study communication practices about global events. Those readers not interested in methodological discussions may wish to skip chapter 1 and move on to the actual analyses and findings.

Overview of the Chapters

Chapter 1 establishes a methodological framework for the critical and rhetorical study of transcultural communication practices by importing theories from rhetoric and composition, critical theory, transnational theory, and complexity theory. The chapter proposes a critical contextualized methodology to examine transcultural construction and negotiation of SARS among key players at global, transnational, national, regional, and communal levels. Such players include nation-states, the World Health Organization, and transcultural communities, including immigrants, foreign workers, and international travelers. Beginning with temporal and spatial dimensions, the new methodology pays particular attention to tipping points (the key transformational moments in the event), power-knowledge relations, contextual factors, and interaction analysis of key players. It offers heuristic tools not only to identify forces at play during transcultural communication about global events but also to analyze the types of interaction among such forces. In addition, it provides analytical tools to navigate through global discourse networks by focusing on tipping points and forces that lead to those key transformational moments.

Chapter 2 focuses on three types of health risk communication channels: mainstream and commercial regional newspapers, expert discourses, and classified governmental discourses. It investigates their respective roles in official risk communication at the early stage of SARS in Guangdong Province. The official and classified governmental risk communication scene provides a rich load of activity for thinking through the interrelations of various media and institutional apparatuses when the new epidemic created utter confusion, panic, and fear of economic disruption. The analysis highlights the need for existing risk communication theories to move beyond ethnocentric tendencies and to pay close attention to the unique cultural, social, material, and economic contexts surrounding transnational risk communication practices of non-Western cultures.

Turning from institutional risk communication to its extra-institutional counterpart, chapter 3 investigates the way anonymous professionals, whistle-blowers, and the general public employed alternative media to disseminate risk messages in participatory and unofficial health risk communication about SARS. It focuses on the rhetorical impact that alternative media had on the leakage of risk information despite rigid censorship and the subsequent production of local resistance. This chapter stresses the materiality and cultural contingency of risk communication practices and alternative media. It examines how, despite the prevailing media control, alternative media facilitated extra-institutional risk communication about the quickly spreading SARS epidemic through the use of overseas Chinese websites, independent and often contending foreign media, and the guerrilla media of text messaging and word-of-mouth communication.

Chapter 4 compares the transcultural rhetorics about SARS as a global epidemic as employed by mainstream and regional media of the United States, China, and WHO. It reveals three rhetorical constructions (ideological, infrastructural, and technological) of the medical event of SARS that were employed by the United States, China, and WHO. It calls attention to the close connection among power apparatuses, national/institutional interests, and rhetorics in global outbreak narratives. In addition, it identifies a question unanswered by the US media, namely, how China managed to eventually eradicate SARS, and attempts to find some clues by examining regional media coverage about the people's war against SARS in affected areas in China. Finally, it explores regional media's and ethnic Chinese media's coverage of SARS in transnational Asian communities, particularly China-towns and international travelers in the United States and Canada, as well as the much-criticized efforts to put an ethnic face to SARS during the outbreak.

Whereas chapter 4 compares the rhetorical strategies of mainstream and regional media from various cultural sites to interpret the SARS-China relationship, chapter 5 investigates transnational risk discourses from health institutions and mass media. It examines the transnational risk management of SARS and the H1N1 flu through the use of travel advisories. Global risks are full of ambiguity and incalculability and, thus, are uncontrollable by any single actor. During the SARS epidemic, China employed technical language in its risk negotiations with WHO despite the country's economic concerns. Toronto, Canada, in contrast, was preoccupied with economic losses and political impacts and brought those issues as legitimate concerns to the negotiating table. Combining technical and economic arguments, Toronto managed to persuade WHO into withdrawing the travel advisory. The CDC issued a downgraded travel advice for Toronto, calling for precaution in travel on the same date that WHO listed Toronto on its travel advisory. Despite WHO's heavy reliance on travel advisories and health screening during SARS, the United Nations agency admitted the limited utility of such measures and, to avoid economic disruption, rejected requests to use them again in the H1N1 flu pandemic. Both the sharp contradiction in SARS risk definitions for Toronto and WHO's reluctance to use travel advisories in the H1N1 flu pandemic highlight the contingent nature of medical knowledge supporting WHO's travel advisories and the contention surrounding global risk management.

The concluding chapter synthesizes the rhetorical forces operating at different cultural and institutional sites about SARS and considers the implications of such forces for future research in rhetorical studies, transcultural communication, media studies, and risk communication. Attention is called to the way rhetoric functioned in heterogeneous cultural and institutional practices and to the need for ethical intervention from journalists, professional communicators, and practitioners to play a more active and participatory role in communicating to the public the risks of new and emerging health crises.

Emerging global epidemics not only affect public health, economies, and political structures but also produce social side effects ranging from panic and stigmatization to overt exclusion. They create heroes, villains, victims, and scapegoats. In response to the uncertainty and ambiguity surrounding such global risks, global agencies, national authorities, medical experts, multinational research laboratories, and affected communities all scramble to provide make-do risk definitions and contingent coping strategies. Institutional and cultural risk responses are often contradictory and confusing, and it takes tremendous time to coordinate risk efforts across countries and regions. What further complicates this havoc is the lack of knowledge about emerging epidemics and different risk management approaches employed by countries and regions with vastly different political and economic priorities. This book attempts to provide heuristic tools and theoretical concepts to facilitate efforts to navigate through the transnational discursive maze surrounding emerging epidemics and to examine the way risk rhetoric emerges and develops as attempts to manage such global risks.

1
Critical Contextualized Methodology
for Transcultural Communication Study

How do we study transcultural professional communication about global scientific or public health events to identify opportunities of civic intervention and ethical action?

Involving multiple players working at different geopolitical, cultural, and institutional sites over a relatively long period of time, intercultural communication about global events poses huge challenges for both researchers and practitioners because of its sheer complexity, interactivity, and richness. Despite its importance, intercultural professional communication about global events remains little studied, and researchers have no existing methodology or analytical tools to guide them.[1] This chapter fills in this gap by proposing what I call *critical contextualized methodology*, a dynamic analytical tool for the systematic investigation of intercultural communication about global events.

In their award-winning book *Opening Spaces*, Patricia Sullivan and James Porter distinguish between methodology and methods. Noting that methodology has been traditionally "equated with particular observational procedures or data-collection strategies and with specific data analysis techniques," they advocate for a revised approach that "calls particular attention to its rhetorical nature" and functions as "an explicit or implicit theory of human relations which guides the operation of methods" (11). In other words, their methodology of "broad, theoretically informed frameworks" serves as "an intervening social action and a participation in human events" to "locate critical research practices in the activity of situated practice" (11). By contrast, methods, for them, are "techniques or specific sets of research practices," that is, discourses analysis, surveys, or ethnographies (11).

My proposed critical contextualized methodology strives to accomplish the goal that Sullivan and Porter set out: providing a theoretically informed framework both to examine transcultural rhetorics and to explore ways for participation and social intervention in global events. Offering an alternative to the current tendency in professional communication research to focus on nation-states as the unit of analysis and to oversimplify other cultures in terms of traits and dimension, I aim to highlight the ways in which global events are shaped by the "complexity and intricacy" of their historical, cultural, and political contexts (Tufte 33). I also intend to counter the ethnocentric tendency in intercultural studies, to offer voices to non-Western cultural actors, and to help invent research methodologies that recognize and take into consideration the full complexity of cross-cultural events. It is dangerous to impose existing Western theories and methods, which are often developed in a monocultural context, on other cultures with vastly different values and material conditions. Such dangers include subjugating and silencing local cultural knowledges and essentializing socially, historically, and politically diverse cultures by depicting them in Western terms. Echoing Sullivan and Porter's call for research as ethical and political actions as well as Arjun Appadurai's emphasis on cultural as differences and contrasts, I develop a methodology that pays particular attention to the changing cultural, political, and material contexts surrounding cross-cultural events.

Critical contextualized methodology gives equal voice to Western and non-Western countries through the acknowledgment of the multifaceted, complicated, and interactive nature of global events. In addition, it promotes a multivocal listening game, as advocated by Michel Foucault and Jean-François Lyotard, and pays as much attention to petite narratives and subjugated knowledges as to grand narratives. Power plays a prominent role in cross-cultural studies; therefore, studies like mine are necessarily political. Tracing negotiations among cultures, I circumvent the temptation to speak about cultures in binary or hierarchical terms so as to better explore the full complexity of the intercultural relations.

The next section explains in detail heuristic tools for critical contextualized methodology. After operationalizing the heuristic tools, I use interaction, context, and power-knowledge analyses to examine how Appadurai's theory of perspectival landscapes can be employed to investigate how the unique cultural and material contexts of China and the United States helped to shape these two countries' interactions during the SARS and H1N1 flu epidemics. The proposed methodology contributes to the fields of transcultural rhetorics and professional communication, as it helps researchers to approach complicated intercultural communication about global events systematically without imposing existing theories or essentializing cultures involved in such global events.

A Critical Approach to Intercultural Professional Communication

Early professional communication studies, or what Jeffrey T. Grabill calls "descriptive and instrumentalist research," examine workplace communication and the production processes of documents and designs (152). Recent efforts to bring the methods of cultural studies to professional communication, however, call for integrating power-knowledge analysis and considering professional communication's "broader conditions, circulations, and effects" (Scott, Longo, and Wills). For instance, Carl G. Herndl criticizes the narrow focus of the professional communication scholarship on the production process of various discourse communities, a focus that "describes the production of meaning, but not the social, political, and economic sources of power which authorize this production or the cultural work such discourse performs" (351). As part of the solution to the problem Herndl identifies, Bernadette Longo calls for the study of technical communicators' involvement "within situated institutional relationships of knowledge" and the way national and international "political tensions shaped the texts" (112–15).

In "Institutional Critique," Porter, Sullivan, Stuart Blythe, Grabill, and Libby Miles highlight the lack of "material punch" and "critique edge" in workplace studies and disciplinary critiques (612). They differentiate institutional actions (i.e., administrative, classroom, and disciplinary critique) from institutional critique, which "employs a rhetorical and spatial methodology as it looks at institutions as discursively and materially constituted" (625). Elizabeth Britt distinguishes the concepts of organization and institution, pointing out that "much technical communication research that examines discourse in context is primarily concerned with how texts and writers operate within organizations" (134). In contrast, institutional critique extends beyond organizational borders "by attending to the power relations inherent in particular spatial and material conditions" (Britt 135). Sharing Porter et al.'s concern with power and discourses, Britt also calls for the consideration of power relations and ideology in the study of the way discourses "function rhetorically and materially within and between institutions" (147).

Following Porter et al.'s institutional critique methodology, I identify gaps in cultural, institutional, and media discourses through the use of Foucauldian genealogy. Foucault's methodology of genealogy, as exemplified in *Discipline and Punish* and *History of Sexuality*, serves as a powerful tool to examine the interplay of power and knowledge. Genealogy identifies accidents, deviations, and errors in the historical conditions of existence, or in Foucault's words, "historical ontology." Foucault stresses that analysis of discursive formation facilitates a better understanding of the construction of knowledge and the power-knowledge interplay; as he puts it, "[i]n stating what has been said, one has to re-state what has never been said" (*Birth of the Clinic* xvi). Genealogy makes discontinuity both an instrument and an object of research.

As my project is driven by the need to explore the power-knowledge interaction within and between cultures, genealogical critique provides a helpful tool. Genealogy questions the historical conditions of the existence of discourses and examines "culturally true discourse's insertion into institutional and other non-discursive practices" (Mahon 105). Foucault sees genealogy as a way to insurrect "subjugated knowledges," namely, "the buried knowledge of erudition and those disqualified from the hierarchy of knowledges and sciences" (*Archeology of Knowledge* 81). Genealogy reveals the practical, historical, institutional, and discursive conditions of the event under study as well as the speakers' dispersion in their statuses, the institutional sites they occupy, and their own positions.

Sharing Foucault's preoccupation with anomalies and gaps, Lyotard advocates the use of local/petite narrative to combat the violence done by the master narrative and to give voice to alternative stories.[2] Replacing Habermasian consensus with dissensus and paralogy (60–67), Lyotard and Jean-Loup Thebaud believe that it is ethical for us to determine the truth value of narratives "on a case by case basis" (28). The concept of petite narrative helps to explore alternative explanations of events and to give voice to the excluded and the silenced. Warning against the use of terror in discourses, or "the attempt to reduce the multiplicity of the games or players through exclusion or domination" (103), Lyotard calls for "judgments of opinion" instead of "judgments of truth" (28). For justice to prevail, one should play the game of listening and allow the maximization of "the multiplication of small narratives" (Lyotard 59) rather than using violence to exclude other competing voices from the game. My study pays great attention to the use of petite narratives by concerned citizens and communities from various cultural sites and the way such small narratives competed with dominant discourses and exerted critical impacts on the development of global and translocal events.

The theories of Foucault and Lyotard can serve as a theoretical guideline for rhetorical and ethical studies of intercultural communication. As researchers of intercultural communication and investigators of power, we must recognize our own cultural positions, assumptions, and biases as well as dominant and petite narratives and official and disqualified knowledges. Foucault's genealogical critique and Lyotard's stress on petite narratives and dissensus can serve as analytical tools to conduct intercultural studies without subordinating one culture to another or transforming particular types of narratives into subjugated knowledges.

Incorporating genealogy, institutional critique, and critical studies in transcultural communication, this book investigates the intersections among individual cultures, local and translocal communities, international agencies, transnational corporations, public health institutions, and mass media to consider the power-knowledge relations that were at work during the global epidemic of SARS. Furthermore, I expand the inquiry about the operation of power and knowledge not only to various institutional sites but, perhaps more important, to extra-institutional sites across cultures. By doing so, I demonstrate how the field of intercultural professional communication can expand its toolkits, explanatory power, and inquiry scope by incorporating issues of power, knowledge, technologies, institutions, extra-institutional forces, and transnational connectivities as possible subjects of study. This expansion of inquiry can also help the field to move beyond its present "commitment to corporate capitalism and high technology"—or its focuses on skill training, efficiency, and profit—and to incorporate humanistic, civic, and ethical concerns (Miller, "Humanistic Rationale" 615).

As mentioned above, intercultural professional communication scholarship is often ethnocentric in nature. Despite their intercultural focus, most studies are conducted by American researchers examining one-way interaction between the United States and other cultures. Moreover, the existing focus on English publications in data collection and analysis inevitably results in the unjustified preferences given to perspectives of English-speaking cultures and the exclusion of cultures where English is not a dominant language.

Several useful attempts have been made by scholars coming from other cultural backgrounds who examine the intercultural communication practices from other cultural perspectives and introduce new knowledge and insights about their source cultures (Ammara and Portaneri; Canagarajah; Chu, "Continuity"; Fukuoka, Kojima, and Spyridakis; Fukuoka and Spyridakis; You, "*Way*"). Such studies can help the field of intercultural communication to grow and flourish by adding fresh perspectives, approaches, and cultural perspectives.

As discussed later in chapter 1, I advocate that we shift our attention to cultural and global connectivities in intercultural communication. To do so, my critical contextualized methodology operationalizes tools and concepts from the proposed theoretical framework of transcultural communication. It explores the way transcultural connectivities function in rhetorical contestations and power dynamics in global events.

To distinguish my approach from those taken previously, I use the term *transcultural communication and rhetorics*. My goal is to bring non-Western perspectives into transcultural studies and introduce discourses previously ignored by and invisible to Eurocentric studies. In addition, I investigate how various cultures, institutions, and transcultural communities communicate about emerging global epidemics, while also considering possible ways to negotiate such different strategies and their implications for future research.

Critical Contextualized Methodology, Transcultural Communication

Critical contextualized methodology is shaped by Sullivan and Porter's discussion of postmodern critical research methodology, Foucault's genealogy method, Appadurai's theory of global cultural flows, and Mark Taylor's complexity theory. Seeing methodology as "broad, theoretically informed frameworks . . . [and] an intervening social action and a participation in human events," Sullivan and Porter view their framework for research methodology as a much-larger term encompassing ideology, practice, and method (9). They also stress that critical practice, or praxis, "acknowledges the rhetorical situatedness [of the research project] and recognizes research as a form of political and ethical action" (15). Despite their focus on writing technologies, their emphasis both on methodology as heuristic, dynamic, and negotiable and on "social change as the appropriate aim of research praxis" are highly relevant to this project (25, 46). Seeing power-knowledge relations as one of the key issues in transcultural communication, critical contextualized methodology investigates knowledges created and legitimized across cultures and the power relations sustaining such legitimizing processes. It also employs Taylor's concept of a tipping point to identify the transitional movement from quantitative changes to qualitative changes and investigates how such changes take place through the mediation of competing discourses.

Here, for convenience's sake, I use the singular form of global *event* to describe what in actuality may exist as a cascade. James Rosenau defines cascades as dynamic action sequences of global macro-events and processes as well as local micro-events that "gather momentum, stall, reverse course, and resume anew as their repercussions spread among whole systems and subsystems" (299). Cascades play an important role in global connectivities because they "work their way into highly localized structures of feeling by being drawn into the discourse and narrative of the locality" and thus "provide material for the imagination of actors at various levels for reading general meanings into local and contingent events" (Appadurai 154). Globalization forces witness the extreme mobility of global capital in pursuit of profit and the "bifurcated play" between "the multicentric system and the statecentric system" that helps to shape the dynamics of the world politics (Appadurai 139). They also bring forth interconnected transnational communication networks, incessant information flow, and transcultural political and economic contacts, conflicts, and compromises. All these forces are constantly in operation, influencing the way cascades of global and local events unfold and develop. For instance, the global SARS outbreak, when viewed as a cascade, consists of participation and interaction among nation-states, intergovernmental organizations, transnational corporations, multinational research teams and public health infrastructure, local communities, professionals and ordinary citizens all over the world.

Critical contextualized methodology employs six dimensions of inquiry to help investigate transcultural communication about global events. I articulate these dimensions, in no particular order, as: key players, time-space axes, tipping points, interaction analysis, power-knowledge relations, and contexts. Transcultural communication analysis can proceed in different ways and focus on various combinations of these six components. These six dimensions work very well with existing transcultural theories as articulated by scholars such as Appadurai, Inderpal Grewal, Aihwa Ong, and Doreen Starke-Meyerring. Indeed, they not only offer analytical tools to apply transcultural theoretical concepts to actual studies but also provide operationalized tools to build on and expand such concepts to better investigate transcultural communication practices. The following sections define these six components and explains the procedures to perform critical contextualized inquiry about global events.

Key Players

One dimension of critical contextualized methodology begins with identifying key players, which can be found on multiple levels, depending on the purpose of the inquiry. After locating key cultural or institutional players, the researcher can move on to identify local communities, individuals, and professional communicators initiating and participating in such communication processes.

The heuristic tool of key players helps to operationalize Appadurai's five scapes in the analytical processes. It enables the multilevel, multidimensional analysis of various forces at play in different cultural sites. For instance, at the ethnoscapic level, we can identify communal, professional, and individual key players. Table 1.1 provides an incomplete list of key players that one may identify in the study of global events, depending on the type of study one

Table 1.1. Incomplete list of key players at the five Appadurian scapes

Levels	Key players
Ethnoscape	Communal, professional, ethnic, individual
Mediascape	Traditional/mass/new media; mainstream/ alternative media, competing discourses circulated in various media
Technoscape	Communication technologies, information technology infrastructure, censorship technologies, manufacturing/industrial facilities
Financescape	Global capital, transnational corporations, investment environment and policies
Ideoscape	Dominant/subversive ideologies, ideas promoted by propaganda campaigns or hidden in tacit messages
Other key players	Global, national, regional, local; institutional; extra-institutional

conducts. It should be emphasized that key players never function in isolation. Instead, they are in constant interaction, communication, and negotiation with one another. Together, they form an interconnected transcultural network that can exert influence not only across cultural and institutional sites but also on other key players.

Time-Space Axes

As the next step, the researcher can use the time-space axes to analyze the temporal-spatial dimensions of the event by mapping key players on the axes. The criteria for such temporal-spatial mapping include the beginning point when individual key players get involved in the event[3]; the duration of their involvement; the geographical, institutional, and cultural sites where their participation takes place; and the full range of geopolitical and cultural sites when the event emerges, develops, and draws to a close. This analysis offers a tool to map out the spatial and temporal elements not only of the global event under discussion but, more important, of the various forces at play in that event. In other words, the time-space axes can be employed at both global and local levels for multiple rounds of mapping to explore the way various players intervene in the event (see table 1.2 for relevant questions for each heuristic tool).

To use my case study as an example, I locate key players and place them on the time-space axes, with a horizontal east-west space axis and a vertical time axis. As shown in figure 1.1, I identify five different cultural/institutional players in the time-space axes, with the United States, Canada, WHO, mainland China, and Hong Kong in the 2003 section of the time axis and Guangdong Province in the 2002 section. The United States and Canada are placed on the left (west) of the space axis, mainland China and Hong Kong on the right (east) section; the international organization of WHO is placed in between.

Tipping Points

Borrowing from Taylor's complexity theory, which can be "used to illustrate social and cultural dynamics," I find the concept of "tipping point" particularly relevant and useful to my discussion (24). It refers to the "critical moment in an epidemic when everything can change all at once," or the "moment of critical mass, the threshold, the boiling point" (Gladwell 10–12). At the tipping point, "the critical transition takes place . . . where quantitative

Table 1.2. Critical contextualized methodology as a heuristic tool

Dimensions	Possible questions to ask
Key players	Who played important roles in the event? From what institutions/cultures/regions/communities/professions were they acting? Whose interests were they promoting? Why? Which of the five global scapes were the key players acting from? What kind of rhetorical messages did the key players create and circulate about the event? For what purposes?
Time-space axes	Where did the event take place? When did the event take place? Where were the key players geographically located? How did the event unfold over time and occur geographically?
Tipping point	What were the transformational moments for the event? When did those transformational moments take place? How did those transformational moments take place? Who played a role in facilitating or impeding the transformations? Why did they do it? How did they achieve their goals? What kind of changes took place during those moments? How did the key players talk about and respond to those changes? How was the event transformed before and after those transformational moments? Who benefited from those changes, and who did not?
Interaction analysis	How did the key players interact with one another? Through what means? What media? Was there any conflict, competition, contradiction, compromise, or collaboration among the key players? How did the changes take place? How did the key players negotiate with one another to accomplish the changes?
Power-knowledge	What power relations were observed surrounding the event? What kind of official and unofficial knowledges were created during the event? By whom? For what purpose? How did the competing knowledge claims function to shape the outcomes of the event? How were they legitimated or excluded? How did power apparatuses legitimate their knowledge claims during the event?
Context	What political, cultural, historical, material, and social contexts did the event have? How did the contexts influence the way people/cultures communicated about the event? How did the contexts influence the way the event under discussion was constructed in various cultural and institutional sites?

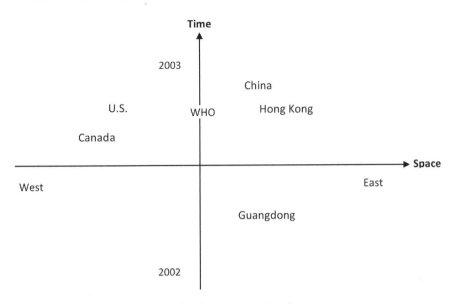

Figure 1.1. Time-space axes for the SARS outbreak

change suddenly leads to qualitative change" (Gladwell 148). Featured by nonequilibrium, instability, and contradiction, the tipping point is a direct result of "the dynamic interaction among individual elements of the system" (Bak 2). In his discussion of the "self-organized criticality" in the nonlinear dynamics of complexity systems, Bak points out that a poised, "critical" state "is established solely because of the dynamical interactions among individual elements of the system," and that in such critical state, "minor disturbances may lead to events, called avalanches, of all sizes" (2). Gladwell pinpoints three critical factors or agents of change in tipping a medical or social epidemic: (1) the Law of the Few, or the extraordinary transmitting capacity of a few selecting carriers or passengers; (2) the Stickiness Factor, or the contagiousness and impacts of infectious agent or messages; and (3) the Power of Context, or the environment in which the infectious agent is operating, or the creation of groups and communities to tip a large word-of-mouth epidemic. Further, there are multiple ways to tip an epidemic, and changes can occur in more than one of the three areas to jolt an epidemic out of equilibrium (Gladwell 19).

Taylor stresses that "the dynamic interaction among individual elements of the system generates [a] global event that requires a holistic description" (148).

Similarly, to study tipping points in cross-cultural events, it is important to take a holistic approach and to examine the complicated dynamics among players, messages, and contexts rather than studying them in isolation. A tipping point, or what Kelso calls "the punctuated equilibrium," may take place in different forms, including "the development from one form, pattern, structure, or system to another" or the qualitative transformation from have-nots to haves and from being negative to positive or vice versa (16).

To understand the complex dynamics of transcultural communication about global events, the investigation of the conflicts, contradictions, and gaps surrounding tipping points can help us to understand rhetorical contestations surrounding such crises and their impact on global and local responses. The search for changes in the development of local and global events can serve as a starting point to identify tipping points in such events. Possible markers include qualitative changes, such as the adoption of new policies; abrupt changes in international and national responses to certain issues, that is, from denial to admission or from nonaction to action; or perhaps the successful eradication of regional or global threats to health or environment. Tipping points can and should be identified at the international, national, regional, and communal levels, a practice that, in turn, facilitates the exploration of interrelationships among global and national politics and the micropolitics of local communities. The use of the tipping point as the entry point, and in some cases, as the focal point of the study, enables the researcher to penetrate the sometimes over-whelmingly complicated discourses surrounding global events and to identify key transitional moments for further analysis. Doing so helps the researcher to engage more productively with various lines of inquiry into the discursive formations about the event under study. For example, it may be productive to analyze how certain tipping points are achieved by kairotic communication, negotiation, and intervention from key players at various levels.

Again, my study serves as an example. Tipping points I examine include the dates when the Guangdong provincial government held the first and only press conference to respond to the widespread panic buying caused by the fear of SARS (February 11), when WHO issued its first travel advisory against traveling in SARS-affected areas (April 2), when China first acknowledged that SARS was spreading in Beijing (April 20), and when Xiaotangshan Hospital was charged with containing the SARS outbreak in Beijing (May 1). These key transitional moments demonstrate the tremendous impact of rhetorical transactions and negotiations on the regional and global development of

SARS, and studying them in depth allows me to explore the power dynamics among the key players.

Interaction Analysis: Dynamic Interaction, Negotiation

Understanding how various actors reach a tipping point requires a holistic approach that examines complex power relations among cultural, economic, political, and ideological forces in various cultures, institutions, and transcultural communities. It is also necessary to explore the interaction, contention, negotiation, and collaboration among various players. In other words, studies should examine not only key texts and local contexts of events but also the ways primary actors negotiate with one another to solve problems. Such work can begin with findings in the key player, time-space axis, and with tipping-point heuristic analyses. Interactions among key players can be examined both at similar levels (i.e., global, national, regional, cultural, institutional, and professional) and across different levels. Understanding the starting and ending points, duration, geopolitical, cultural and institutional sites, and key transformational moments about the global event allows for further investigation of interactions ranging from exchanges, negotiations, and competition among key players; to compromises and collaboration; to new disagreements, conflicts, and contradictions. Individual players may participate in such interactions with their own motivations and goals, yet the ultimate outcomes are usually determined by complex global, local, and translocal power dynamics.

Interaction can take place not only among key players but also within and across Appadurai's five scapes. For instance, both ideological contestations and interactions between global and local discourses—two core features of economic globalization, according to Starke-Meyerring—can be identified and investigated through mediascapic and ideoscapic analyses. Another type of interaction, the cut-throat competition for profit and productivity, results in swift deterritorialization and reterritorialization as global capital responds to local policies and conditions. Financescapic and technoscapic analyses are particularly well-suited to examining such interaction processes.

Again, in addition to interaction among key players, scholars must examine the interaction between key players and the larger contexts shaping their responses, that is, the five scapes and global and local environments. These investigations can focus on different things: for instance, types of interaction; quality of interaction; groups, key players, and environments involved in such interactions; cultural and institutional sites in which such interaction takes place; media delivering and recording such interaction; and the consequences and side effects of such interactions.

Power-Knowledge

Returning to my study as an example, I employ Foucault's genealogy method to examine the forms of power operating in various cultural and institutional sites; the relations between power and knowledge; and the gaps, ruptures, and breaks in the knowledges created in and about certain events. My analysis considers cultural and institutional practices, competing networks of power, apparatuses of knowledge, and interactions between power and discursive and nondiscursive practices. Investigations of power help to analyze the way epidemics are "insert[ed]" into cultural, "social, political and economic space" (Mahon 6). The genealogy method is "both the reason and the target of analyzing discourses as events," which shows "how those discursive events have determined in a certain way what constitute our present—either our knowledge [or] our practices" (Jay). Foucault's genealogy aims to insurrect "subjugated knowledges," namely, those disqualified from the hierarchy of knowledges and sciences (*Archeology of Knowledge* 80). However, such discourses and knowledges do not exist alone but, as Mahon puts it, are "embedded in social, cultural, and institutional practices" and carry with them "institutional bondage," or the power relations in their social, cultural, and historical existence (118).

Power-knowledge analysis requires the investigation and critique of the conditions, production, circulation, and consumption of discursive and nondiscursive practices in their cultural and institutional contexts; the way discourses are embedded in a social/cultural matrix and employed in struggles of knowledge legitimization; and the social, political, and economic sources of power that authorize the production of meaning and the legitimation of certain knowledges. In other words, power-knowledge analysis focuses on the "politics of knowledge legitimation and the exclusionary effects of power," which, as J. Blake Scott, Longo, and Katherine V. Wills point out, are missing in technical communication research (12). By adding a transcultural perspective to power-knowledge analysis, critical contextualized methodology goes beyond the institutional approach and enables the investigation of the impacts of international and national political, ideological, economic, and cultural tensions related to discourses and knowledge legitimation as well as the interrelatedness among them.

Contexts

Viewing culture as unifying, concrete, and abstractable, theories of inter-cultural communication have focused their discussions on variables and dimensions of cultures, that is, individualism versus collectivism, power dis-tance, high and low context, masculinity versus femininity, face negotiation, and nonverbal codes, such as proxemic and silence (for a literature review of intercultural communication, see Gudykunst, Lee, Nishida, and Ogawa). Many studies of intercultural professional communication use these cultural variables and dimensions as the theoretical support for their research, even though such approaches run the risk of oversimplifying and essentializing other cultures by studying them as objects with empirically identifiable and universally applicable variables.

To avoid the oversimplification of transcultural events into readily appli-cable stories about cultural variables, scholars must pay attention to cultural differences and contrasts (Appadurai; Hunsinger). More specific, we must take into consideration the historical, cultural, political, economic, ideolog-ical, and economic forces at play in transcultural communication and nego-tiations about global events. To achieve this goal, the heuristic dimension of context both calls attention to and enables detailed analysis of the materiality of those global events. The starting point is to examine the historical, cultural, political, economic, and material conditions in all cultures that are involved in such events. Sullivan and Porter stress that research is situated and rhe-torical (41). We as researchers should make explicit not only our ideological positions and beliefs and values but also the particular historical situatedness of the event under study. In other words, to uproot cross-cultural events from their proper historical and material contexts is to impose our own power as researchers on such events and to deprive them of their unique features as individual events through the violence of decontextualization. Doing this is dangerous because it leads us to essentialize or homogenize other cultures.

Table 1.2 presents critical contextualized methodology as a heuristic tool, listing six dimensions and possible questions to guide the inquiry for each dimension. Figure 1.2 portrays critical contextualized methodology as a pen-tagon tool with five dimensions, namely, key players, time-space axes, tipping point, interaction analysis, and power-knowledge relations.[4] This forms a core pentagon, which is encompassed in a large square, or the larger and constant inquiry about the contexts surrounding the event under discussion.

Contexts

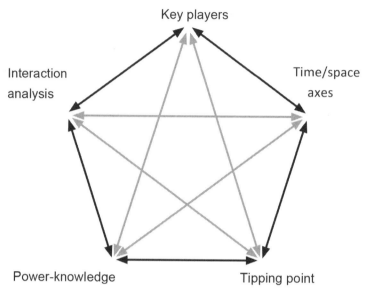

Figure 1.2. Critical contextualized methodology

Accommodating Existing Research Methods

In discussing his rhetorical-cultural approach, Scott calls for "the development of new hybrid approaches that focus on different dimensions and functions of rhetoric," or "alternative methodologies as supplements to [rhetorical studies'] established and valuable strands" (34). Sharing his methodological interests and concerns, this chapter explores possible methodological frameworks for the critical and rhetorical study of transcultural communication about global epidemics. Critical contextualized methodology is not a linear or rigid analytical tool but is instead highly flexible and dynamic. Rather than following rigid procedures, any of the six dimensions can serve as a starting point for investigation, and various combinations of part or all of the six dimensions can be used to go through the investigation recursively until comprehensive examination about the global event can be accomplished. Critical contextualized methodology draws on existing research methods, including those employed in rhetorical studies, critical studies, and cultural studies, but goes beyond what those methods have to offer. Starting with ways to trace and analyze transnational discourses about global events, it moves beyond rhetorical theory's conventional concern with well-defined rhetorical

44

situations (Bitzer), with rhetorical ecologies within one locale (Edbauer), and with international rhetorical fields consisting of similar discourse communities (Queen). Using tipping-point analysis to identify transformational moments in global events, critical contextualized methodology provides a means to tackle overwhelmingly complicated and widely dispersed discourses about such events. Focusing on radical changes in the development of such events, it maps participating key players at the global, regional, and local levels and analyzes discourses they produce; institutional and cultural sites from which they speak; political, economic, and material contexts surrounding their rhetorical moves and their interactions with one another; and the power dynamics surrounding their knowledge claims. Critical contextualized methodology pays equal attention to participating key players, without emphasizing the global, the national, or the institutional over the communal or the individual. Doing so allows the mapping of a full spectrum of contesting forces at play. It asks different questions about grassroots participation, civic intervention, and bottom-up collaborative action—what Appadurai calls *grassroots globalization*—and helps to solve research problems with an innovative and theoretically sound approach. Both my study of the guerrilla media in chapter 3 and my analysis of transcultural risk tactics in H1N1 flu in chapter 5 illustrate this methodology's explanatory and heuristic power to study global events.

In addition, critical contextualized methodology serves as a platform accommodating existing research techniques, such as rhetorical analysis (e.g., analysis of rhetorical situations, topoi, enthymemes, and tropes, among others; see chapter 2), discourse analysis (see chapter 4 for corpus-assisted discourse analysis), historical study, and empirical research. Serving as a broad, theoretically informed framework to guide such research projects, the methodology helps to identify possible entry points and approaches to investigating past or ongoing transcultural communication about global events in various cultural sites (see the appendix for more in-depth discussion about the invention processes of the methodology as well as chapter-by-chapter descriptions of how I applied the methodology in each historical case). The following sections examine the way critical contextualized methodology, particularly its heuristic tools of context, interaction, and power-knowledge analysis, can work together with Appadurai's theory of global cultural flows to examine how mediascape, ideoscape, ethnoscape, technoscape, and financescape unfolded and functioned in transcultural communication about SARS.

Transcultural Interactions among
Mediascapes and Ideoscapes

Appadurai coins the terms *mediascape* and *ideoscape*, or "closely related landscapes of images," to study the way cultural imagination works (35). Mediascape refers to

> the distribution of the electronic capacities to produce and disseminate information (newspapers, magazines, TV stations, and film-production studio). . . . These images involve many complicated inflections, depending on their mode, their hardware (electronic or pre-electronic), their audiences (local, national, or transnational), and the interest of those who own and control them. (33)

As a result, people around the world experience the media as "a complicated and interconnected repertoire of print, celluloid, electronic screens, and billboards" that produce "scripts [and fantasies] of imagined lives of their own and others" (35). As "concatenations of images," ideoscapes are often political and relate to ideologies of states and to counterideologies (36). They consist of "elements of the Enlightenment worldview" using "a chain of ideas, terms, and images," such as freedom, democracy, rights, representation, and sovereignty (36).

In their edited collection *New Media for a New China*, James F. Scotton and William A. Hachten call newspapers, magazines, radio, and television "traditional media" because of the tight control held over them by the ruling Communist Party. As economic reforms change China from "Marxist communism to authoritarian capitalism," traditional media gain more freedom in terms of content and management, but the government still retains firm control over them (3). By contrast, Scotton and Hachten categorize the Internet, "bi-directional" cell phones, and blogs as "new media," whose "impacts are rapidly changing the economic, political, and social landscapes of China" (9). In 2008, China had 350 million cell phones, 250 million Internet users, and 30 million blogs (3)—reflecting a population of new media users so large that its constant activities are overwhelming even to the roughly fifty thousand Internet censors that China employs to control information and delete "unhealthy" content related to pornography or politics (Macartney). These new media help to bring a new "openness," function as a bridge between the government and the public, and may "[develop] into 'public sphere' that Habermas says is essential to any democracy" (Scotton and Hachten 40).

Scotton and Hachten believe that both traditional and new media provide news and entertainment. My study is more interested in news media than entertainment media (film or TV shows) because of the prominent roles played by print media and the Internet in news making. It is important to distinguish these newer alternative media, or what Scotton and Hachten call "new media," from the more traditional media controlled by either nation-states, as in the case of China, or by leading media corporations, as in the case of the United States. To do so, I define *alternative media* as nonmainstream media that implicitly or explicitly contest the dominant power in individual nation-states and cultures, including a wide range of independent overseas Chinese websites, contesting foreign media, and guerrilla media. I consider *guerrilla media* as interpersonal communication technologies widely used by and easily accessible to the general public, namely, technology-assisted media that include mobile-phone text messages, phone calls, Internet forums and chat rooms, traditional word-of-mouth media, and popular social media applications, such as personal blogs, instant messaging, and equivalents of Facebook and Twitter in various countries.

Transcultural mediascapes and ideoscapes played significant roles in communicating to the public the magnitude of and the risks posed by SARS. To understand these functions, one has to investigate how media structures and communicative practices operate differently in individual countries and how such cultural differences, in turn, influence the ways those countries communicated about SARS to the local and global communities. Scrutinizing the historical, cultural, political, and economic contexts surrounding mediascapes and ideoscapes allows us to better study the production, circulation, and consumption of widely dispersed, continuously evolving, constantly contesting, and highly ambiguous knowledges of new, emerging epidemics.

Comparison of Chinese, American Media Structures

Media play different roles in the United States and China because of different political systems, ownerships of media organizations, communicative practices, and media policies. In the United States, newspapers and periodicals are "preeminently profit-making organizations" controlled by private entrepreneurs rather than state or local governments (Fairclough 42); accordingly, they depend on revenue to function and stay in the market. Because of this structure, systematic media control or overt censorship by the government seldom takes place, and members of the press frequently issue self-congratulatory claims of freedom of speech. Norman Fairclough describes a "form of complicity between the media and the dominant social classes or groups," a function of media texts that reinforces social control and social reproduction (47). Meanwhile, media texts also "operate as cultural commodities in a competitive market" and are "caught up in—reflecting and contributing to—shifting cultural values and identities" (Fairclough 48).

However, the lack of systematic censorship does not prevent American media from being propagandistic or from serving the interest of the privileged. In *Manufacturing Consent*, Edward S. Herman and Noam Chomsky identify three reasons that turn the media into propaganda tools: the reliance on advertisement revenue for profit, the corporate structure of news ownership and production, and the acceptance of information from biased sources. Their case studies demonstrate that the American media distort domestic and international events to serve the interests of the privileged at the expense of minorities and the underclass. David A. Schultz also warns that "news is increasingly what will entertain, sustain the status quo, and maximize corporate profits" (24).

Deeply embedded in a vastly different political system and historical context, the structures and functions of Chinese media tell a completely different story. The media-control system in China was originally borrowed from the former Soviet Union, where media claimed to represent mass will by upholding the Party creeds (Hong and Leow; C. C. Lee, "Ambiguities"; Schell). Calling the media the "tongue of the Party," the Communist Party of China (CPC) has been controlling the media as an "ideological vehicle and propaganda tool" since the foundation of the People's Republic of China in 1949 (J. Zhang 165). The CPC functions concurrently as the owner, manager, and operator of the media (Chu). For many years, Chinese media was financed by the government rather than by advertisements as the primary source of revenue (Hong and Leow). Print media in China can only operate after obtaining official licenses from the State General Publishing Administration, which is subordinate to the Central Propaganda Department (Schell). Any production and circulation of politically or economically sensitive information may put the publisher at risk and may result in license suspension.

As governmental subsidies are withdrawn from most media organizations except for a few national ones, ongoing economic reform in China, in addition to invigorating China's economy, is unintentionally liberating China's media system. Since the 1990s, driven by the need to commercialize the media so that they can make profit to survive, the Chinese government has "actively promoted corporatization of the media industry [by] forming 47 large state-owned media groups" (J. Zhang 167). Each group owned up to a dozen newspapers and magazines ranging from the Party's mouthpieces to affiliated trade newspapers and tabloids. Like other state-owned enterprises, these media corporations must compete for customers. In other words, they must maintain profitable margins to survive financially, or they will wither and die. This change creates a lively, realistic, and contesting atmosphere in the media industry because journalists constantly push the limits of the CPC by reporting on sensitive political and economic issues (Hong and Leow; Zhao). In response to such challenges of censorship orders, the CPC's propaganda departments at the provincial, municipal, and prefectural levels take measures to control the information flow in China. They closely monitor the content of the media through a "three-level post-publishing punishment," such as "internal criticism and warning, changing the staff and suspending license, and closedown" (J. Zhang 170).

Interaction, Contestation between the Two Systems

Despite the seemingly drastic difference between the media systems in the United States and in China, they share a long history of competition and contestations as national news media in the era of cultural globalization. In the United States, the Voice of America (VOA) started to offer Mandarin- and Cantonese-language shortwave broadcasts in 1942. Part of the impetus for offering foreign-language news programs was the liberation and independence of previous colonies in Africa and Asia and the establishment of communist countries, such as China and Cuba. The mission of VOA's Chinese program, for instance, was to disseminate unfiltered, "prodemocracy" information, to subvert the dominant propaganda, and to peacefully sabotage the communist regime in China (Gertz). Although China's domestic media were tightly controlled before the 1990s, shortwave broadcasts, such as VOA and the BBC, had long been providing politically sensitive news in the air to anyone with access to a transistor radio. VOA has been broadcasting anti-China views and discussing politically sensitive topics, such as the Pearl Harbor attack in 1941, the US atomic bombings against Hiroshima and Nagasaki in 1945, Japan's decision to surrender at the end of the World War II, the liberation of China in 1949, and the 1989 Tiananmen Square event. Chinese popular movies about the anti-Japanese War (1937–45) or the Chinese Civil

War (1945–49) often feature influential military leaders, spies, and ordinary people anxiously listening to VOA or BBC radio broadcasts to learn about the latest developments in both wars.

With increasing exchanges between China and the United States and with the rise of the Internet, radio broadcast services gradually lost their popularity and their international impact over time. Technically savvy Internet users now circumvent e-surveillance in China to read and disseminate news published on the official websites of major foreign media. Because of a dramatic decrease in shortwave listening and a shrinking budget for foreign broadcasting in the United States, the Barack Obama administration decided in 2011 to shut down VOA's shortwave broadcasts to China, which are considered "relics" of "a Cold War–era propaganda playbook" (Landler 4). VOA will modernize and streamline its programs for delivery "via television, the Web, social-media services, and mobile phones" (Landler 4). Meanwhile, to promote the use of digital media to disseminate unfiltered news to "repressive countries," the State Department devoted about $70 million to develop so-called circumvention/liberation technologies, such as "stealth wireless networks" and mobile phone–based "trusted networks of citizens" (Glanz and Markoff 1).

In their book on media globalization, David Machin and Theo van Leeuwen observe "a trend towards global domination by transnational media conglomerates," with local media copying "modes of production, formats and technologies that originated in the USA" (169). Asian media often accuse their Western counterparts of monopoly, intentional distortion, and slandering. According to this view, Western media dominate international public opinion because of their ability to release over 90 percent of daily news in international news coverage in traditional print-based media, mass media, and the Internet (Meng and Fang). To counter Western media's global impacts, leading editors and managers of news groups in East Asia urged media organizations in the region to "pool resources and cooperate" both to "break the monopoly held by Western media giants" and to avoid being "squeeze[d] out" as regional players ("Call for Media Group").

The global media market is full of competition, contestation, and fragmentation. Both global players and regional players compete for transnational audiences, regional subscriptions, and impacts on global and regional public opinions. The year of 2011 witnessed not only the US government's major reduction in its overseas propaganda machine but also "Sino-cast expansion"

(Gertz). Beijing expanded its "propaganda footprint" in the United States both by launching sixty affiliates and by making the China Central Television (CCTV) widely available on US cable networks (Gertz). In addition, Hong Kong–based Phoenix Satellite Television established a global presence at the beginning of the new millennium to "shorten the distance between the Chinese around the world" ("Major Roles for Mass Media"). Despite this expansion, overseas Chinese media still function mostly as "niche media" targeting "the expatriate Chinese community," thus exerting limited impact on the global media market ("Tackle Western Media").

Alternative Media: Integral Force

Although Appadurai is more concerned about print and televisual media in his discussion of mediascapes, the recent rapid development of communication technologies further complicates the existence and function of the term. As sites of contention among media powers, alternative media challenge dominant power structures and communicate to a large audience across geographical and media boundaries. As a more flexible, mobile, and accessible force in alternative media, guerrilla media function as "weapons of the weak" that open up media spaces to marginalized groups and help define new political situations (Chin-chuan Lee 163).

During the SARS outbreak in China, these alternative media were particularly active, presenting inside stories, anonymous personal narratives, and contradictory messages about the nature and magnitude of the outbreaks and possible preventive measures—functions that stood in stark contrast to more official Chinese media outlets, which either printed occasional success narratives about the containment of local outbreaks or remained silent about the epidemic before WHO's intervention in mid-March. Because this mixture of risk messages presented a significant challenge to the official narratives state-controlled mass media told, no study of local and global SARS discourses would be complete without examining the roles played by alternative media. To better understand the different rhetorics surrounding SARS, it is not enough to focus on the mainstream rhetorics of SARS from China or the United States, as existing studies have done (Fidler; Kleinman and Watson).

With the introduction of the Internet and the World Wide Web, a wider terrain for media production has been made available both to power apparatuses and to the public. Nick Couldry and James Curran define alternative media as "media production that challenges, at least implicitly, actual concentration of media power" ("Paradox" 7). Manuel Castells, Mireia Fernandez-Ardevol, Jack Linchuan Qiu, and Araba Sey see mobile communication as a means of supporting insurgent politics because its mobility and multimodality enhance both the "speed of information flow" and the spread of "rumors, inaccurate information . . . and truth" through interpersonal networks (209–12). The use of text messages, mobile phones, and social media helps people to "gain new forms of social power, new ways to organize their interactions and exchanges just in time and just in place" (Rheingold xii). Given the heterogeneous nature of alternative media in terms of form, style, content, perspective, and means of production and distribution, the study of alternative media should be "alert to historical or geographical contingency" and should "pay attention to hybridity" (Atton 29).

The use and impacts of alternative media are determined not only by the nature of the technology itself but, more important, by the local cultural and political contexts within which they are embedded. For instance, spammers have been using various types of online tools to exploit worries about the H1N1 flu outbreak in the United States. Such tools range from newly registered Internet domains and spam e-mails with provocative titles to links to phishing or malware sites. These spammers aim to infect computers, to steal personal information, and to promote online pharmacy sales. At the early stage of the H1N1 flu pandemic, when online webcasting services and social-networking sites were flooded with swine-flu messages, the US Centers for Disease Control and Prevention (CDC) generated news alerts via its Twitter accounts and its YouTube channel to distribute authoritative and fact-based information (Ding and Zhang). In China, official censorship makes it extremely difficult for alternative media to operate as independent newspapers or websites, which have been the main formats of alternative media in the United States. The Central Propaganda Department constantly exerts media surveillance to control both print and digital media. The use of Internet policing and the "Great Red Firewall" to filter out "unhealthy" content reveals China's political co-option of the Internet in monitoring media output and in shutting down dissenting voices (Hermida). Driven by commercial interests, major Internet service providers, such as Yahoo or Sohu, comply with governmental requirements by filtering politically sensitive news and by monitoring user-generated content on their websites.

As a result of this close monitoring of print and digital media, the Chinese public turns to other, less regulated channels for information. Bulletin board systems (BBS), with their themed forums and mechanism of participation and reward, provide urban middle classes and the younger generations with integrated leisure activities. More important, as public spaces for the construction and negotiations of "indigenous [People's Republic of China] identities," they function as "an alternative model competing with [Chinese Communist Party] orthodoxy" (Mengin 9). By 2005, China became the largest cell-phone market with nearly 350 million users, with a total of 100 million Internet users, which grew at 30 percent per year. The use of "chain letter" e-mails and text messages helped not only to circumvent existing censorship but also to sustain underground conversations about SARS risks. This undercurrent of unofficial risk messages resulted in widespread panic buying in Guangdong and Beijing. In early April, Chinatowns in North America and other parts of the world also witnessed rapidly declining businesses because of rumor mongering (Yardley A1).

These details illustrate that the study of transcultural communication requires close examination of media structures and communicative practices in different cultures. Only by doing so can we understand how and why individual cultures communicate differently about the global epidemics. Moreover, this approach helps to expose the cultural, political, economic, institutional, and historical forces that drive and shape communication practices as well as the power apparatuses that authorize or silence media production.

Interrelated Financescapes, Technoscapes, and Ethnoscapes

Transnational connectivities at work during global epidemics involve not only networks of discourses circulating in mediascapes but also disjunctive global human movements (ethnoscapes), technology flows (technoscapes), and financial transfers (financescapes) (Appadurai 35). Appadurai emphasizes that "the global relationship among ethnoscapes, technoscapes, and financescapes is deeply disjunctive and profoundly unpredictable" because each of them is "subject to its own constraints and incentives at the same time as each acts as a constraint and a parameter for movements in others" (35). The economic and public health interests of developing and developed countries are simultaneously overlapping and competing. Starting in the 1970s, contemporary globalization led to trade expansion, the growth of investment, the "migration, relocation, and reorganization of private businesses," and rapid international travel (Schaeffer 2). However, "shared global developments" may mean different things and have different impacts on people in different places (Schaeffer 16). Moreover, individual countries have their own "specific concerns in the context of global institutions and interdependence" (Lampton 161).

Middle-income and lower-income countries are ill-prepared for flu pandemics ("Developing Countries Ill-Prepared"; "Swine Influenza" 1495). Using Christopher J. L. Murray, Alan D Lopez, Brian Chin, Dennis Feehan, and Kenneth H. Hill's data from the 1918–20 Spanish flu pandemic, a *Lancet* editorial in 2009 predicts that the next flu pandemic would "kill 62 million people, with *96% of those deaths occurring in low-income and middle-income settings*" ("Swine Influenza"; emphasis added). Contributing to this disparity of pandemic impacts is the unbalanced distribution of the global stockpile of antiviral drugs (i.e., Tamiflu and Relenza and flu vaccines), with most of them held by "governments of wealthy countries such as the United States, Britain, Canada, France, Italy, and Japan" ("Developing Countries Ill-Prepared").

In his analysis of the impacts of the H1N1 flu on Asian countries, Mark MacKinnon points out that the Asian economy is more vulnerable because of its heavy reliance on international trade and tourism as well as the high density of population and inadequate public health infrastructure in many countries (A13). The same is true for Mexico, the origin country of the H1N1 flu, and for many other developing countries. Compared with the United States, Mexico suffers from a much higher mortality rate owing to inadequate medical facilities, insufficient funding, densely crowded cities, comparatively low nutrition levels, and people's delay in seeking medical treatment.

Graduated Sovereignty in China

Many countries, including Malaysia and Indonesia, "have responded to market demands and political resistances through a strategy of graduated sovereignty that subjects different segments of the population to different mixes of disciplinary, caring, and punitive technologies" (Ong, "Graduated Sovereignty" 22). Ong invents the term *graduated sovereignty* to refer to

> the differential treatment of populations according to ethno-racial differences, and the dictate of development programs. [. . .] Segments of the population are differently disciplined and given differential privileges and protections, in relation to their varying participation in

globalized market activities. [. . .] Such variegated citizenship is greatly reinforced when the state reorganizes national space into new economic zones that promote international trade and investments. ("Graduated Sovereignty" 65)

In other words, graduated sovereignty manifests itself not only in "the ethno-racial discriminations of populations" but also "the rise of production and technological zones which have required certain legal compromises in national sovereignty" ("Graduated Sovereignty" 65). It offers "differential treatment of populations that differently insert them into the processes of global capitalism" ("Graduated Sovereignty" 62). To apply this concept in the context of China, I adapt Ong's definition to describe packages of rights, privileges, and duties assigned to different populations, classes, and regions with vastly different levels of economic development. Such privileges and duties are determined by the outdated *hukou* system of internal passports that perpetuates the urban-rural divide, by class structures that are increasingly determined by citizens' professions, and by solidified social structures that pay more attention to "who your father is" than "who you are." Exploring these aspects of graduated sovereignty helps to illustrate the disjunctive and unpredictable relationship among the financescape, the technoscape, and the ethnoscape.

Outdated Hukou System and the Ever-Widening Urban-Rural Gap

Modeled after the Soviet Union's internal passports, China's hukou system was introduced in 1958 to prevent the flow of poor rural residents to cities and to keep track of people. A kind of household registration permit, the hukou contains not only all identifying information of any household but, more important, the city, town, or village to which anyone belongs (Richburg A08). Hukou records "arbitrarily divide Chinese citizens into two categories, urban and rural, not according to where they live, but on a hereditary basis"; by using inherited birthplaces as the criteria to determine the rights and duties that various types of citizens can claim, it perpetuates an ever-widening urban-rural divide ("Rural Economies"). The hukou system has been criticized as "one of the most strictly enforced 'apartheid' social structures in modern world history"; it treats farmers as second-class citizens (Luard) and creates "gaping discrepancy between the level of services offered in rural and urban China" (McCabe A16). As rural migrants travel to big cities to find jobs in construction and in other low-wage, labor-intensive industries, this dual residential structure denies them subsidized housing, free education and medical care, unemployment benefits, and pensions. As a mechanism of differential treatment, the hukou system provides city residents with education, housing, and social security while marginalizing rural migrants who have little economic, political, or cultural resources. To some extent, it is a type of discrimination based on the geopolitical urban-rural division. After the 2003 SARS epidemic, the government did take some measures to partially address these gaping discrepancy by adopting a pension system and a new rural health care cooperative, but even these accommodations offer much less than their counterparts for city dwellers. It is estimated that China would have to spend an additional 1.65 trillion RMB, or about US$25 billion, every year to ensure that all of its 1.3 billion people enjoy standard social security (E. Zhang 06).

Social Status, Profession-Based Social Classes

Before the economic reform that started in the late 1970s, China had three social classes: workers, farmers, and intellectuals. The last thirty years have witnessed the adjustment of economic structures from state ownership to a variety of ownerships as well as changes in modes of distribution of wealth. Currently, most of the country's wealth is concentrated in big business owners and directors as well as high officials controlling key decisions, such as the distribution of land titles and bank loans.

In their influential book *Study of Contemporary Chinese Social Strata*, Xueyi Lu and his research group divide Chinese populations into ten social classes, mostly determined by professions and the subsequent ownership of institutional, economic, and cultural resources. These ten classes, ranking from the highest to the lowest, are

1. governmental officials (1 percent)
2. upper- and middle-level managers of large and mid-sized enterprises (1 percent)
3. private enterprise owners (1 percent)
4. professionals with expertise in science and technologies (5 percent)
5. office staff (5 percent)
6. self-employed small-business owners (10 percent)
7. employees of tertiary industries (8 percent)
8. manufacturing workers (20 percent)
9. agricultural workers (40 percent)
10. unemployed or underemployed urban residents (9 percent)

Figure 1.3 maps out the varying types and degrees of resources that these social classes own, as indicated both by the locations of the numbers in the three circles representing the three resources as well as the font sizes of the numbers representing the ten classes. Governmental officials, private-enterprise owners, and professionals with specialized expertise own the greatest percentages of institutional, economic, and cultural resources, respectively. By contrast, employees of tertiary industries, workers, and farmers own few, if any resources.

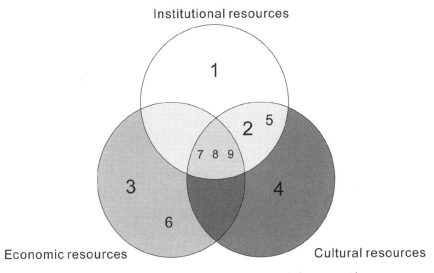

Figure 1.3. Ownership of resources by the ten social classes in China

Lu also defines five social statuses: upper class, upper-middle class, middle class, lower-middle class, lower class (*Study*). Members of various social classes, depending on their status in their own professions, may fall into several different categories (see fig. 1.4). For instance, senior and best-connected professionals with specialized expertise may belong to either the upper class or the upper-middle class whereas novice professionals may still strive simply to join the middle class. Farmers, depending on their skills and their land ownership and use (i.e., building houses for rental purposes near big cities), may belong to either the lower-middle class or the lower class. China provides very different packages of rights and duties to the ten social classes. While the first five classes enjoy high salaries as well as access to child care, public education for their children, medical care, and pensions, the lower five classes often receive very low salaries and have little access to other benefits.

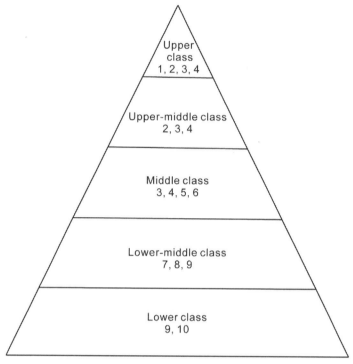

Figure 1.4. Five social statuses and ten social classes in China

Era of "Competition among Fathers," Inherited Poverty

An article in *Study Time*, a publication owned by the Central CPC's College, warns of "the accelerating solidification of all social classes, the resistance against further reform toward equity, and the lack of mechanism for vertical mobility among the social classes" (Cai). The lower classes have little opportunity either to benefit from economic reforms or to move up the social ladder. With the majority having little access to resources, equal services, or equal opportunities for development, the unequal social structure becomes increasingly solidified.

To make things worse, China's educational system is losing its capacity to facilitate mobilization among social classes and to build a more equal society. Feudal China relied on the *keju* mechanism, which used annual national examinations to identify future officials and serves as the traditional, albeit limited, channel for kids from poor, lower-class families to acquire social mobility. Often translated as "imperial civil service examinations," the keju mechanism lasted for over thirteen hundred years in China and exerted tremendous influence on the way other Asian countries, such as Vietnam, Japan, and Korea, elected their own public officials (Miyazaki). With keju functioning as the mechanism of meritocracy for numerous dynasties, many famous leading officials spent many years "farming on sunny days and studying on rainy days" before they succeeded in the national examinations and got promoted to junior officials. However, as the national education system became industrialized and the job market became increasingly competitive, poor students began to suffer from their inability to pay tuition before graduation. After graduation, many now find themselves jobless or underemployed because of their lack of connections in the city. Accordingly, Cai claims that China is now in an era of "competition among fathers": "[I]t is who your father is, not who you are, that determines your life after college." Students from rich and powerful families get the best-paid jobs and become what Chinese Internet users commonly call the "rich second generation." Students from poor families, however, suffer the fate of "inherited poverty" and become the "poor second generation." Some may be lucky enough to join the middle class of professionals or office staff, but most are stuck in tertiary or manufacturing industries. With "segments of the population differently linked to global circuits of production, competitiveness, and exchange," those who play important roles in national economic and political activities may rise as the privileged elite, and those who play peripheral roles become disarticulated from and thus less legitimate in the national political and economic order (Ong, "Graduated Sovereignty" 69).

One of the most highly desired means of escape from this solidified class structure is to obtain financial support from foreign universities to pursue advanced degrees abroad. Applicants are required only to take standard tests, to put application packages together, and to apply for different programs in foreign universities. This is one of the few things that "who your father is" does not determine; thus, obtaining advanced degrees abroad serves as a shortcut to social mobility. With many students finding jobs in science and engineering and staying in countries such as Canada or the United States, Chinese government officials at various levels regularly go abroad to recruit foreign-educated Chinese talent as a means of bringing international technologies, expertise, and investments back to China. These recruits then serve in middle management or play leading technological roles in various enterprises.

Special Zones, Global Intellectual Citizenship

In China, zones of graduated sovereignty range from special economic zones in coastal areas to economically deprived countryside in the inner provinces. Deng Xiaoping designated four coastal cities as special economic zones in 1979, granting them greater autonomy and privileges, including preferential policies regarding taxation, duties, and foreign exchange. Heavily subsidized by the government, special economic zones were expected to develop export-oriented industries and to serve both as receptors of foreign investment and as generators of foreign-exchange earnings. The same policies of openness and reform encouraged "certain areas and some people to get rich first through honest work and legal operations"; as Deng declared in his famous southern tour in 1992, "To get rich is glorious." In this influential tour, Deng visited special economic zones, such as Shenzhen and Zhuhai, and called for further economic reform and opening up, which later became China's national policy (Y. Wang). Such national policies aimed to "maximize the inflow of international resources for [China's] modernization" (Lampton 62). Global financial flows to China not only brought "technologies, modern management techniques, growth, and jobs" but also created economic interdependence and risks (Lampton 189). For instance, coastal provinces, such as Guangdong, Jiangsu, and Fujian, developed export-oriented economy and attracted about 86 percent of foreign direct investments (FDI) in 2003 (E. Zhang). With the inflow of low technologies and the high concentration of labor-intensive, export-oriented industries, such as garments and electronics, the Guangdong Province alone attracted twelve million migrant workers from the countryside of numerous poorer provinces in 2003 (P. Wang). Therefore, the constant inflow of foreign investments, orders, and migrant workers became an essential condition to the continuous prosperity and development of export-oriented provinces.

Because of increasing labor costs in China, foreign investments in labor-intensive industries have gradually shifted to other countries, such as Vietnam and Cambodia, with cheaper labor. To enhance national competitiveness for foreign investments, China initiated so-called high and new technology zones, or what Ong calls "technology parks," in metropolitan areas, such as Guangzhou, Shanghai, and Beijing. Such high-tech parks aim "to promote local research and development and to link up with the transnational technological research and development communities" (Ong, "Graduated Sovereignty" 68).

As a driving force to change transnational configurations of technoscapes, these zones attract both top talent produced by Chinese universities and others returning from overseas with management and professional backgrounds and/or high-tech products and investments. The zones also become the hot zones that produce upper and middle classes of upper- and mid-level managers and private-enterprise owners as well as middle classes of specialized professionals and office staff, further demonstrating the close interconnectedness among technoscapes, financescapes, and ethnoscapes in China.

Françoise Mengin explores the creation of the "Silicon Valley model" and the rise of informational capitalism in mainland China, Taiwan, and Hong Kong. This Siliconization strategy mobilized "high-tech development" discourses in private and public actors both in the region and in the overseas Chinese communities (Mengin 5). Taiwan built its first science-based industrial park in Hsinchu in the early 1990s to better integrate the nation into the global circuit of capital, knowledge, and expertise. The government employed economic incentives to appeal to its diasporic networks of engineers and venture capitalists. Silicon Valley returnees functioned as the key transnational links and "brought back with them technical skill, organizational and managerial know-how, entrepreneurial experience, and connections to [information and communication technology] markets in the United States" (Sum 212). Like Malaysia and Singapore, Mainland China and Hong Kong started to catch up in the "Silicon Wave" after the 1998 Asian Crisis. High-tech industrial development zones, including software parks, bioengineering centers, cyber-hubs, and medicine valleys, were established not only in the Pearl River Delta but also in Shanghai and Beijing as a part of China's national development project. The quick rise of Silicon Valleys in "Greater China" resulted in intense competition "to lure talented personnel from other provinces within China, from among the diasporic entrepreneurs, and from overseas–Chinese student community to work in the parks or elsewhere in the economy" (Sum 226). A "transnational silicon coalition" emerged across the trans-Pacific region, with "clusters of Silicon Valleys in 'Greater China' functioning as part of the longer Silicon production chain that stretches to the heartland of informational capitalism in the United States" (Sum 227). This creation of the "transnational silicon coalition" not only facilitated intense interaction among global technoscapes, financescapes, and ethnoscapes but also resulted in "brain circulation," allowing the most desirable knowledge workers to cross national borders as well as the borders among various sectors (Sum 216).

Ong coins the term *globalized intellectual citizenship* to describe a globally mobile knowledge population for whom states and regions compete to accumulate intellectual capital ("Urban Assemblage" 252). For instance, Singapore's "quest for global city status depends on a policy of 'opening borders to brains'" and requires "leveraging [of] managers and knowledge workers across industries, regions, and cultures" (Ong, "Urban Assemblage" 241). Singapore employs "fine gradations" in its immigration process to attract talented expatriates: "The top criteria are for foreigners with professional qualifications, university degrees, or specialist skills. They must either be entrepreneurs or investors, or hold professional or administrative positions" (Ong, "Urban Assemblage" 248). These global business and professional classes enjoy a transnational intellectual citizenship that "cuts across different political domains of social rights," and they are "treated as a special class of urban citizens regardless of their actual legal status" (Ong, "Urban Assemblage" 250). Expatriates from Europe, North America, and Australia—known to local Singaporeans as "citizens without local roots"—often have five-year contracts in business, finance, and academic fields, but many leave sooner. The expatriates most likely to apply for citizenship are mainland Chinese and Indian students who earn undergraduate degrees from local universities before locating jobs in the high-tech sector. Nevertheless, Ong wonders whether this group constitutes a "flow-through" population who views taking jobs in Singapore as a step in their career paths before they move on to better jobs in China or in the United States ("Urban Assemblage" 250). Although China employs far fewer North American or European expatriates in its high-tech and finance industries, it places equal emphasis on the global recruitment of talents. Like Taiwan, it employs preferential policies to lure diasporic entrepreneurs and professionals as well as overseas students to return and work for its Silicon Valleys.

Regional Disparity, Global Capital, Compromised Sovereignty

In addition to huge influxes of foreign investments and thriving regional economies, Chinese coastal regions, such as Guangdong, also enjoy strong public health infrastructure, world-class medical facilities, and a concentration of medical experts. Thus, even in February and March 2003 when little was known about the mysterious pneumonia, Guangdong medical experts made quick progress in both clinical treatment and anti-infection measures, which was highly valued by WHO.

Whereas coast provinces enjoyed strong public health infrastructure, personnel, and funding, poor central and western provinces had minimal public health infrastructure because of their poor local economies. One instance is Qingxu County in Shanxi Province, which witnessed not only the first SARS case in the province but also an explosive outbreak because of its poor medical infrastructure and subsequent high infection rate among medical care workers. Qingxu's disease-prevention station was so severely underfunded that it received from the county only one-fourth of the budget needed to cover staff salary and operational expenditure; to survive, it relied on public health monitoring fees. Worse, in the entire province of Shanxi, only a few hospitals had specialized respiratory divisions, each with only thirty to forty beds (Hu, Luo, and Li). Shanxi's medical and public health systems became so overwhelmed by SARS that the provincial government issued an unusual alert titled "Urgent Notification of Strengthening the Treatment and Control of SARS," which requested "rigorous case reporting and strict control of the transfers of patients across cities" to prevent further spreading across the province (Hu, Luo, and Li). Unsurprising, Shanxi was listed in WHO's April 23 travel advisory along with Beijing and Toronto.

This huge disparity of economic and health resources contributed to a widespread fear that the SARS epidemic would be impossible to contain once it reached the underdeveloped hinterland. The countryside was even less prepared, since most farmers had little or no medical resources and no medical insurance. Villages in provinces and near municipal cities with ongoing infections took radical measures to protect themselves. Nearby highways were blocked, facilities designated to become SARS clinics were destroyed, and migrant workers returning from SARS-affected areas were quarantined for two weeks. In addition, volunteers employed health registration forms and thermometers to monitor visitors' health conditions before admitting them into the community.

In sum, the existence of special economic zones resulted in severe economic disparity among regions, which worsened the increasing urban-rural divide. In 2005, two hundred million migrant workers, the so-called floating population, left their hometowns to search for temporary jobs in big cities. Therefore, China's ethnoscape has been profoundly changed after the economic reform. Every year before the Spring Festival, the equivalent of Christmas in the United States, hundreds of millions of migrant workers travel home for annual family reunions. Then after the Spring Festival, they take trains or long-distance buses to look for new jobs and better pay in rich coastal provinces. Such massive flows of people produce great strain not only on the transportation system but also on the labor market in China.

Unprecedentedly mobile because of the "transnationalization of production," capital and production are in constant search for maximal profit while avoiding any social, political, or biopolitical disruption (Wilson and Dissanayake 28). With transnational corporations dominating the flows of production, capital, and commodity, the nation-state has only limited power to regulate the economy internally. Moreover, "regions and region-states increasingly override national borders and older territorial forms and create special economic zones of uneven development and transcultural hybridity" (Wilson and Dissanayake 2). This weakened sovereign power results in economic fragmentation and global economic interdependence.

As one of the leading recipients of foreign direct investment in the world, China received US$60 billion in 2005. The total number of employees in foreign-invested enterprises exceeded 23.5 million, representing 10 percent of the nonagricultural working population nationwide ("Attracting Foreign Investment"). China's reliance on foreign investments has become so heavy that the withdrawal of global capital would not only damage the national economy but also threaten the economic survival of some of its population. For instance, Guangdong, the province where SARS originated and the home manufacturing base for the Pearl River Delta, accounted for one-tenth of the gross domestic product of China in 2002. However, because of SARS, Guangdong "trade fared down eighty percent in terms of its contracts" ("Impact of SARS").

As a developing country offering cheap labor, China was one of the most popular destinations of foreign investment in the 1990s. During the SARS epidemic, this investment placed a significant burden on its government. Maintaining the health of its population required China to declare itself as affected and to engage in stringent measures, such as quarantine or health screening. But such measures would, in turn, disrupt local economic activities and result in huge losses of foreign investments. In other words, in the short term, the preservation of reproductivity (health) could be achieved only at a huge cost to productivity (work and profit), leading to inevitable economic losses. Thus, during the initial stage of SARS, China's biopolitical concern with the reproductivity of its citizens was subordinate to its larger concern with productivity, or social and economic stability, because of the important role that global capital plays in the country's economy (Lampton).

2
Risk Communication about
an Emerging Epidemic
in Guangdong, China

How can we study health risk communication about emerging global epidemics in non-Western countries when the urgent need to acquire preliminary understanding about the new epidemics is further complicated by media control and self-censorship?

With avian flu posing a catastrophic pandemic threat capable of breaking out in any part of the world, the study of global risk communication practices, particularly that of risk communication practices in non-Western cultures, becomes increasingly important. Only with the understanding of various risk communication practices can the global community collaborate more effectively in pandemic outbreaks. Such studies help to identify gaps in and possible ways to expand existing risk communication theories. This chapter examines the way risk communication operated during the initial stage of SARS in its origin, the Guangdong Province, from November 2002 to February 2003, right before SARS grew from a regional epidemic into a global one.

Concerned with the communication practices between experts and the public, most risk communication theories focus on the interaction among industry, scientists, technical communicators, interest groups, and the public (Grabill and Simmons; Leiss and Powell; for a comprehensive review of risk communication theories, see Simmons). William Leiss and Douglas Powell, for example, define risk communication as "the process of exchanges about how best to assess and manage risks among academics, regulatory practitioners, interest groups, and the general public" (33). Risk communication practices surrounding SARS in Guangdong, China, however, pose questions that existing risk communication theories neglect or cannot address. Some such issues include the relative absence of interest groups or technical communicators as a specialized profession; strong governmental intervention; the simultaneously ongoing processes of risk assessment and risk communication as attempts to understand the unknown and spreading epidemic; the use of two distinct communicative channels, that is, partial disclosure[1] in publicly released governmental discourses in the media and full disclosure in classified governmental discourses; and the creation of the official "no risk" narrative through the use of cooption, selective coverage, and partial censorship. Specifically, this chapter addresses the following questions:

1. How did risk communication practices in non-Western cultures differ from those in Western countries, such as the United States and Great Britain?
2. How did rhetoric operate to facilitate the acceptance of the official "no risk" narrative amid uncertainty and confusion about the emerging epidemic of SARS?
3. What implications does the study of health risk communication about SARS in China have for the theory building of global risk communication?

This chapter examines the way health risk communication about SARS operated in the media and in governmental institutions amid uncertainty and fear at the early stage of SARS. First is a review of the issue of information vacuum in risk communication and the possible impacts of selective censorship on the creation of less-visible risk vacuums and the false impression of honest reporting. What follows is a historical review of the development of the regional SARS outbreak. My study of these risk communication processes reveals the existence of two distinct and noninteracting channels of risk communication: the mass media claiming that the SARS outbreak was under control in order to prevent mass panic and the classified governmental discourses addressing the severity of the local outbreak and coordinating institutional efforts to fight against SARS and its social side effects of panic buying, inflation, and economic losses.[2] Using enthymemic analysis, the chapter examines the way the official rhetoric of "SARS is under control" operated in the regional media. Then investigated are the roles that co-opted expert discourses, reviews, and critical commentaries played in convincing the public that the local epidemic was truly under control.

The next section explores the heightened sense of uncertainty, urgency, and action demonstrated in classified governmental discourses and the real-time risk communication deployed among the government, medical institutions, and regional media. The chapter concludes by proposing a critical contextualized model to study risk communication practices in non-Western countries that pays close attention to local power relations, material conditions, and values and beliefs instead of oversimplifying risk communication as an easily abstractable and universal practice across cultures. My analysis calls attention to the larger issues of culture, institutions, power, and knowledge in global risk politics. It also shows how professionals, including journalists and practitioners, played the dual role of subject-area experts and risk communicators and were deeply enmeshed in power relations among governmental apparatuses, media, economic interests, and cultural communicative practices.

Risk Communication Vacuum and Selective Reporting

Leiss and Powell's theory of risk communication failures examines the role media play in the risk communication processes and the interaction among experts, governmental institutions, and the media. It offers insights complementary to Jeffrey T. Grabill and Michele Simmons's discussion of contexts, power, and user knowledge in risk communication. Leiss and Powell examine expert risk assessment in technical documents from scientific journals and governmental reports and employ media accounts as "source[s] of clues to the public perception" of risk (39). They trace and compare "the parallel tracks of the two dimensions" of expert risk and perceived risk, which reveals the way these two dimensions influence each other. Their collection contains numerous case studies that examine risk communication exchanges and the formation of public risk perceptions through the analysis of media coverage and technical documents. Their cases draw lessons from risk communication failures in the United States, Great Britain, and Canada, particularly focusing on the negative impact of risk information gaps, or the risk communication vacuum, between experts and the media.

However, the presence of risk communication vacuums does not necessarily mean that there is a lack of communication between experts and the public, but that *there is something amiss in the nature and types of risk information being communicated*. In fact, this study shows that *excessive and selective reports about nonessential aspects of a particular risk may create false impressions of ongoing active risk communication. Nevertheless, the risk communication vacuum may still exist* unless information about the actual nature and scope of the risk is passed on to the public. For instance, in Guangdong's media coverage about the local atypical pneumonia outbreak in February, most reports focused on what I call *social side effects* of the local epidemic:

mass panic; increasing prices of health and food products; widespread panic buying of antibiotics, masks, and food; and governmental intervention and measures to control overpricing and mass panic. Little was reported about the *substances* of the outbreak, that is, its extent, the number of patients, infection and death rates, and locations where new cases were found. As a result, the excessive coverage of the side effects of SARS and the successful control of mass panic and price hikes helped to create and sustain the false impression that the epidemic itself was under control.

The Panicked Public Trope and
Containment Rhetoric of Epidemics

In addition to analyzing official risk communication efforts, this chapter also explores a secondary yet intertwining theme, namely, the construction of containment discourses through narratives about the panicked public who calmed down after official interventions. As official risk discourses repeatedly claimed that SARS was brought under control, in-depth analysis of the containment discourses can help to shed light on how these risk discourses helped to persuade the panicked public, at least temporarily, that the epidemic was indeed contained by clinicians and researchers.

Despite existing claims of mass panic as common responses to crises, studies of people's responses to disasters and fire situations reveal that the trope of the panicked public is inaccurate (Quarantelli, "Panic Behavior," "Sociology"; Wenger). Paul Slovic, Melissa L. Finucane, Ellen Peters, and Donald MacGregor emphasize the interactive relationship between emotion and reason, the wide range of meanings conveyed by such emotions, and, thus, the need for risk analysts to take the emotions of the public seriously. Similarly, Sabine Roeser argues that instead of connecting reason and emotion with rationality and irrationality, respectively, emotional responses to risks are rational, and they range from "choice, control, and responsibility as well as uncertainty and insecurity" depending on the "serious consideration of [individual] responsibilities" and of future reactions (xi).

Citing examples of ad hoc volunteers working after the September 11 attacks and public responses in the 1918 Spanish influenza pandemic (Barry, "Determined Volunteers"; Crosby), Thomas A. Glass and Monica Schoch-Spana argue that public responses to crises have been examples of "resourcefulness, civility, and mutual aid" (218). Therefore, characterizing people's crisis responses as irrational is counterproductive. In addition to bringing no benefit, it also "lead[s] public health professionals and emergency managers to miss the opportunity to harness the capacities of the civilian population to enhance the effectiveness of a large-scale response" (Wenger; Glass and Schoch-Spana 217). Glass and Schoch-Spana emphasize the context sensitive nature of behavioral responses because in times of disaster, "the action of emergency managers may determine the extent and duration of panic" (218). In addition, because of the dominance of the "'command-and-control' model of disaster management," "behavior that is not sanctioned by officials is erroneously defined as panic, rather than as an effective response of resourceful people acting in concert" (Glass and Schoch-Spana 218). The fact that mass panic took place in Guangdong before the official press conference indicates the close connections between the panicked public and the lack of timely official risk communication in this case. Beijing witnessed a similar pattern of mass panic following official denial: "Unable to rely on government reports, Beijing's citizens were forced to depend on the rumor mill, which was turning at 1,000 R.P.M." about quarantining the capital and shop closure in late April (Beech).

Several studies investigate how media and medicine employ rhetorical strategies to produce containment discourses and to dispel public panic about emerging epidemics. Sheldon Ungar examines what he calls a "containment package" employed by American media to frame the hot crisis of Ebola virus outbreak in Zaire in 1995. Such a package consists of the following components: citing authorities to play down the anxiety and to offer assurance to counter public panic, resorting to the metaphor of otherness to create distance between people in the United States and those living in Zaire, blaming a failed poor state as the origin of the disease, stressing protection offered by local strict infection-control measures, and finally offering disease detective narratives about intervening foreign experts and about the search for its host. Priscilla Wald adds a few more elements for containment discourses: offering advice against panic, predicting the curative power of science, stressing personal responsibility, and reinforcing safety practices.

The analysis here of the containment strategies employed in governmental and media discourses suggests the use of some common strategies and reveals some radically different approaches. Governmental authorities and medical experts were cited repeatedly to offer assurance that all-out efforts had been made and that desirable outcomes had been achieved in the battlefield against SARS. Collaborative institutional efforts of disinfection, cleansing, and rumor dispelling received prominent media coverage. In addition, the media used two terms, *containment* and *control*, simultaneously to provide different and confusing claims about the success of the local anti-SARS campaign. The term *under control* quickly became adopted as the official way to describe an all-out victory in the regional battle against SARS.

Interesting but perhaps not surprising, with SARS being a novel disease originating from a province, little scapegoating took place in risk discourses. In addition, because of the widespread panic, much emphasis was placed on the containment of social side effects of SARS: overpricing, rumormongering, and panic buying. Indeed, the institutional policies of selective censorship and partial disclosure helped to successfully transfer the impression of the success control of side effects of SARS to that of a total success in containing the epidemic of SARS itself.

Early History of Guangdong's SARS Outbreak

The SARS outbreak began on November 16, 2002, when the first SARS patient was found and treated in Foshan No. 1 Hospital, Foshan, Guangdong, and infected eleven people, including nine medical workers (Pan). On December 15, two SARS patients were hospitalized in Heyuan, Guangdong, and five medical workers were infected. Driven by a rumor claiming that Heyuan was attacked by an unknown and highly contagious virus, the city of Heyuan saw the first panic buying of vinegar and antiviral drugs in late December (Chen, Wang, and Duan). The "atypical pneumonia" cases were reported to the Guangdong Health Administration on January 2, 2003.[3] The next day, the Heyuan Center of Disease Control and Prevention came out as the first official voice discussing the outbreak by publishing a notice in *Heyuan News*, denying the existence of an "epidemic virus" (C. Taylor, "China"). It suggested that the symptoms, caused by "the unusually cold weather," could be cured with immediate medical treatment ("Analysis of Reasons"). This brief story was the "first media reference, and the last for more than a month, to a disease that appeared from nowhere in southern China" before the mysterious epidemic reached Hong Kong two months later (C. Taylor, "China"). On January 5, *New Press* published the first report about the mass panic buying in Heyuan (J. He, "Test in Spring"). On January 16, Zhongshan witnessed its first panic buying of anti-viral drugs after the rapid circulation of rumors about a mysterious infectious pneumonia that "infected doctors in the morning and killed them that evening" (Wang and Ji). On the same day, a patient from Zhongshan whose symptoms were similar to Heyuan's atypical pneumonia cases was transferred to the Guangzhou People's Liberation Army Hospital. On the next day, this patient infected seven or eight medical workers, including "an emergency room physician and a resident physician, [who] took no protective measures because they had no idea that the disease was communicable" (Qiang).

The newspapers *Nanfang Daily* and *Information Time* in Guangzhou published reports about outbreaks in Zhongshan, a city fifty-five miles south of Guangzhou, on January 17and January 18, respectively. Administrators and medical workers of Zhongshan People's Hospital refused requests for interviews: "We [had] received administrative orders from the Health Administration. We [could] not say anything about it" ("Unexplained Pneumonia"). The reporter's visit to Heyuan's CDC and the Health Department of Zhongshan as well as hospitals in Zhongshan and Shunde, another city thirty miles south of Guangzhou, yielded no findings. However, *Nanfang Daily* pointed out in its mid-January report that the "unexplained pneumonia" in Zhongshan shared similar onset symptoms with the "atypical pneumonia" in Heyuan, which caused mass panic in both cities. The report also listed the symptoms: quick development, prolonged fever, no effective antibiotic treatment, severe lung damage, and frequent use of respirators to sustain patients' lives ("Unexplained Pneumonia"). Meanwhile, local hospitals in Zhongshan started to provide free preventive antibiotic drugs to their medical staff ("Unexplained Pneumonia"). Despite the early and invaluable warning signals sent by both reports, CDC officials in Zhongshan denied the existence of any pneumonia cases in the city and called the news a "mere rumor" ("Heyuan Zhongshan"). To some extent, this official silence and denial exacerbated public concerns about rumormongering, which eventually resulted in panic shopping, a grassroots risk reduction measure during times of uncertainty and fear.

On January 21, a government expert team sent by Guangdong Health Administration developed a full-scale report on the situation of the SARS outbreak. However, because of the weeklong Spring Festival break from February 1 to February 8, that report was not released until February 11. This twenty-day delay resulted in serious medical and material consequences. Forty-five medical workers from No. 2 Hospital and twelve from No. 3 Hospital of Zhongshan University were infected and isolated in Guangzhou for treatment on January 30 and February 3, respectively. By the end of January

2003, SARS cases had been found in the cities of Zhongshan, Guangzhou, Shunde, and Dongguang ("Events"; Q. He, "Background"). Rampant rumors travelled more quickly than the mysterious pneumonia, with people claiming that the mysterious disease was "extremely contagious and resulted in lung puncture" and that it would soon "turn Guangzhou into a dead city" ("Pestis in Guangzhou").

Guangzhou witnessed the first wave of panic buying from February 8 to February 10, during which local residents waited in long lines in drugstores to purchase ban lan gen, vinegar, and masks.[4] On February 11, the municipal government of Guangzhou and the Guangdong Health Administration held the first and only press conference to release official statistics about the SARS situation in the province. They also condemned rumors that claimed the outbreak was caused by a bio-attack or alien viruses: "Over one month after the start of the outbreak, all patients [had] been effectively treated and the outbreak [had] been brought under control" ("Announcements").

The next day, different sets of rumors were widely circulated through text messages and by word of mouth, predicting an upcoming "food shortage caused by the War in Iraq" and "city closure" (Ying and Lee 1). Citing leading international experts and genetic codes of the virus as supporting evidences, various conspiracy theories attributed the outbreak to a "well-planned" bioterrorist attack from the United States, which aimed to "ruin China's economy" ("Ten Questions"). Such theories claim that an academician from Russia's Academy of Medicine announced that atypical pneumonia was "a bioterrorist weapon that had leaked from secret U.S. laboratories" because the virus was "a hybrid of measles and mump which could only be genetically engineered in world-class laboratories" (Chen, "SARS May Be"). These rumors produced a second round of mass panic buying of rice and salt in Guangzhou. *Guangzhou Daily*, the only newspaper authorized to report about the panic buying, condemned the rumors and reassured the public that everything was perfectly under control ("Disease under Control").

The ten days from February 11 to February 20 witnessed a huge increase in reports and commentaries about SARS and its social side effects. This temporary peak in news coverage did not last long, however, because of the quick intervention of official censorship and internal disciplinary measures, including changes of personnel in news agencies. With little news about the outbreak from late February to early April, the topic of atypical pneumonia seemed to be forgotten until increasing international pressure forced the

Chinese government to address the issue again in April. This chapter focuses on risk communication practices about the emerging mysterious pneumonia taking place at institutional sites and in regional media. Chapter 3 investigates the roles played by rumors, gossips, and other extra-institutional forces in the unofficial risk communication processes about the unknown pneumonia around the same time in Guangdong.

Real-Time Risk Communication
in Classified Discourses

The prevailing "hierarchy of access" determines not only who enjoys privileged and substantial access to the media but also who decides what to include and exclude in those media (Glasgow University Media Group 245, cited in Atton, 11). My analysis shows that the governmental discourses in Guangdong were produced for two types of audiences through two different channels. To prevent mass panic and economic losses, the publicly released official discourses in the regional media repeatedly reassured the public that things were under control and that the public was safely protected from the outbreak. I call this subgenre the *governmental discourses for public consumption*, or the publicly released governmental discourses. Power apparatuses, namely, the regional governments and other governmental institutions, produced and circulated a completely different set of discourses in the forms of oral and written orders, meeting minutes, and inside circulars for the internal use of governmental officials, medical experts, and the media. This subgenre, which I call *classified governmental discourses*, conveyed messages completely different from and, in some cases, contradictory to those produced for public consumption. Invisible to the public, the latter was employed to direct various power apparatuses to play their roles in the fight against SARS.

One example of the classified discourses is the earliest "Investigation Report about the Unknown Pneumonia in Zhongshan City." On January 21, Guangdong medical experts and experts from China's CDC worked together to examine patients in three hospitals in Zhongshan City, officially named the disease "atypical pneumonia (unknown)" and collaboratively produced the expert investigation report ("November 2002"). On January 23, the government health committee issued its report as a "top secret" document to Guangdong Health Administration (Hong and Leow). However, having "no one with sufficient security clearance" to open the document, the Health Bureau "did nothing about it for three days [. . .] and when it finally sent a circular to all Guangdong hospitals, most of their staff had gone on holiday to celebrate the Chinese New Year" (Hong and Leow).

Providing an initial consensus amongst the experts on the atypical pneumonia cases, the January 23 report covered topics such as diagnosis, epidemiological features (including clustered cases), clinical features, prevention measures, and treatment guidelines, which served as a foundation for future diagnosis and treatment. It also suggested that the "Health Department in the province should advise all provincial areas of the need to monitor the situation closely" and to "enhance the capacity and management of" intensive-care facilities (SARS Expert Committee). Despite the significance of the expert report, the Guangdong Health Administration did not notify the Provincial CPC Bureau, the Provincial government, or the MOH of the investigation results of the local outbreak until February 3, when it issued "Report on the Unexplained Pneumonia in Guangdong" ("Side Report").

Hong Kong's official review of the 2003 SARS outbreak, the SARS Expert Committee's *SARS in Hong Kong: From Experience to Action*, contains a small section titled "Forewarned Is Forearmed: A Critical Consideration." That section reviews the production and dissemination of Guangdong's January 23 investigation report, then laments that "the Hong Kong authority was not a recipient of the report, neither was WHO" (14). It concludes, "The expert report contained information of significant value to decision makers for disease control and prevention. Owing to the limited circulation of the report, others were not forewarned, and therefore forearmed" (14). The same thing can be said not only about local hospitals and frontline medical care workers who contracted SARS because of the lack of knowledge about the mysterious epidemic but also about hospitals and medical care workers outside Guangdong. On January 30, Guangzhou Health Bureau received the first report about atypical pneumonia cases in the city of Guangzhou. Without a mechanism to coordinate immediate efforts of risk notification, invaluable risk messages became private weapons owned by the privileged few instead of serving as a public resource readily available for medical facilities fighting SARS on a daily basis.

The risk communication processes among the government, medicine, and regional media functioned like a closed-circuit system, with the government on the top and the communication channels between medicine and the media severed by administrative orders (see fig. 2.1). As a result, the

medical institutions and the media reported to the government the imminent risks that SARS posed to local communities. In contrast, nothing other
than administrative orders forbidding discussions about the outbreak was
passed down from the government. My investigation of the circulation of
early public health notifications reveals that the communication processes
within the government were centralized, hierarchical, unidirectional, and
closed circuit. With strict restraints not only on who could speak but also on
who could hear, the intragovernmental risk communication created a rigid
hierarchy of speakers, knowledge, and audience. It excluded not only local
publics but also public health officials and clinicians in other parts of China
from the classified risk communication processes.

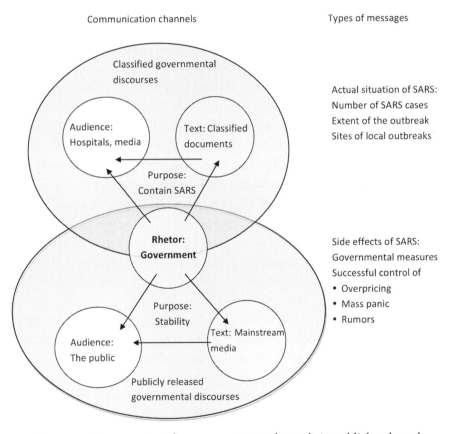

Figure 2.1. Two separate risk communication channels in publicly released
and classified governmental discourses

Creating False Impressions of
Active Risk Communication

Some rudimentary knowledge about Guangdong's economic structure is necessary for one to understand the governmental risk decisions. As a popular destination for foreign direct investments with an export-oriented economy, in 2002, the province attracted foreign investments of US$13.1 billion and ten million migrant workers, about one-third of the national total. The annual gross domestic product (GDP) of the Guangdong Province was US$14.2 billion, about 10 percent of the total GDP of China.

In 2003, rural residents still had no health or retirement benefits. Millions of migrant workers in low-skilled, labor-intensive industries spent long hours in crowded factories and lived in poor-conditioned dormitories. Such poor working and living conditions enhance the possibility of local mass outbreaks. Concerned about the lack of medical insurance and low salaries, migrant workers tried to go back home to reduce risks of contracting the mysterious pneumonia and being denied medical treatment because of poverty. For instance, the State Council News Office announced in its press conference on May 15 that altogether, thirty-six million to forty million migrant workers traveled across provinces to look for jobs in 2003, and by mid-May, around eight million migrant workers had returned to the countryside ("News Press"). A regional epidemic like SARS would seriously disrupt the regional economic stability and would result in the mass exodus of not only foreign investment but also sick migrant workers. Therefore, forces driving risk decisions included financescapic concerns about the outward movement of global capital and export orders and the subsequent ethnoscapic disruption, namely, job losses and cross-country travel among millions of migrant workers.

At the early stages of SARS, risk communication approaches were directly influenced by the regional government's preoccupation with economic and social stability. In late April, a Shanghai health official expressed the same concern about the central-government officials' directives demanding that local bureaucrats maintain Shanghai's "reputation as essentially SARS free": "Sometimes the reality can be different from the image, but if you want to attract foreign investment, image is the most important thing" (Beech). As a result, Guangdong authorities only released the least-alarming risk messages and partial information related to SARS. Meanwhile, administrative orders were issued requiring medical workers and journalists to refrain from disclosing any SARS-related figures.

Forbidding regional newspapers from publishing anything about the outbreak and denouncing any outbreak reports as rumors, local governments cut off the top-down flow of credible information. This decision created a gigantic information gulf during a period of heightened uncertainty and confusion. In addition to blocking the media from accessing news about the outbreak, the government further restricted what the media could say by issuing explicit orders against the publication of certain types of news and against the use of sensitive words. An undisclosed journalist posted online one example of administrative orders from the Provincial Propaganda Department, which was then widely circulated online, with some orders also recorded in the book *SARS Investigation*. The post states:

> February 8 (the first work day after the Spring Festival): The unknown pneumonia has been brought under effective control; February 10: to keep the outbreak secret, no reports or interviews are allowed; February 12: Urgent notification about the order not to report the panic buying in parts of the province; except the official arrangement, no news agencies should send journalists to hospitals; don't use the phrases "outbreak/epidemic" or "avoid going to crowded places"; February 13, 14, 17: Never frame the discussion about the outbreak as the so-called "slow responses of the government" or "the public's right to know the truth"; February 23: from today on, the decision about whether and what to report about atypical pneumonia will be made by the propaganda department. Nothing should be reported without official approval. ("Notifications")

Serving as one of the primary sources of risk information for the public, journalists relied on governmental institutions and medical experts to obtain risk messages (M.-l. Hsu, "Reporting an Emerging Epidemic"). Constrained by administrative directives, however, regional media could only obtain from medical authorities less relevant and politically safe information, such as preventive tips and patient-recovery stories.

In the 1990s, China witnessed the corporation of the media industry and the graduate severance of governmental subsidiaries. The news media's subsequent reliance on profit for survival in the market brought unprecedented changes, at least in terms of Chinese media's financial operations (Huang and Hao 94). Only major newspapers at the national and provincial levels continue to obtain governmental subsidies and serve their traditional role as the Party's "mouthpiece" to propagate the official Party lines and policies (C. C. Lee, "Ambiguities and Contradiction"). Newspapers without governmental subsidies became commercialized and learned to attract more readers and to expand their circulation through exposure and critique of sensitive social, economic, and political issues. Since then, the corporatization of the press and the market competition have turned many Chinese newspapers from "dry broadsheets devoted to the government's line into daring and living newspapers with news articles that expose the negative side of the society" (J. Zhang 170). Moreover, commercialization has created some opportunities for relative autonomy where party control and market imperative intertwine (Zhao 94). As a response, the government employs administrative measures, such as "internal criticism and warning, changing the staff and suspending licenses, and closedown" to "tighten its ideological control and to streamline the press" (J. Zhang 170).

As serious risk communicators, progressive journalists and editors working for market-oriented newspapers made numerous efforts to circumvent the official censorship by investigating local outbreak situations. Sometimes, such risk communication efforts escaped the immediate attention of power apparatuses and reached the public. On several occasions, however, newspapers carrying radical risk messages were recalled and destroyed, and key editors of the South Press group were removed as administrative punishment (H. Shi). Among these newspapers were South Press Group's *Southern Cosmopolitan, Twenty-First Century Globe,* and *Southern Weekend,* three of the most popular and outspoken commercialized newspapers in China ("Thorough Cleansing"). In fact, Zhang Mindong, director of the news division of Guangdong's Propaganda Bureau, was appointed as the associate editor of the South Press Group and the editor-in-chief of *Southern Weekend,* which demonstrates the CPC's principle of "the Party directing the media" ("Thorough Cleansing").

Because of the partial disclosure offered by officials and experts after February 11, little real-time risk communication took place despite the large number of SARS reports. However, regional newspapers, particularly commercialized newspapers like the *New Press* and the *Yangcheng Evening,* published numerous retrospective reviews about the development of the SARS outbreak, reflective commentaries on communication practices, public psychology, and commercial ethics, and, in some cases, strong critiques about governmental responses to the outbreak. These reviews and commentaries were originally published to reflect on and critique governmental performances during the SARS outbreak. They, nevertheless, became another contributing force that helped to create false impressions of transparent, honest reporting about SARS risks. Contrary to their original intentions, the reviews and commentaries facilitated the public's acceptance of the official rhetoric of "SARS is under control."

Official Rhetoric and Risk Control Measures

This chapter defines the official rhetoric about SARS as the rhetoric employed by governmental institutions to convey information about SARS to the public, which was primarily published and released in reports about governmental announcements, policies and responses in regional mainstream and commercialized newspapers.[5] Focusing on social stability and economic development, the official rhetoric started with silence and denial about the SARS outbreak but, after waves of mass panic buying, acknowledged the existence of the outbreak and repeatedly stressed that "SARS [was] under control" and that "[there was] no need to panic." Publicly released governmental discourse employed regional newspapers, radio, and television to reach a mass audience. Whenever the official rhetoric made its way to the regional media, it repeated the same claims to reassure the public of their safety and of the government's ability to bring the epidemic under control. The official rhetoric operated to calm down the public with partial disclosure about SARS situations. To achieve this goal, it focused on the positive changes and progresses while remaining silent about the actual magnitude of SARS. In other words, instead of communicating SARS risks to the public, the official rhetoric replaced substantial risk information with governmental measures to contain SARS and its social side effects (e.g., mass panic and price fluctuation) as well as prevention tips and recovery stories.

The official narrative employed three strategies in Ungar's containment package, namely, citing authorities to play down anxiety, stressing protection offered by local infection-control measures, and reinforcing safety practices. Selective censorship created an overflow of less threatening and less relevant information about the side effects of SARS in the media. This strategy helped to create a false impression of active and honest risk communication. Repeatedly reinforced by local media and supported by the successful control of panic buying and price hikes, the official claim of "SARS is under control" became the official containment narrative and was gradually accepted by the public. Two randomly sampled surveys conducted by a Shenzhen survey company revealed the public's confidence in the government. Their results showed that "seventy percent of the citizens were satisfied with the response of and measures taken by the government" and that "over eighty percent of citizens did not believe in rumors" in Guangzhou ("Investigation").

Official Rhetoric before, after
February 11 Press Conference

Official rhetoric took different approaches in dealing with SARS before and after the February 11 press conference. Beforehand, commercialized regional newspapers alerted the public about health risks posed by SARS through focused reports about the early panic buying ("Mass Panic"; "One Thousand People Waiting in Line"). Progressive newspapers, such as *New Press*, sent journalists to investigate the actual scope and nature of local outbreaks in hospitals with SARS patients in Zhongshan City. On January 16, *New Press* reported responses ranging from absolute silence to open sharing of information about the number of SARS patients ("Unknown Pneumonia"; "How Rumors"). Most of these reports were immediately followed by official "clarifications" denouncing outbreak reports as rumors and denying the existence of any such outbreak, which seriously damaged the rhetorical impact of early alarming reports. Concerned about the social upheaval that the epidemic could cause and the lack of knowledge about the emerging epidemic, the government took a highly proactive approach to control the risk communication processes.

After the February 11 press conference, official rhetoric focused on the governmental performance in the SARS outbreak to achieve the following goals:

- to declare that SARS was under control
- to condemn rumors
- to publicize official policies and measures to fight against SARS and price hikes
- to distribute information about the positive impacts of the anti-SARS campaign on various aspects of life
- and to reassure the public that the government was making every effort to combat SARS, that life would go on as usual, and that SARS was under effective control

Employed by various governmental institutions, this containment rhetoric aimed to calm down the public and to reassure the people that they could continue to live normal lives because of successful governmental intervention.

Overuse of Undefined Terms, Inappropriate Analogies

The explicit declaration of SARS being under control appeared in the mainstream media as early as February 12. At the February 11 press conference, Qingdao Huang, the head of the Provincial health administration, used the phrase "under preliminary containment" in his description of the SARS situation (Shiyuan Li, "Guangdong"). On February 19, the head of the health bureau of Guangzhou used the same phrase to describe the SARS situation in a meeting about disease control and prevention. In contrast, other officials and regional media employed various terms indicating a larger scale of success and created much confusion. While the only report dealing with SARS in *South Press* claimed that "SARS is preventable," *Guangzhou Daily* was more aggressive in its reports. Some claimed that "SARS is preventable and treatable" and that atypical pneumonia had been brought "under preliminary control" or "effective control" (Yan, Fu, and Xu). Others announced that Guangdong had "a strong mechanism to prevent the further spread of atypical pneumonia" and that "no new cases were found" in several cities in the province ("Rumor Denounced"). The terms *contain* and *control* suggest two very different things. The *Oxford Dictionary* defines *contain* as "prevent (an enemy, difficulty, etc.) from moving or extending." *Control*, meaning "the power of directing, commanding, dominating, or regulating," suggests a much larger success. Although governmental discourses and news reports used different phrases (for instance, "under preliminary containment," "under control," and "under effective control"), none of them clearly defined the terms or explicitly explained their criteria for using those terms. Announcing that the disease was "brought under preliminary control," several reports claimed that the average number of new cases per day was "in gradual decrease after February 6" and that "no new cases" were reported from three of the six cities where the SARS cases were found (Chen, Wang, and Duan).

Such statements, among others, provided a hidden definition for the term *effective control* and created a false impression that "under control" meant "few or no new cases." Meanwhile, whereas the public health officials used the phrase "under effective containment," the Provincial and local officials and the media chose to use the phrase "under effective control," which implied a greater degree of success in terms of disease control and prevention. Ambiguous and undefined key terms were used interchangeably and inconsistently to describe the outbreak's scope and the effects of governmental efforts, which exerted a significant impact on the public understanding of the situation. Whenever the mainstream media reported anything about the actual scope or development of the SARS outbreak, those reports would be considered partial definitions, or at least pieces of evidence for the official claim of "SARS is under control."

These contradictory claims worked together to create "a fiction of containment" (Wald 240). How can a virus be contained in early patients and infected close contacts when it can survive and spread via airborne droplets and bodily secretions? The later discovery of transmission routes of SARS reveals hard-to-contain "dangers of spatial promiscuity," which later led to aggressive nonpharmaceutical public health interventions, such as medical isolation, quarantine, and contact tracing. Well protected by this mix of containment narratives, the mysterious virus continued its rapid spread to Shanxi, Beijing, Hebei, and Hong Kong before it exploded into a global epidemic in mid-March.

In early April, Beijing witnessed the juxtaposed use of "control" and "containment" again by officials and medical experts. On April 3, Health Minister Zhang Wenkang declared that SARS in Beijing had been "under effective control" and that it was safe to travel and live in Beijing. Zhang's claimed was criticized by Dr. Zhong Nanshan, the leading medical specialist in Guangdong's anti-SARS campaign, on April 10. At a State Council press conference, Dr. Zhong contested the use of the term of *control* for providing false assurance. Recommending the use of "containment" instead, he asked, "How can you control a disease without knowing anything about its sources and pathogen?" (Bi). On April 25, *Face to Face*, an extremely popular program hosted by Central China Television (CCTV), interviewed Dr. Zhong about his heroic leadership in Guangdong's anti-SARS campaign. Dr. Zhong distinguished the two terms in the interview:

> The conditions for the control of any disease include the discovery of
> the pathogen, the identification of its route of infection, and effective
> treatments. Even in late April, we [knew] a little about the pathogen, but
> we [had] no idea where it came from and how it spread. All we [could] do

now [was] to alleviate its symptoms, shorten its course, reduce its death rates and reduce the number of SARS patients. This is containment, and it is more scientific to say that the situation is under containment. (Bi)

The resurfaced disputes about those two terms vividly illustrate the huge impacts carried by the terms employed to define the magnitude and severity of the SARS outbreak.

Selective Coverage, Inferential Leaps through Enthymemes

The regional media publicized and sang high praise for anti-SARS policies and measures, for instance, the regular disinfection of public transportation vehicles, the thorough cleaning of public facilities, and the timely start of all schools ("Railroad Strengthened Sterilization"; "Dismissing Rumors"; "Thorough Cleaning"). Policies taken to fight against inflation and panic buying were reported to inform the public of ways to report cases of overpricing and to warn merchants of punishments for those who wantonly raised prices of drugs and food ("Dial 12358"). Other reports denounced widespread rumors related to the epidemic and urged the public not to panic ("Legion Disease and Pestis"; "Rumor Denounced"; see chapter 3 for more detailed analysis about rumors).

One award-winning commentary, "Calm Response to Settle the Crisis," fully exemplifies the way the official rhetoric operated through selective censorship and inferential leaps in a series of enthymemes.[6] Publicizing the so-called insider information revealed by officials, it stated that "under the leadership of the Provincial Committee of the CPC and the Provincial government, various governmental divisions collaborated closely, carried out their duties, and won a great victory in the battle against atypical pneumonia and rumors"(Chen, Wang, and Duan). It claimed that the anti-SARS efforts were very successful and listed numerous evidence to describe a comprehensive victory: "school started on time; mass panic vanished; the number of recovered patients kept increasing whereas that of new cases kept decreasing; rumors about SARS were quelled down; the social order was restored; and people's work, life and study went on as usual" (Chen, Wang, and Duan). The report well exemplifies the official containment rhetoric by focusing exclusively on the implementation of infection-control measures and successes achieved in the official fight against the side effects of SARS. The official rhetoric vaguely equated the control of panic buying, the most visible social side effect, with the control of SARS itself while reporting little about the magnitude of SARS. Selective reporting strategies highlighted what had been done to combat the side effects of SARS and its positive outcomes. It created an umbrella enthymeme that consists of the basic lines of movement for the argument, that is, rigorous governmental measures against SARS brought its side effects under control; therefore, SARS was under control (see diagram 2.1).

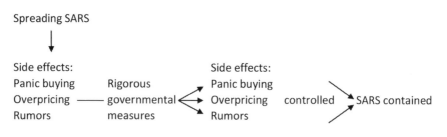

Diagram 2.1

To some extent, the official containment rhetoric and the full coverage of successes of anti-SARS measures in combating the social side effects were mutually reinforcing. The successful control of overpricing and panic buying was portrayed as evidence for the effectiveness of official anti-SARS measures and, thus, as evidence of SARS being brought under control. In reality, however, only social side effects of SARS were brought under control when the actual epidemic spread swiftly to other parts of China. One key difference between the SARS outbreak and its social side effects was their differing degrees of visibility. Whereas mass panic and overpricing were highly visible because of their direct impact on people's daily lives, the actual development of the epidemic was far less visible: the public was only granted limited access to medical and epidemiological information. In addition, it was difficult for anyone but medical care workers and SARS patients and their families to sense its immediate impact. Therefore, although it is impossible to hide mass panic and overpricing from the public, information blackout can easily though temporarily prevent the public from realizing the actual existence and development of epidemics.

Numerous enthymemes were employed to support the umbrella enthymeme about SARS containment. One of the most frequently used enthymemes claimed that if the quickly spreading SARS caused overpricing and if overpricing was brought under control, then SARS was under control (see diagram 2.2).

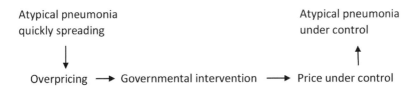

Diagram 2.2

This enthymeme omits a generalization and disguises a huge inferential leap it makes. Although SARS caused price hikes, the causal relationship between the control of overpricing and the subsequent control of SARS is a false one. Many other factors could have stopped overpricing: for instance, rigorous administrative measures and governmental intervention. Therefore, the attempt to establish the reverse causality indicates the huge inferential leap taken in such an enthymeme. The official containment rhetoric operated with the implementation of numerous enthymemes using the same false reverse causal relationship. Parallel enthymemes focused on the disappearance of the SARS side effects, that is, school disruption and sharply reduced tourism, which all came to the same conclusion that SARS was under control (see diagram 2.3).

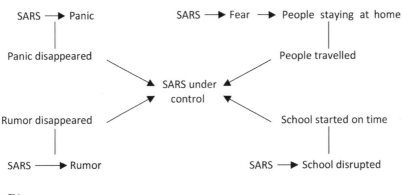

Diagram 2.3

When combined together, the four frequently cited observations can be represented in another umbrella observation, one often seen in official discourses, which claims, "Life goes on as usual." The four generalizations accompanying them can be converted into a second umbrella generalization, namely, "because the outbreak of SARS had greatly disrupted people's lives and because life then went on as usual, SARS was brought under control" (see diagram 2.4).

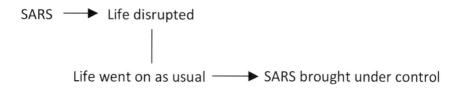

Diagram 2.4

The actual statement should be "the *knowledge* about the outbreak of SARS had greatly disrupted people's lives," since mass panic did not result directly from the actual medical consequences of the epidemic. Instead, panic buying took place after official denial and rumormongering. Because of selective censorship, people had no direct access to knowledge about the magnitude of SARS. Once selective censorship and partial disclosure severed the information flow among the medical institutions, the media, and the public, the media started to equivocate between the effects of the anti-SARS campaign and those of the anti-overpricing efforts. Therefore, the causal relationship between "SARS is under control" and "Life goes on as usual" was a false one. The equation of the containment of SARS with that of its side effects is a huge inferential leap. That logical leap was masked, however, by the overreporting about governmental efforts to control SARS and its side effects, by the commercialized media's strong criticism of governmental performances, and by the subsequent false impressions of honest reporting. The Guangzhou Epidemiological Team conducted a random sample survey of three hundred residents and found out that over 90 percent of interviewees believed that Guangdong had the capacity to eradicate atypical pneumonia ("Over 90% Guangdong Residents"). This survey result indicated that the enthymeme widely used in the official rhetoric helped to calm down the public and to persuade them of the success of the anti-SARS campaign. The official no-risk narrative undermined serious risk communication efforts made by the commercialized newspapers and resulted in the public's acceptance of the official "risk contained" narrative.

Closed-Circuit Communication
between Government, Medicine

This section analyzes governmental and official intracirculated documents to examine the rhetorical interactions between the government and medical institutions. Some of the documents circulated within the public health institutions were mentioned in news reports and witness narratives from independent websites, but none of these documents were publicly available online.[7] Altogether, twelve official notifications were issued by the Provincial Health Administration of Guangdong from February 3 to March 27. As early as February 3, the "Report on the Unexplained Pneumonia in Guangdong" was sent by the Guangdong Health Administration to the Provincial government, saying as follows:

> Cases of unexplained pneumonia were found in Heyuan, Zhongshan, Fushan, and Guangzhou last month. According to incomplete statistics, till today 90 cases have been hospitalized and 2 deaths reported. . . . Some cases were clustered in families and medical workers treating such patients. . . . This disease falls into the category of atypical pneumonia, is caused by some unknown pathogen, and can be transmitted through the respiratory route[s] and close contact. The Health Administration has sent experts to investigate the cases and to offer guidance for prevention and control. Reports have been sent to all cities in the province, asking medical institutions to pay attention to the situation, to strengthen the management of the disease, and to establish a reporting system.

The document demonstrated the tremendous pressure SARS had produced in the public health system, the immense anxiety caused by its novelty and uncertainties, and the great attention it had attracted from public health officials, researchers, and medical experts in early February. Unfortunately, as an important document of emergency health risk communication, the report was not distributed until the end of the Spring Festival break because of the weeklong holiday. As the earliest official evaluation of SARS, the report was then circulated within governmental divisions and health administrations instead of being shared with hospital administrators, medical personnel, or local media for prevention purposes. The uncoordinated risk responses failed to inform frontline medical workers of the highly infectious disease and resulted in multiple in-hospital cross-infection events.

Several important anti-SARS events took place on February 3. A notification titled "On the Control and Prevention of Unexplained Pneumonia" was issued that provided a retrospective investigation of hospitalized unexplained pneumonia (UP) cases, diagnostic criteria, a preliminary description of the disease's characteristics, and tips on patient management and treatment. The notification was sent to regional health departments, hospitals under the direct administration of the health departments, the Ministry of Health (MOH), the Chinese CDC, and the Provincial Municipal Office of Guangdong. The decision to inform health institutions at the national, provincial, and local levels reveals the tremendous pressure on and the constant risk communication efforts made by medical institutions.

In the 2001 anthrax scare, the public health system in the United States, particularly the US CDC, was also under enormous pressure to respond quickly to the public health emergency and to assess the risks in real time. Wading through uncharted waters like China did during SARS, the public health sectors experienced similar problems, such as "a back-logged written clearance system" and the uncertainties surrounding intentional anthrax exposures, which differed greatly from natural outbreaks (Robinson and Newstetter 27). At the beginning, much confusion and fear resulted from the lack of coordination among CDC scientists, governmental officials, Federal Bureau of Investigation investigators, non-CDC researchers involved in anthrax investigations, "nonscientific sources," and reporters covering the event (Robinson and Newstetter 27). Leaks, prematurely released information, misspeaking officials, and speculation forced CDC scientists and communication staff to "chase the rumor rather than [to] make the news" (27). All these challenges lead to flurries of media requests and complaints that overwhelmed the CDC's response capacity, caused delays in timely information release, and resulted in the eventual communication breakdown (Robinson and Newstetter). The CDC quickly lost its credibility as an institution of scientific authority because of its inconsistent risk messages. Emergency risk communication about health crises is multifaceted and complicated. It is often characterized by uncoordinated institutional responses, political intervention, confusing media messages, and competing expert claims. It also provides opportunities to improve emergency-response mechanisms, procedural innovations, and communication capacities in future emergencies, as demonstrated by the limited progress in Guangdong's emergency responses discussed below.

The Guangdong Health Administration established one working group to lead the UP prevention and control work and three working groups for medical research, epidemiological investigation, and etiological research. On the same day, the construction of a systematic UP epidemiological database was started for the entire province, and retrospective investigation was conducted for every new case to obtain information about symptoms, treatments, contacts, and living environments (Shiyuan Li, "Guangdong"). On February 19, another inside flier, "Notification of Further Improvement of UP Prevention and Control," was issued after China's CDC declared on February 18 that *Chlamydia* bacteria was the pathogen of UP. That report contained two appendixes, one on the laboratory analysis of the antibody and the second a new form for the daily reporting of new UP cases. As one of the most important epidemiological tools, the daily reporting form should be filled out by individual hospitals before being submitted to local health departments and to the Guangdong Health Administration on the same day.

Power directs the transmission of knowledge and determines the relationships among people, institutions, and knowledge. To understand the risk communication approach taken by medical institutions at this stage of the outbreak, one must consider not only the position of medicine but also the practical and historical contexts surrounding medical discourses, for "medicine is not just affected by cultural, social, economic, and political variables—it is embedded in them" (Brandt 5). In other words, it is important to engage questions of cultural, power, and political contexts and to examine the insertion of medical discourses into institutional and other nondiscursive practices. Driven by the larger concern with local economic development, the power apparatuses in the Guangdong Province strove to convert SARS into an object of knowledge only within public health and medical institutions and rendered the disease highly invisible to the public by forbidding medical workers to discuss the outbreak with the media or the public.

In addition, both health institutions and the local government operated under the legislation restraints. Tony Saich points out the following:

> According to the 1996 implementing regulations [on health-related issues], SARS would have fallen under the category of highest-level secret (jia lei),[8] since it was a widespread infectious disease, like viral hepatitis. As a result, it could not be disclosed until the Ministry of Health or those organs authorized by the ministry had made the disclosure. (77)

Considered a top-level secret, SARS would require official approval to be released to the public. Medical workers would break the law if they chose to reveal such risk information. Moreover, as Joan Kaufman points out, SARS was "not a mandatory reportable disease and did not fall under the requirement for surveillance and reporting" as stipulated by the 1989 Law on the Prevention and Control of Epidemics (10).[9] By keeping the initial outbreak from the public, the Guangdong Provincial government complied with the legislative requirement because SARS did not belong to the mandatory reporting of class A, class B, or class C epidemics.

Drafted and adopted in an era when migration and air traffic were much less prevalent, this outdated legislation functioned as the guideline for the entire risk communication process and imposed severe institutional and material restraints on the outbreak management. Precious time was spent on bureaucratic communication and coordination, and the poor crisis-response system further impeded the official reaction to the outbreak.

Experts: Minimal Risk and No Need to Worry

Because of the relative nonexistence of the technical communication profession in China, medical workers treating SARS patients acquired great authority and functioned as highly credible risk communicators during the outbreak. Administrative orders silenced most medical experts by forbidding them to discuss SARS cases and in-hospital infection. As a result, medical experts widely employed self-censorship, which appropriated medical discourses to reinforce the official containment rhetoric. Regional newspapers publicized expert opinions about the living and working conditions of medical workers and SARS patients, about research findings and preventive tips, and about the progress made in SARS prevention and treatment. As officially sanctioned knowledge, expert discourses selectively presented perspectives of leading medical scientists and practitioners. They added another layer of credibility to the official rhetoric of "SARS being under control" and became the authoritative voice that provided further assurance in the containment package (Ungar).

To start with, analogies were used to downplay health risks SARS caused. Because of the lack of understanding about the etiology or pathology of SARS before March, numerous existing names for the disease were employed, changed, and then discarded as more knowledge was acquired about the disease. Medical workers named SARS "unexplained pneumonia" at the beginning of the outbreak. With increasing understanding of its pathological and epidemiological features, the disease was renamed "community-acquired pneumonia" because of its tendency to occur in clusters in families and hospitals. Finally, the disease was renamed as atypical pneumonia "because of its clinical flu-like symptoms and its lack of response to commonly used antibiotics" (J. Chen, "Hot Topic"). A Guangdong medical expert challenged the use of this term as early as February 13 during an interview with *New Press*: "Previously defined 'atypical pneumonia' is mostly caused by viruses, and can be effectively treated with antibiotics. Many patients can recover without being hospitalized. Therefore, atypical pneumonia is an imprecise name and is seldom used in clinical diagnosis" (Q. He, "Scientific Definition"). Such confusion is reflected in a physician's letter reporting his "previous experiences with and quick recovery from atypical pneumonia in the 1970s" ("Tips from Physician"). The writer explains that the reasons for "the regional outbreaks of this common disease" in Guangdong was viral mutation, radical temperature changes around the Spring Festival, and people's weakened immunity due to excessive partying and lack of sleep during the holiday ("Tips from Physician"). The MOH's intentional use of an existing name to downplay the health risks SARS posed was accidentally revealed by Zhong Nanshan at a press conference on April 11 when he explained,

> After some cluster cases in hospitals and families, the epidemic spread quickly and attracted serious attention from the provincial government and the health bureau. It was defined as a special pneumonia, one that might be contagious. The name we used back then was unknown pneumonia. It was changed to atypical pneumonia because the previous name sounded very frightening. (Q. He, "Scientific Definition")

He Qiang argues that it works better to give new contagious diseases a new name to differentiate it from existing ones, as WHO did with SARS. He believes that the intentional use of atypical pneumonia was "politically driven and aim[ed] to confuse public opinions inside and outside China," which, in turn, brought unnecessary ambiguity and challenges to medical and epidemiological work ("Scientific Definition").

Widely used in the media, atypical pneumonia was often compared to other common types of pneumonia to make the new killer disease less threatening. One of the most widely cited analogies compared the disease to another type of pneumonia in the United States, which "was acquired by around 5.6 million patients and resulted in a five percent death rate" and was "the sixth most common disease that results in death and one of the most common fatal hospital acquired infections" (Liang). Other widely cited general statements about pneumonia claimed that "in developing countries, lower respiratory tract infection was the second main reason leading to deaths, following diarrhea" and that China has an annual average of "2.5 million pneumonia patients and 0.125 million deaths" (Liang). Coming from physicians with actual experience treating SARS patients, these analogies functioned as an intentional piece of the containment package that emphasized protection provided by existing knowledge when in reality none of the existing treatments worked for SARS. In addition, such co-opted expert claims downplayed the unusually high infection rate, the quick development of lung failure, and the lack of response to antibiotics in SARS patients. Such misleading analogies caused the public's transfer of existing understanding of common pneumonia to that of SARS and the subsequent underestimation of SARS risks and its fatality rate.

Most reports of expert opinions adopted a complimentary and reassuring tone. Lauding the altruism of medical workers, heroic narratives were published about "angels in white" who "put their self-interest aside and worked around the clock to save pneumonia patients" ("Angels in White"; "Twenty Days' Continuous Work"). Patients and medical workers infected with SARS told recovery stories, which functioned as witness narratives, claiming that "the disease was not at all as fearsome as imagined" and that "taking good rest worked much better than taking excessive amount of drugs" ("Tips from Physician"; "Experience of a Recovered Doctor"; "Stories from Recovered Patients"). Expert tips focused on the preservation of stability rather than on disease prevention. Quite a few medical experts reminded the public that "they could lead a normal life and go out traveling, shopping, and dining as usual" because of the minimal risk of contracting the disease (Deng; "Expert Reminded"). They warned people against "blind use of drugs" and against "unfounded suspicion or self-diagnosis just because of mild cough" ("Experts: The Cause"). They also predicted a period of two weeks for those without complications to recover from SARS. Such expert discourses reassured the public that "doctors were capable of killing any type of virus," that "there was no need for citizens or even medical workers outside the emergency rooms to wear masks," and that "hospitals were safe enough for patients to seek treatment" (Deng; "Expert Reminded"; "Experts Denounced

Rumors"). Li Limin, the director of the Chinese CDC, claimed on February 13 that no new cases had been found in Guangdong in the past four days, that most patients had recovered, and that 80 percent of hospitalized patients were cured and released from the hospital ("Experts: The Cause"). As most experts were cited using their real names, such practice boosted the ethos of various expert claims.

As we would later learn, before late April, hospitals often functioned as the hot zone of infection because of the lack of appropriate infection-prevention measures. After being transferred from Shanxi to Beijing for treatment on March 1, the first SARS case in North China caused huge outbreaks in 301 Hospital and 302 Hospital in Beijing, two of the best hospitals in China ("First Imported Atypical Pneumonia Patient"). Reporting to the Department of Defense instead of the MOH, these two military hospitals later became not only the site of investigation for Dr. Jiang Yanyong, the retired veteran physician who exposed the SARS outbreak in Beijing to Western media, but also the key evidence for MOH's underreporting that Yanyong describes in his open letter to *Time* magazine (see chapter 3). With the setup of fever clinics and the shutdown of hospitals with superspreading incidents, in-hospital infection rates started to decline after early May.

It was difficult to tell whether experts' overoptimism resulted from the media's selective coverage or whether it actually came from the experts themselves. Even if such reassuring stories came from the experts, it is hard to tell whether they really believed what they said or if they thought that telling success narratives would calm down the public, which, in turn, would promote the overall anti-SARS campaign. However, as professionals with direct access to SARS information and with daily exposure to the risks of contracting the disease, the medical experts cited in regional newspapers chose either to passively obey administrative orders of censorship or to actively comply with the official ideology of stability by reinforcing the official "no risk" narrative.

Analysis of the expert rhetoric also shows the indelible impact of official censorship on what can be said and how it should be said in the experts' discourses: only prevention tips and research findings about SARS were reported. Expert discourses were filtered to reinforce the official "SARS is under control" narrative. Experts were caught in the middle of their institutional positions as professionals hired by and subordinate to governmental apparatuses, their limited access to the media, and their secondary roles as risk communicators for both the government and the public. As Grabill and Simmons point out, the meaning and value of risk are determined by multiple competing discourses. Although leading medical experts enjoyed quick access when communicating SARS risks to the government, their public communication attempts were largely impeded by official censorship and the active co-option of their messages. As a result, the expert discourses became quickly subsumed by the official containment narrative and became another consenting voice.

Reviews, Strong Critique in Commercial Newspapers

Amid the government-lauding choir jointly produced by the mainstream media and co-opted expert discourses, one dissenting voice of serious critique and reflection came from regional commercialized newspapers. They published reviews of the SARS development and commentaries on the government's performance in communicating the SARS risks to the public. Whereas mainstream regional newspapers focused exclusively on governmental anti-SARS measures and its side effects, commercialized newspapers paid great attention to what had happened before the official admission and why a two-month delay in communicating SARS risks took place. Such reviews and commentaries analyzed reasons for the risk communication failure before February 11 and concentrated on possible ways to avoid making similar mistakes in future.

Commercial newspapers published systematic reviews of panic buying, rumor dissemination, and governmental responses. Some urged the government to be more open with risk communication and to better meet the public's information needs, and others either criticized the purposeful manufacturing of false text messages to promote sales of products or urged the public to take a more rational attitude toward rumors. Such reviews revealed for the first time the way rumors followed traces of atypical pneumonia before they became the targets of official clarifications. For instance, Wang and Ji reviewed the entire SARS outbreak from its beginning in November 2002 to official interventions in mid-February 2003. They focused on the development, growth, and containment of rumors as well as governmental measures taken to fight rumors. Their commentary shows that rumors and panic accompanied the trail of the SARS virus from Heyuan City in December 2002 to Guangzhou in February 2003 and argued for more-transparent risk communication practices.

The ten days from February 11 to February 20 witnessed a temporary trend of serious criticism of governmental performance and of open discussions about more effective ways to deal with public emergencies. For instance, *Yangcheng Evening*, a highly influential independent newspaper in Guangdong, published a series of reflective commentaries on the issues of mass communication, mass media, ethical business practices, public psychology, and crisis-response systems. One article openly criticized the government: "The culprits are the governmental slow response and slow release of information" ("Guangdong Media's Reflection"). Ping Xiao considers the leading causes of mass panic to be information blocks "the long-standing practice of reporting good news while withholding bad news," the inadequate social-security system and emergency-response mechanism, and the lack of public trust ("Reasons Leading To"; "Lack of Trust"). Another *New Press* commentary advocated the investigation not only of mistakes made by officials but also the accountability of governmental departments that "clarified rumors" about the outbreak ("Accountability of Officials"). The commentary states, "Those in charge should be held responsible for their decisions for two reasons. First, they sent out false information and caused mass panic which could have been avoided; second, their poor judgment did great harm to the image of the government." The same newspaper continued its critique in another commentary on February 16:

> Atypical pneumonia was found in Zhongshan and Heyuan as early as the end of last year. *New Press* published the first report about the outbreak on January 5. However, instead of releasing reports about the outbreak and searching for ways to deal with it, the government in charge responded by denouncing the report as rumors, denying the facts, and treating true information from the media as true lies. As a result, an important channel of information was blocked and the public expectations to learn about the authority's viewpoint from the media were let down. (Su)

This unusually strong critique of the official censorship marked commercialized media's engagement in serious risk communication and the frustrations caused by repeated official denials. Working together, however, the reviews and commentaries reinforced the official containment narratives because of their focus on the strict control measures for mass panic and overpricing as well as their critique of the government's early risk communication approaches. Suggesting that "we can now talk about all the mistakes and problems," the highly critical reports in commercial media created a false impression of transparent risk communication and promoted the official containment rhetoric by suggesting that the epidemic, like its side effects, was indeed brought under control.

The Provincial Propaganda Department soon issued numerous administrative orders warning against further reporting on SARS risks and governmental responses. It eventually stopped this temporary trend of criticism by the "cleansing" of the South Press Group, one of the most progressive press groups in Guangdong, removing key editors and changing its personnel. Little reporting, let alone criticism of the government, appeared in regional newspapers after February 20 or during the entire month of March. Although commercialized newspapers enjoy more freedom in their coverage of social events, they are still subject to official supervision and control in times of crises. With more-stringent restraints and administrative personnel changes, these commercialized newspapers lost their previous, limited coverage freedom and were forced into compliance with the official orders of censorship.

Success of Official Rhetoric

Subject to official censorship and disciplinary control, the media were only allowed to discuss certain topics and to disseminate filtered information for governmental institutions. Therefore, they functioned more as official communication tools than as public information outlets. Figure 2.2 presents a modified technocratic model of risk communication approaches that reflects the top-down and one-way flow of risk messages and the impact of censorship on risk communication. A careful examination of the risk communication process shows that one key component about the risk of SARS was completely missing: the actual development of SARS, namely, the numbers of new cases, places where such cases were found, and their infectious rates. Several strategies helped to create and maintain the false impressions of honest reporting, that is, the highly selective overreporting of governmental anti-SARS measures, effectively implemented orders of partial censorship, and the subsequent silence about SARS spread in hospitals and communities. Behind the false impression of honest reporting lay a glaring information vacuum that was carefully masked by the power apparatuses.

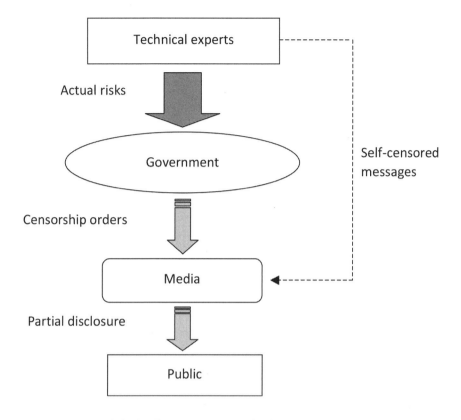

Figure 2.2. Modified technocratic model of risk communication approaches

Figure 2.3 adds more detail about the way risk communication operated at the early stage of SARS in Guangdong. It shows the multilayered influences from self-censored experts, consenting mainstream media, and critical commercial media. It demonstrates the way the government controlled risk communication processes by appropriating expert discourses and by forcing regional media into compliance through censorship orders. Measures taken and progress made by governmental divisions were covered comprehensively. Commercialized newspapers made serious attempts both to question the development of local SARS outbreaks and to reflect on lessons learned from the event about media-government-public relations. Such interrogation was thwarted, exploited, and appropriated by partial disclosure and by the gradual implementation of censorship that forbade any communication about the cumulative number of SARS cases or the infection rates in hospitals and communities.

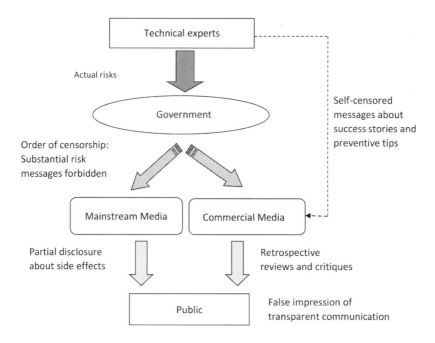

Figure 2.3. Application of the revised model to the SARS outbreak in Guangdong

With "dynamics of capitalogic moving across borders" and eroding the economic and political independence of nation-states, risks become incalculable, indeterminable, and uncontrollable (Wilson and Dissanayake 1; Beck). Chapter 3 focuses on the uncontrollable aspect of transnational risk communication. It shows that the modified technical model is idealized and that governmental apparatuses can never achieve complete control of risk communication processes. Conscientious technical experts and ordinary health and news workers with access to inside risk information resorted to alternative media to circumvent official censorship. In other words, when the researcher goes beyond government-controlled print and broadcast media and investigates the less credible yet more accessible alternative media, a completely different story unfolds. One would witness an unexpected undercurrent economy of leaks, cracks, subversions, contradictions, and seething rumors about local risks. This undercurrent of leaks got to its peak in Guangdong in mid-February and reached the tightly controlled capital of Beijing in late March. It was the extra-institutional risk communicators who managed to break the official silence and released key SARS data to the transnational communities.

Consequences of Limited Risk Communication

Guangdong's decision to employ limited risk communication brought both positive and negative consequences. Because of the lack of understanding about the etiology, epistemology, and treatment of SARS in early February, the official containment rhetoric functioned to calm down the public and to prevent widespread mass panic. In addition, Guangdong had a huge number of foreign and joint ventures and labor-intensive and export-oriented industries. The province attracted twelve million migrant workers in 2002 as compared with three million in Beijing and ninety million in China in the same year. If a mass exodus to go back home of migrant workers had occurred in February or March, as happened in Beijing in late April and early May, it would have most likely brought the SARS virus to the poor countryside. Complicated by the lack of clinical or surveillance knowledge about SARS, such a mass exodus may have resulted in a much larger SARS outbreak throughout China and a much more intricate challenge for containing the epidemic throughout the world.

The concerted efforts made by the regional medical expert team, led by Dr. Zhong Nanshan, yielded great progress in diagnostic criteria, patient management, in-hospital infection prevention, and clinical treatment from February to April. The numbers of new cases and deaths for each month show a clear declining pattern, and those for cured cases constantly increase. For instance, in March, Guangdong witnessed 361 new SARS cases and 507 cured cases, which meant a 47.5 percent decrease and an increase of 133 cured cases, respectively, when compared with those of February ("Experts Predict"). By mid-May, 86 percent of SARS patients in Guangdong were cured and released from the hospital. As one of the regions that treated SARS most effectively in all outbreak areas, Guangdong boasted of a low death rate of 3.5 percent. The clinical treatments were "based on previous experiences with [other] respiratory infections and evolved over the course of the epidemic" (Donnelly et al. 676). On May 23, WHO removed its April 2 recommendation for people to postpone nonessential travel to Hong Kong and Guangdong province because of the successful containment of local outbreaks.

Susan Sontag eloquently argues that epidemic control relies on mass education and mobilization: "With an epidemic in which there is no immediate prospect of a vaccine, much less of a cure, prevention plays a larger part in consciousness. . . . [M]ass mobilization [should be employed] to confront an unprecedented menace" (76–85). Such mass mobilization, however, never took place at the early stage of the SARS outbreak. Despite the intense pressure and sense of crisis within governmental institutions, little information was released to the media or to the public. The official rhetoric of "SARS is under control" was the only authorized knowledge. Forbidden to communicate with the media about the outbreak, medical institutions took a rather reactive approach and relied solely on the clinical treatment of patients within the hospital and gave up the more important battlefield of epidemiological surveillance and prevention through public education. Only partly severed, the person-to-person chain of SARS transmission expanded in public places and community settings, particularly in crowded and poorly ventilated places, such as airplanes, trains, classrooms, and hospital halls. The cutoff of this chain would require the early identification and isolation of cases, mass mobilization, and the mandatory implementation of comprehensive preventive measures, which did not take place until late April. Moreover, medical facilities outside Guangdong knew nothing about either symptoms of SARS or effective ways to prevent in-hospital outbreaks. Guangdong's invaluable, hard-acquired knowledge about SARS was confined within the province instead of being widely shared with medical workers elsewhere in mainland China and in Hong Kong. During this period of media silence and limited medical efforts within hospitals, the epidemic silently yet quickly travelled across regional and national borders, finally becoming a global epidemic in March.

Risk Communication in Non-Western Cultures

Leiss and Powell argue that "problems in communicating about risks originate primarily in the marked differences that exist between the two languages used to describe our experiences with risks: the scientific and statistical language of experts vs. the intuitively grounded language of the public" (26). They emphasize the importance of effective communication practices between scientists and the public that "seeks to break down the barrier between the two languages [of experts and layman] and facilitate the productive exchanges between the two spheres" (29). Interested in user participation in decision-making processes, Grabill and Simmons's critical rhetoric of risk communication relies on technical communicators' symbolic analyst role to introduce more-democratic risk communication practices. Both models leave out confounding problems, such as governmental interests and agendas, "the interrelationships between political economy and public health practices"

(Barnes 15), and the complicated negotiations among institutions, media, experts, and the general public.

Risk communication operates differently in different cultures because of local power structures, cultural beliefs, communication practices, and media functions. It is dangerous and reductive to assume that risk communication is a universal, generalizable process, for culturally based risk communication practices are multifaceted, and their development is constantly shaped by changing social and cultural conditions and historical circumstances. Therefore, the cross-cultural study of global risk communication calls for a critical contextualized approach that stays away from imposing existing Western risk communication theories on cultures with vastly different conditions. This critical contextualized approach aims to understand risk communication practices in local contexts and raises questions about the target culture's political system, power structures, dominant cultural values and beliefs, media functions, technical communicators' roles and positions, and the relations among governmental institutions, media, science, and the public. For instance, through analysis of media discourses, I show containment rhetoric at operation in regional media, official governmental messages, and expert discourses in Guangdong. My analysis reveals completely different messages, or the anxiety about "noncontainment" and strategies to cope with the spreading epidemic, in the secretive, classified governmental discourses. Well-disciplined experts and medical care workers provided prevention tips and recovery stories, discussed the successes in the official anti-SARS campaigns, and cited the containment of side effects of SARS as the evidence for the containment of SARS itself. Therefore, the political economy surrounding media and classified SARS discourses helped to promote the containment rhetoric and the success narratives in the region.

This volume calls attention to some key issues and problems that are understudied in existing risk communication theories, particularly those related to power, knowledge, institutions, and cultures:

1. The intricate relations and interconnectedness between institutional risk communication practices and the larger political, cultural, economic, and ideological contexts
2. The possibility that various risk communication approaches may exist in different cultural and institutional sites or different communication channels

3. The intervening role of governmental institutions and the media in risk communication
4. The false binary between risk assessment and risk communication as being clearly separate practices rather than simultaneously ongoing
5. The possibility that practitioners, rather than technical communicators, may function as risk communicators in emerging crises
6. The need to move beyond the expert-public binary to examine institutional and cultural forces at work in risk communication processes

Researchers of risk communication should pay attention to the possibility that various risk communication approaches may exist in different cultural and institutional sites. Consequently, to better understand risk communication practices, one has to explore various communicative channels to identify attempts of risk communication from different stakeholders and key players and the motivations driving such attempts. Because of differences in cultural contexts, communicative practices, and media structures between Western and non-Western cultures, governmental institutions and the media may play different roles in risk communication.

I agree with Grabill and Simmons that the binary between risk assessment and risk communication is a false one. My analysis differs from theirs, however, because of my focus on the timing of and key players involved in risk assessment and risk communication rather than on the sites of knowledge production. Under the constant threats of new health risks, institutions and scientists may play the dual roles of risk assessors and risk communicators because of the urgent need to take action. They may also employ different communicative channels and media to send different risk messages to diverse audiences. Thus, the investigation of knowledge production, circulation, and consumption has to engage the issues of power relations, institutional functions, communicative practices, communicative channels, and audience types.

Many risk communication studies done in the United States take it for granted that technical communicators play a key role in delivering risk messages to the public. They ignore that in other cultures, professional communication and the practices for communicating scientific and technological issues to the public may still have to establish themselves as regular and legitimate needs. In such situations, practitioners, rather than technical communicators, may function as risk communicators in emerging epidemics or other types of crises. Moreover, because of the more dominant roles institutions and governments play in risk communication processes and the exclusion of the general public from any decision-making processes, researchers may have to move beyond the expert-public binary to examine institutional and cultural forces at work in risk communication processes.

The vastly different cultural and material conditions in different cultures make the critical application of existing risk communication theories to non-Western cultures an absolute necessity. The critical contextualized approach to risk communication stresses careful examination of the unique contexts of individual cultures and their power relations when studying risk communication practices in non-Western cultures, which may help us to better understand the variety of risk communication practices across cultures and possible ways to better study such diverse phenomena.

3
Rhetorics of Alternative Media, Censorship, and SARS

How does emergency health risk communication operate amid scientific uncertainty and official silence? What role does public communication play in such risk politics?

To help address these questions, this chapter reports the results of a rhetorical study that examined health risk communication about SARS in China during a period of utter confusion and official silence. The initial stage of the SARS outbreak, which occurred between November 2002 and March 2003 in Guangdong Province, was characterized by little official media coverage. However, my research demonstrates that alternative media were anything but silent about SARS during that stage of the epidemic. As early as January 2003, speculations, rumors, official clarifications, and confusion pervaded SARS reports from alternative media, such as independent websites and word-of-mouth communication. As a response to these messages from alternative-media sources, waves of mass panic buying took place on February 8 and February 10 in numerous cities in Guangdong.[1] These two waves of mass panic buying were followed by the first and only official press conference that the Guangdong municipal government offered; in this press conference, government officials claimed that the local epidemic was under control. The panic buying also produced an anomaly in the silence about the SARS outbreak in Chinese print media prior to April: an unusual, closely clustered wave of intensive reports (altogether, 605) took place in Guangdong regional newspapers from February 11 to February 20 (see fig. 3.1).[2] In contrast, *People's Daily*, the official tongue of the Communist Party of China, remained silent about the outbreak from January to March.

This anomaly in the news reporting pattern was preceded and followed by media underreporting and, most of the time, official silence. However, numerous rounds of panic buying in Guangzhou and neighboring cities took place, and the rampant rumors about a mysterious, fatal epidemic, perhaps a mutated type of avian flu, soon caught the attention of not only transcultural media in Hong Kong, Singapore, and Western countries, such as the

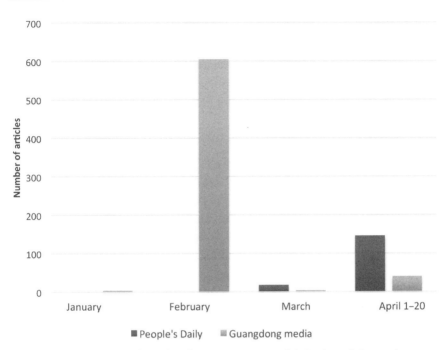

Figure 3.1. Number of articles about SARS in *People's Daily* and Guangdong regional newspapers, January to April 20, 2003

United States and Great Britain, but also the United Nations health agency WHO. As a result, the outbreak of mysterious pneumonia in Guangdong entered the transcultural risk communication network and became the focus of international biopolitical surveillance. How can rhetoric function to communicate the risks of an emerging health crisis to the public when the dominant power structure imposes censorship? What role did rhetoric play in the production of the two rounds of mass panic buying, and how did risk communication operate in Guangdong amid official silence?

Many rhetorical and critical studies have been conducted to analyze how public health crises were constructed in public discourses (Barnes; Brookey; Leiss and Powell; Rosenberg; Scott; Treichler). Scholarly attention has recently focused on the coverage of the global epidemic of SARS in international mainstream media (Kaufman; Kleinman and Watson). However, the ways in which alternative media can function as extra-institutional channels to challenge and contradict official media and to communicate imminent risks to the public have been largely neglected in the previous work on health crises. In the case of China, alternative media include independent overseas Chinese websites, contesting foreign media, and guerrilla media, such as text messaging and word-of-mouth communication. Alternative media function as sites of conflict and contention that challenge dominant power structures and communicate to a large audience across geographical and media boundaries.

The classification of contesting foreign media, which may be mainstream in their own countries, as alternative media in China is based on their historical functions of disseminating dissenting viewpoints and subverting the dominant propaganda in China, as discussed in chapter 1. During the global epidemic of SARS, foreign media functioned to facilitate transnational risk communication about the epidemic and to penetrate China's censorship by obtaining and publicizing unauthorized risk messages from people with access to such information. The examination of the rhetorical and cultural potential of alternative media is particularly significant in the study of unofficial risk communication practices in countries that strategically control print and online media through constant surveillance.

In his discussion of tactics and strategies, Michel de Certeau defines *tactic* as "a calculated action" without a place or "a spatial or institutional localization." As "an art of the weak," a tactic depends on "a clever utilization of time" and always watches for "the precise instant of an intervention [which can be] transform[ed] into a favorable situation" (xix, 39). Tactics "vigilantly make use of the cracks that particular conjunctions open in the surveillance of" the dominant power (37). *Strategies*, in contrast, are "systems and totalizing discourses" created by an institution with a "place of its own power and will," such as a business, an army, or a city. Strategies are used to influence, guide, or manipulate human society (de Certeau 36–38; for more-detailed analysis, see Kimball). In the media contestation in China during the SARS outbreak, the state apparatuses maintained strategic control of both traditional mass media and the Internet through constant policing. To circumvent the state surveillance, the public resorted to the tactical use of alternative media to distribute and receive unauthorized risk messages and dissenting political views.

Interested in the interaction among "technology, discourse, and people's lives," M. A. Kimball calls attention to the need to study both safe and dangerous extra-institutional documentation practices. My study extends Kimball's concern with tactical extra-institutional technical communication beyond the genre of technical documentation. Specifically, the study traces various forms of tactical extra-institutional risk communication practices through the use of alternative media, particularly guerrilla media, such as text messages, phone calls, and word of mouth. As a more flexible, mobile, and accessible force in alternative media, guerrilla media function as "weapons of the weak" that open up media spaces to marginalized groups and help define new political situations (Chin-chuan Lee, "Liberalization"). For instance, China had two hundred million cell phone users by the end of 2002; most of these people used text messaging regularly because of its low cost (0.1 RMB per message, or about 1.5 cents, compared to 0.5 to 1 RMB per minute per call) and because of the technological capacity of sending one message to multiple contacts (J. Liu, "False Text Messages"). As one type of guerrilla media, text messaging played an important role in interpersonal communication. For instance, altogether, seven billion text messages were sent in China during the 2003 Spring Festival (Liu, "False Text Messages").

This chapter analyzes how alternative media facilitated tactical extra-institutional risk communication during the SARS outbreak by allowing transmission and diffusion of gossip and rumors.[3] The discussion starts with the use of critical contextualized methodology in this study and then examines two types of rhetoric employed in the risk communication processes. The first type is the rhetoric of proclamation, which anonymous rhetors use to make short, dramatic, decontextualized, and often exaggerated proclamations to large, attentive, and receptive audiences. The content of these proclamations during the SARS outbreak was often unverified, and the anonymous rhetors who disseminated them relied on guerrilla media. The second type is the rhetoric of personal narratives, which anonymous professionals and individual whistle-blowers employ to tactically reveal information, in this case, about health risks SARS caused. Finally, I explore this study's implications for both professional communicators and professional communication classrooms.

Health Risk Communication about SARS in China

Chapter 2 investigates the coexistence of three separate channels of risk communication during the SARS outbreak: a channel of classified risk communication within the government, an official risk communication channel from the government to mainstream media and then to the public, and an unofficial channel through which the public resisted media control and underreporting during the early stages of SARS. Classified official risk information about SARS was restricted to medical institutions and the government, and administrative measures and policies were issued to limit SARS information to medical settings. In mainstream media, the government repeated and reinforced the official rhetoric of "SARS is under control" to maintain regional economic stability and to prevent a drain of foreign investments.

Because of the closed-circuit nature of China's official communication about SARS, the public was excluded from the information-sharing process and was deprived of access to knowledge about emerging risks. Concerned with individual survival, Chinese citizens used alternative media to learn and communicate about the actual SARS situation and its immense health threat (A. Wu, "Reflection"; Z. Wang, "Over 55 Million People"). Alternative media helped break down the information blockade by giving voice to individuals with access to more-or-less-credible insider information and by allowing such information to be widely disseminated. The discursive machine that produced unofficial information about SARS risks was decentralized, nonhierarchical, interactive, tactical, resilient, and dynamic. Professionals from various institutions disseminated information about the outbreak, and citizens received, circulated, and sometimes reinvented such information about the risks. The lack of centralized structures both in alternative media and in the communicative processes posed great difficulty for the government to co-opt these tactical, unofficial forms of risk communication.

Decentralized Tactical Risk Communication

Rumors about the SARS outbreak did not simply arise out of nowhere but were disseminated through various layers of actors in extra-institutional communication before reaching demographically diverse audiences. Jenny Edbauer's theory of rhetorical ecology conceptualized rhetoric as a public creation with processes of "distributed emergence and ongoing circulation and transformation" that add "the dimension of movement back to the discussions of rhetoric" (13). This emphasis on circulation, movement, and transformation applies well to the participatory risk communication about SARS in Guangdong. Risk messages emerged as insider information from widely distributed sources. Such information usually leaked from the first layer of actors, professionals "working in public health and medical institutions" (Xiao and Lin). This layer of actors used guerrilla media to disseminate what they considered important information about the mysterious pneumonia to the second layer of actors—their immediate social circles—to warn them of the publicly unknown threat. At this stage, risk information was disseminated on a small scale and with low frequency. However, what started out as partially true information grew in both volume and scope as it was circulated and eventually "changed in shape, force, and intensity" (Edbauer 17). Fueled by the material reality of the quickly spreading SARS epidemic and the official silence, risk messages from anonymous professionals were quickly disseminated, changed, mutated, and expanded by a panicked and receptive audience.

Rhetoric of Personal Narratives from
Anonymous Professionals

As early as January 2003, risk messages about local in-hospital outbreaks in small cities in Guangdong were already reported in commercial regional newspapers as journalists investigated various rounds of small-scale panic buying of antiviral drugs in the cities of Heyuan, Fushan, and Zhongshan. Despite local governments' quick denunciation of such reports as baseless rumors, official silence did not disrupt the underground economy of spreading infection and its accompanying anxiety and speculations. In late January, frightened patients sought treatments at leading hospitals specialized in infectious disease in Guangzhou, and, thus, the SARS epidemic was spread to that city.

Several narratives were recorded in alternative media about the roles played by professionals, such as journalists, police, and medical workers, who created and disseminated rumors about the mysterious pneumonia at the beginning of the SARS outbreak. For instance, a journalist working for a Guangzhou newspaper learned about the atypical pneumonia on February 9, two days after the seven-day Spring Festival break:

> Several hospitals had found over 100 cases of respiratory infection, with several deaths and over 20 doctors and nurses infected in one of the hospitals. Most newspaper agencies had learned about the situation, but without official verification, none of them dared to report about the disease. What they could do was to watch the situation closely and send journalists to investigate the situation in hospitals. (Lan, "Deliberate Downplay")

Realizing the huge gap between the quickly spreading outbreak and the silence of the media, this journalist, like many others, rushed to purchase antiviral drugs and to call or text message friends and relatives to warn them of the outbreak (Lan, "Journalists in Panic"). For this reason, Manuel Castells, Mireia Fernandez-Ardevol, Jack Linchuan Qiu, and Araba Sey characterize cell phone users as "instant media reporters of their experiences," who "share

[news] in real time with their friends and through them, with the world at large" (212). Because official communication channels were blocked, those who had access to credible information resorted to guerrilla media and became active reporters and distributors of true or partially true information.

Another anonymous personal narrative on February 10, 2003, tells about the inside news that a policeman in Guangzhou learned from an urgent inside circular. This unofficial document claims that SARS had "resulted in 280 deaths and over 100 cases in Guangzhou, with half of them being medical workers" and that "suspected cases would be sent to specialized hospitals or wards for infectious diseases" ("Newest Report"). The document states that because the causes and viral sources were unknown, "there was no effective treatment" for the disease ("Newest Report"). It also confirmed that vinegar and immunity-enhancing herbal drinks were in such a huge demand that "in most stores they were either sold out or increased to twenty to fifty times" of their usual prices ("Newest Report"). A final source of information came from medical workers who had direct contact with and knowledge about the atypical pneumonia cases in local hospitals. Many medical workers "sent out warning mobile messages from hospitals, which were further distributed to the social circles of their friends and relatives" (A. Wu, "Reflection"). Such messages revealed inside news about the SARS situation and emphasized the widespread infection of medical workers in local hospitals. They also described SARS symptoms and warned people against going to crowded public places.

As demonstrated in the three narratives previously mentioned, professionals made use of informal and private transmission channels to anonymously distribute unverified information to the public. Such risk communication tactics relied largely on personal narratives and depended on participation from both narrators and audiences. Professionals with access to knowledge about the outbreak were not sanctioned to speak publicly about it from their institutional sites. As de Certeau explains, professionals with privileged access to insider information are "already caught in the nets of discipline," and, thus, they must resort to clandestine "procedures and ruses" to "compose the network of anti-discipline" through the use of "tactical and make shift of creativity" (xiv–xv). Despite their limited access to traditional mass media, professionals resorted to direct person-to-person texting or phone calls to circumvent censorship and to send warning messages via interpersonal networks. In other words, official censorship worked well in regulating conventional media, but the officials could not prevent information leakages through the use of easily accessible antidiscipline tools, such as cell phones. Thus, most anonymous personal narratives started as insider information sent by professionals to warn their immediate social circles of the emerging epidemic and its accompanying health threats. Such information was soon transformed into gossip and rumors that traveled rapidly among acquaintances and interpersonal networks and eventually reached the wider public.

Rhetoric of Proclamation in Guerrilla Media

As the rhetoric of anonymous personal narratives spread, it was quickly adopted, transformed, and, in some cases, co-opted by various audiences to serve their own purposes. At the same time, a second type of rhetoric, which I call the rhetoric of proclamation, was also widely employed by the immediate social circles of the anonymous professionals and the wider public. With viral intensities, this rhetoric quickly circulated as short, dramatic, anonymous, and often decontextualized proclamations. Such proclamations were repeatedly forwarded and transformed by a quickly increasing number of people, many of whom used cell phones. This rhetoric helped to produce numerous rounds of panic buying not only in Guangdong but also in neighboring areas, such as the Hainan Province, Hong Kong, and the more distant cities, such as Shanghai. Panicked people rushed to drugstores and grocery markets to stock up on masks, antibiotics, vinegar, and traditional Chinese medicine. Driven by wild speculations and unchecked rumors, numerous cities also witnessed brief periods of panic buying of salt, rice, and vegetable oil. The high visibility of such widespread panic buying served as the earliest warning signals in the transnational risk communication networks about the growing epidemic of the atypical pneumonia (August, "Fear Spreads" 20; Ying and Lee 1; Ng; Gittings 26).

Confounding Factors Surrounding the Outbreak

Contributing to the rampant rumor mills in both Guangdong and Hong Kong were the utter confusion surrounding avian flu cases taking place in Hong Kong in late January and early February, the possible connection between the Guangdong outbreak and Hong Kong's avian flu cases, and disputes about the nature of the mysterious pneumonia. Three cases of avian flu were found in a Hong Kong family after they travelled back about eight hundred miles to the Fujian Province on January 26. The young daughter died on February 4 in

Fujian, and the father died on February 17 after returning to Hong Kong on February 8. Hong Kong found the H5N1 (avian flu) virus in the man's nine-year-old son, who was hospitalized for treatment, and reported the avian flu cases to WHO on February 19. This incident "led WHO to issue a global alert on Avian Flu on the same day" (SARS Expert Committee 15). Questions were raised about the connection between the unexplained pneumonia outbreak in Guangdong and the Hong Kong avian flu cases. In addition, Guangdong health authorities claimed that no new pneumonia cases had been reported in the province since February 10, which Hong Kong media later claimed was the official misinformation that expedited the export of the SARS virus from Guangzhou to Hong Kong (Bradsher, "Flu's" A1; "Official Denies"). Another event adding to the confusion was China's CDC's official announcement of *Chlamydia* bacteria as the cause of Guangdong's mysterious pneumonia outbreak. As discussed earlier, Guangdong medical experts challenged this officially supported theory, using their rich experience treating SARS patients as the counterevidence.

Rumors and Proclamations Surrounding the Mysterious Pneumonia

Starting on January 16, rumors about the infectious pneumonia were widely circulated and resulted in panic buying in Zhongshan of erythrocin, an antiviral drug (Yan and Pan). Some rumors described a frightening transmission channel of the strange disease: "[A]ny face-to-face meeting or even taking the same bus with the patient may result in getting the same disease." This same message claimed, "Many medical workers who had contact with the patient got the disease in the morning and died at night" (Wang and Ji). Exaggerating the magnitude of the outbreak, these rumors helped to create widespread fear. The disease was described as incurable with a 100 percent death rate and characterized by fever, pathological lung change, a short incubation period, and quick development of respiratory failure ("Entire History"). Some rumors claimed that their information was inside news revealed by medical workers, with one instance stating that "an extremely contagious disease causing lung puncture almost turned Guangzhou into a dead city" ("Pestis in Guangzhou").

In such messages, the disease was identified as avian flu, *Pestis*, the plague, Legionnaires disease, and anthracnose. Some versions of the rumors attributed the disease to mutation of imported pollen. Others claimed it was bioattacks from the United States or Taiwan. Numerous Internet posts were widely reprinted online, and books were published to offer biological, historical, or sociological arguments for the bioterrorist nature of the SARS outbreaks in China and Hong Kong ("Ten Questions"). Several Internet posts and news reports cited evidence, such as the 0 percent death rate in the United States and the claim from a member of the Russian Science Academy that the SARS virus was artificially manufactured and genetically combined in laboratory settings. Analyses of the unusual RNA codes of the SARS virus were presented as further evidence to support the theory that SARS was the result of bioterrorist attacks from the United States (Y. Ren, "SARS").

Similar rumormongering took place during the 2001 anthrax scare in the United States. As the first lethal bioterrorist attack on the United States, the anthrax incidents carried with them a lot of unknown factors in terms of penetrators, motivations, routes of delivery, and the scope of the attack. Public health experts and police faced unprecedented challenges posed by bioterrorism, which resulted in uncoordinated institutional responses and the overflow of inconsistent, and oftentimes contradictory, risk messages. What further complicated the emergency risk communication scenes were thousands of anonymous anthrax threats and hoaxes both in the United States and in Great Britain, which involved either suspicious powder or claims of released anthrax into air conditioning or water systems (Barry, "Anthrax Pranks" 4.2; Hoge B6). Rumormongering swept numerous cities, announcing local positive testing of people with contact of anthrax or speculating on the terrorist nature of attacks in various incidents. Circulated via Internet posts and e-mails, other rumors claimed that garlic could effectively treat anthrax, that ironing or microwaving letters would kill anthrax, that people died from opening deadly perfume or detergent samples that they received in mail, and that in a test of Coca-Cola cans, arsenic and anthrax had been found in one fifth of them ("Croak a Cola").

The flourish of rumors in SARS and anthrax threats "offered metaphors for the invisible and fatal contamination that spread like fear, like terror, and like resistance [. . .] within the body politic" (Grigsby 31). Official silence and inconsistent risk messages only further intensified the public alarm. For the suspicious and powerless public in search of truth, "any sign could signify" and any available information would be taken to interpret the extent of the imminent risks (Grigsby 31). Darcy Grimaldo Grigsby's claim that "the way plague [and poisoning] produced misleading rumors" made an "imagination feverish" is highly applicable to both SARS in China and the anthrax threats in the United States, even though he used it to described an event that took place over two hundred years ago in Egypt and Europe. In 1799, Napoleon's army suffered from the plague after their bloody massacre of surrendered prisoners in Jaffa, Egypt. Soon, France, Great Britain, and Egypt reverberated with transnational rumors about the French army's mass poisoning of sick soldiers. Despite the French government's rigorous surveillance of national media, "censorship is never complete" (Grigsby 30). Narratives about the atrocity gained currency in the British press, and memoirs, caricatures, paintings, and novels were produced about the mass poisoning. In fact, London-based publications about the massacre and alleged poisoning circumvented the censorship and became "a clandestine literature to a portion of the population" in Paris (Grigsby 30).

One prominent difference in channels of rumor dissemination between the 1799 massacre and SARS and anthrax threats, however, is the shift from hard-to-access print sources to online sources and text messages that can be freely and constantly accessed, exchanged, and distributed. Indeed, during the SARS outbreak in Guangdong, informal proclamations about the unknown pneumonia were usually written as short statements that could be sent freely by text messengers and arrive at receivers' cell phones at a cost of 0.1 RMB per message to the sender. The recipients could then easily forward such alarming messages to all their contacts, again, without any charge on the senders' part. Some people sent out mass text messages in the name of police departments and health bureaus, "officially claiming" that a novel virus was found in Guangzhou and that there was no cure for the disease ("Gossip and Rumor").

Because of its "distributed ecological spread," this rhetoric was quickly co-opted and transformed across purposes and cultural spaces (Edbauer 19). Driven by profit, greedy merchants took advantage of the technology of mass text messaging, or spam messages, to exploit the already heightened fear of the shortage of medical supplies and to promote the sale of their products. Panic buying of rice, cooking oil, and pure water was triggered by carefully crafted and massive disinformation (Wang and Ji). Different versions of rumors fueled public fear, dramatically changed the visibility, impact, and contour of the rhetoric, and resulted in the widespread panic buying of salt and rice on February 12. Such rumors made various claims, including the following:

- SARS was caused by a lack of iodine in the body.
- The upcoming War in Iraq would result in a shortage of food.
- Salt manufactured after October 2002 was below the required quality standard, so one should buy salt produced before October.
- Salt water can be used for indoor disinfection when one runs out of vinegar.
- Salt water can kill germs and viruses.
- Guangzhou banned the import and export of goods, so there would soon be a shortage of food. (Shi, Li, and Zhu)

In addition to the multiple sources that made these proclamations, the technology of text messaging also further complicated the issue. Because of the lack of supervision and the geographical distribution of cell phone numbers, with some technical skills and simple tools, individuals worked like small broadcasting services and sent mass text messages to thousands of cell phones within seconds. Text messaging allowed messages to reach multiple users with constant access to their mobile phones all at once. As the "always-on tool of communication within everybody's networks," text messaging enabled the instantaneous dissemination of proclamations at a speed much faster than that of traditional word of mouth (Castells, Fernandez-Ardevol, Qiu, and Sey).

Although many of the early rumors entirely lacked a foundation, dismissing them as mere rumors ignores their huge social and political impacts on the development of SARS and its risk communication processes. This informal set of discourses was important because it was produced, accumulated, circulated, and consumed by Chinese citizens and thus served as counter-messages to the government's official discourse. It functioned as an informal site of public participation and produced various forms of resistance, such as leakage and dissemination of insider information, a widespread mistrust of the official narratives, and, finally, panic buying.

Growing from half-true gossip about in-hospital infections to misleading rumors about massive deadly outbreaks and food shortages, the rumors widely circulated in Guangdong and other parts of China exemplified a "non-information" explosion, where the ever-growing black hole between data and information exacerbated the public's existing information anxiety (Wurman 14). Although governmental institutions repeatedly dismissed such proclamations as nonscientific rumors, their refusal to offer any substantial information only further fueled the already heightened mass panic. An information asymmetry existed between the absence of credible official information and the overwhelming number of rumors. Because of rigid restrictions for the media coverage, the public was denied access to quality information and was forced to make use of any available information to ensure their survival in the SARS outbreak. Less concerned with what actually happened and more concerned with ways to prevent potential damage, composers of proclamations resorted to widely accessible communication channels to send the public messages about the imminent risks. This focus on health risks catered to the public concern about physical survival when people had no access to substantive information about the scope or severity of the local SARS outbreaks. In other words, for the rhetoric of proclamation, the low credibility of its claims interfered little with its rhetorical success. Aiming to alert the public as the epidemic unfolded, the rhetoric of proclamation achieved its goal through the quick, resilient, and dynamic guerrilla media and through active audience participation and dissemination.

A survey has confirmed the important role that guerrilla media played in communicating SARS risks to the public: before Guangdong's February 11 press release, 80 percent of Guangzhou residents learned about SARS from unofficial channels, such as mobile text messages and the Internet ("Huge Traffic Jam"). From February 8 to February 10, a total of 1.26 billion mobile text messages were sent by users of Guangdong Mobile Communication Co. (Wu, "Reflection"). In addition to text messages, another guerrilla medium, phone calls, also played an important role. On February 11, the average phone connection rate in Guangdong dropped to about 20 percent, and text messaging also frequently "dropped the line" because of a "traffic jam" and "temporary systemic paralysis" caused by people trying frantically to call their relatives and friends about SARS ("Huge Traffic Jam"; "Failing Connection"). The resilient, dynamic, and inexpensive guerrilla media allowed the means of production to be redistributed and thus increased public participation in communicating health risks. Enabling public production, circulation, and consumption of information, these media posed great challenges for timely governmental supervision and provided both professionals and the public with forums in which they could communicate about upcoming risks.

Tamiflu Netmercials and Changing Contours

In early February, some widely circulated, anonymous Internet forum posts claimed that atypical pneumonia was actually avian flu and that Tamiflu was the only effective cure. As manipulated Internet commercials in the guise of forum posts, or what I call *netmercials* here, this round of proclamations serves as a particularly interesting case of the Internet and texting use of proclamations with unexpected impacts on transnational extra-institutional risk communication.

The manufacturing of panic buying of Tamiflu was achieved through the combined use of official product promotion, forum posts, and mass text messaging, which demonstrate the potential of alternative media as a highly exploitable marketing tool. The product manager of Tamiflu and the public relations manager of the manufacturer, Roche Corporation, announced in a press conference in Guangzhou on February 9 that the supply of Tamiflu for major hospitals in Guangzhou had been sold out as early as January 31 and that the executive of the National Flu Research Center suspected that the atypical pneumonia was "actually a potentially deadly bird flu that could be treated with the Roche-made antibiotic," Tamiflu ("Drug Firm" A1). The rumors surrounding Tamiflu started with two netmercials published online on February 11. The first post announced that the executive of the National Flu Research Center said that avian flu should be the first suspect for the atypical pneumonia outbreak because of similar symptoms and high death rates and that the only cure was Tamiflu. The author of the second netmercial claimed that his message had been issued by the Third Affiliated Hospital of Zhongshan Medical University in Guangzhou and originally published on the official website of the Guangdong Health Bureau. According to this post, the atypical pneumonia was "avian flu B-2," and medical experts identified Tamiflu as the only effective drug and cured many patients with it ("Questioning Tamiflu"). A reinforcing mass-distributed text message stated, "Latest update: the mysterious pneumonia was identified as the mutation of avian flu B-2, and the only cure is Tamiflu. . . . Don't eat chicken or chicken-related products" ("Questioning Tamiflu" A5).

From February 9 to February 13, the sales volume of Tamiflu in Guangdong increased by ten times, and most sales were requested by self-paying patients from doctors rather than prescribed by doctors. Given the high price of Tamiflu and its limited clinical use, the increase in sales helped to bring huge profit to the company. After the publication of numerous news reports questioning Roche's role in producing the panic buying of Tamiflu, health officials and medical experts started to denounce the rumors of avian flu and explained that Tamiflu only cures common flu, not avian flu. In this case, it is not clear whether the rhetoric of proclamation about Tamiflu and avian flu was actually sponsored or initiated by the Roche Corporation, as no follow-up reports were produced about the police investigation of the case. However, the rhetoric was both supported and reinforced by the simultaneous, ongoing marketing campaigns and the deliberate equivocation between flu and avian flu as well as avian flu and the ongoing unknown pneumonia outbreak, which resulted in the identification of Tamiflu as the only cure for the unknown pneumonia.

The combined use of netmercials and mass text messages in the promotion of Tamiflu highlights the ambiguous and potentially manipulative use of alternative media in new outbreaks and participatory risk communication. Because of technical capacity of sending one message to hundreds of users via online forums and text messages, anyone with adequate technical skills can broadcast his/her "risk messages" to a large audience, which results in the abuse of such media by greedy merchants and malicious individuals. As channels that bypass official control, these alternative media allowed the quick flow of rumors and, in this case, netmercials through interpersonal networks.

In transnational rhetorical networks, key risk messages may change their contours and functions when circulating through various networks (Scott, "Kairos"; Edbauer). The netmercials about Tamiflu as the only cure for atypical pneumonia were no exclusion. With Internet posts and text messages warning against a mutant influenza virus and promoting effective cures, the messages not only resulted in panic buying in Guangdong but also triggered international alarm about possible avian flu outbreaks. A routine online search conducted by the WHO global influenza surveillance network picked up the rumors, and WHO's regional office in Manila sent a message to the Ministry of Health (MOH) on February 10, asking for more information about the epidemic. The Tamiflu netmercials were transformed from one isolated incident of rumor dissemination for profiteering purposes into an important event in the transnational risk management of avian flu and potential pandemics.

Adding to the confusion caused by Tamiflu netmercials were the three avian flu cases identified in a Hong Kong family after their return from the Fujian Province around the same time. The Hong Kong Health Department confirmed their avian flu (H5N1) infection on February 19 and notified both WHO and the MOH about the cases. On the same day, WHO issued a global pandemic alert on avian flu and urged Chinese authorities to provide more information about the possible link between the bird flu cases in Hong Kong and the Guangdong pneumonia outbreak.

Rhetoric of Personal Narratives from Whistle-Blowers

Many professionals who had access to information about the outbreak resisted the official censorship by sending out anonymous personal narratives about SARS via guerrilla media. In addition, patients and medical experts also strove to communicate with domestic and international media by appealing to their own credibility as SARS survivors or physicians who had treated SARS. Such personal narratives told by individual whistle-blowers were mostly reported by independent overseas Chinese websites and contesting foreign media.

The most influential whistle-blower during the SARS outbreak was Dr. Jiang Yanyong, a seventy-six-year-old veteran physician from the People's Liberation Army General Hospital, also known as the 301 Hospital, in Beijing. Dr. Jiang, who was in charge of the hospital's surgery division before he retired, heard about the widespread infection of 301 Hospital medical workers in late March. He was infuriated when Health Minister Zhang Wenkang claimed in a press conference on April 3 that SARS was under control, that Beijing had twelve cases and three deaths, and that it was safe to travel and work in Beijing (Zhu). On April 4, Dr. Jiang spoke with his colleagues and learned that the number of SARS cases in the 301, 302, and 309 military hospitals was forty-six, forty, and sixty, respectively ("People's Interests").

The efforts to circumvent official censorship worked both ways. While Dr. Jiang mobilized his interpersonal networks to gather information about SARS cases in Beijing, numerous transnational media agencies were also busy investigating the SARS situations in China. Despite their suspicion and partial information, transnational media could not report their informal findings because they needed a whistle-blower to validate those data. Karl Taro Greenfeld, who worked as the general editor of *Time Asia* magazine during 2003, describes in his book how journalists of the *Time* Beijing office followed traces of rumors to conduct personal investigations about atypical pneumonia cases in various hospitals in Beijing and found out at least a total of thirty-seven cases when "the official tally was still a dozen" (290). He explained the difficulty surrounding the reporting and verification of their unofficial data:

It was a legitimate issue. What would happen if we ran a story about Beijing hiding cases, and it turned out these were not SARS cases but some other pneumonia? More likely, if the government came out and said we were wrong, how could we refute them? We didn't have virus growing in cell lines. We didn't have a doctor backing us up. (290)

Dr. Jiang served as the critical connector between China's unreported yet quickly spreading SARS outbreak and transnational media trying frantically yet in vain to uncover the truth about that epidemic. He accomplished this by attaching his name as a well-respected medical expert to the incomplete SARS data he gathered about Beijing's outbreak. Instead of being a privileged insider content to share risk messages only with family members and friends, as most professionals had done, Dr. Jiang was compelled to send the risk message to media at home and abroad: "As a physician, I have to intervene whenever people's survival is at stake" (Jakes). On April 4, he faxed his open letter to the government-controlled China Central Television (CCTV-4) and Hong Kong's Phoenix Satellite TV, two of China's most influential news disseminators, criticizing "lies told by officials from Ministry of Health and wild talk of Zhang Wenkang" (Mu 33). Not surprising, neither of the TV stations responded. On April 8, Dr. Jiang met with Susan Jakes, a journalist from *Time*, for an interview and issued a signed statement discussing his personal investigations about the SARS situation in Beijing. His statement was published on *Time*'s official website on the same day (Jakes). Almost immediately, Dr. Jiang's story was picked up by major media all over the world. The next day, Dr. Jiang was phone interviewed by representatives from leading media in the United States, Germany, and France to confirm his data. Meanwhile, the *Time* report was "translated and quickly disseminated through chat rooms and text messages" in China despite official silence (Greenfeld 308). Because of the rumormongering surrounding SARS cases in Beijing, people worldwide speculated about the reliability of the *Time* story in China. However, "*Time*'s name attached to the story added credibility," and on April 9, Henk Bekedam, one of the leading WHO officials working in Beijing, offered a rare open critique of his Chinese counterpart: "There seems to be some question over when the central government knew about SARS in Beijing and what they actually knew" (Greenfeld 307).

Dr. Jiang made tactical entry into transcultural networks of risk communication because he moved quickly in selecting and contacting possible media outlets. He seized the opportunity to critique the latest official data, and he courageously cited results from personal investigations as counterevidence for the official SARS updates for Beijing. Speaking as a medical expert, Dr. Jiang greatly enhanced the credibility of his narrative with his professional authority and his ability to circumvent the censorship of SARS data in Beijing. He resorted to personal connections to obtain data about SARS cases in local military hospitals. Considering the utter confusion about Beijing's SARS situation and WHO's thwarted efforts to gain access to Beijing's medical facilities, Dr. Jiang's release of the clinical data helped publicize more reliable information and reveal "the gulf between the truth and the official truth" (Jakes). In addition to obtaining access to reliable and urgently needed medical data, Dr. Jiang managed to use another sort of alternative media, the contesting Western newspapers, to send out warning messages to the rest of the world. As discussed by Greenfeld earlier, a signed statement from Dr. Jiang and its publication with *Time*, one of the leading transnational media, worked together to refute any suspicion of credibility of the incomplete SARS data. Dr. Jiang's tactical entry into the larger transnational media network circumvented China's strategic media control and became one of the most influential moments of transcultural risk communication during SARS. Dr. Jiang employed a quality that de Certeau describes as "metis," or "a principle of economy," to "obtain the maximum number of effects from the minimum force" (82). Dr. Jiang faced "a hostile composition of place," or forces strategically controlling both media access and the type of messages to be spoken (de Certeau 82). However, he "count[ed] on an accumulated time" by attempting to contact first the most influential domestic media and then those abroad, demonstrating an ability to use "its treasure of past experiences and to inventory multiple possibilities" (de Certeau 83). His attempt to test and manipulate various media sites helped him to temporarily occupy a media outlet that was "encountered by chance, on the other's ground" (de Certeau 86).

In addition to his ability to gain tactical entrance to international media, Dr. Jiang also achieved maximum rhetorical impact by choosing to publicize a signed statement rather than relying on the usual format of interviews, which enhanced the credibility of the incomplete data he had gained through personal investigation. Because military hospitals only reported to the military system and did not share any SARS statistics with the MOH in the first half of April, they remained both one of the focal points of international negotiations with the MOH and a source of uncertainty and anxiety. Dr. Jiang's signed statement helped to "concentrate the most [urgently needed] knowledge in the least time" (de Certeau 83). He bridged the huge gap in the MOH's SARS updates and offered a much more complete picture about the SARS situation in Beijing. Moreover, under his influence, "other doctors at Beijing's hospitals came forward (though on condition of anonymity) to corroborate and elaborate the details of Jiang's letter," further strengthening the credibility of his risk message (Jakes). Therefore, Dr. Jiang's kairotic intervention helped to transform his data, despite its weakness and incompleteness, into critical, valid evidence to prove that SARS was, indeed, underreported in Beijing. As Jakes correctly points out, in China, "to openly dispute official information can mean risking career, reputation, even personal safety." Dr. Jiang's decision to disclose SARS risks resulted in negative personal consequences: for more than six months, his family was subject to supervision by the national security force, and his activities were seriously confined.

Dr. Jiang's statement had great impacts on the Beijing's anti-SARS campaign. He spoke at a kairotic moment: WHO issued a travel advisory recommending the postponement of nonessential travel to Hong Kong and Guangdong on April 2. Because access to Beijing medical records or facilities was denied, Dr. Jiang's clinical data helped to bridge the information gap and pushed WHO to take more-aggressive measures. Once Dr. Jiang's data entered the transnational risk network, it was rhetorically transformed and functioned as one of the most critical risk messages that radically altered the way China and the rest of the world responded to SARS. On April 10, WHO openly criticized the disease-reporting system in Beijing and sent another specialist team to investigate the SARS outbreak: "Only a few hospitals reported SARS cases on a daily basis" ("People's Interests"). The next day, WHO's travel advisory again listed Beijing as one of the cities that travelers should avoid. This travel advisory not only offered a fatal blow to the MOH's claim that "Beijing is safe" but also resulted in a quick exodus of foreign investments and businesses from the capital that materialized Beijing's worst fear. Although the MOH did not publicize this decision, changes were taking place, and starting on April 20, Beijing dramatically raised its official count of cases from 37 to 339 and took resolute measures to combat the SARS outbreak ("People's Interests").

Hong Kong: Extra-institutional Risk Messages to Institutional Practices

Another unique case of participatory risk communication is presented by the Hong Kong citizens' use of independent websites to collect and distribute messages about specific locations where SARS infection took place. The Hong Kong health authorities originally rejected the public requests for location-specific risk information. However, the popularity of and media exposure about bottom-up, location-specific risk messages forced the authorities to adopt the practice of offering building-specific information about SARS cases on a daily basis.

It should be stressed that Hong Kong's political system is very different from that of mainland China because of Great Britain's colonial rule from 1847 to 1997. On July 1, 1997, Great Britain returned Hong Kong to China under the condition of what Deng Xiaoping envisioned as "one country, two systems." Designated as a Special Administrative Region, Hong Kong maintains its political system and administrative structure to ensure minimal disruption to its economic prosperity and its function as a world financial and transportation center. Its government reports directly to the Chinese central government, and Hong Kong enjoys more independence and freedom in speech and politics than other Chinese provinces and municipal cities.

Given this historical context, it is not surprising that Hong Kong's media structure shares more similarity with those in Western countries than that of China. Little systematic censorship exists for print and Internet media. Citizens enjoy freedom of speech and can use alternative media to express dissenting viewpoints without worrying about governmental persecution. This more relaxed media policy enabled the highly prominent media coverage of the participatory risk communication taking place in a civilian website sosick.org and the eventual governmental adaptation of similar practices to better meet the public's information needs.

Sosick.org, SARS Cases, Locations

Starting in early March, when atypical pneumonia cases were found in the larger community, pressure "began to build on the Hong Kong government to publish details of where infected cases had been recorded" (Lais 6). On March 24, it was rumored that the chief executive of Hospital Authority, Dr. William Ho, might have been infected. Meanwhile, the Hong Kong government remained reluctant to release its list of infected locations because of its concerns with patients' privacy and possible mass panic. This information gap quickly resulted in rumormongering in Hong Kong. A series of widely circulated rumors claimed that Hong Kong had been declared "an infection port," that the virus was an "experiment in biological warfare intended to target Saddam Hussein," and that SARS cases were "being underreported in Hong Kong" (Philips 1). On March 31, Hong Kong's Department of Health (DH) took the unprecedented step of quarantining all residents of Amoy Gardens, a housing estate in Kowloon, Hong Kong, after a total of 329 atypical pneumonia cases was reported in the residential building (Pomfret and Weiss A02). Thirty-three residents died from the disease. The event was "one of the most baffling and worrisome outbreaks in the epidemic" because it suggested that the virus could be "transmitted in ways other than close person-to-person contact" (Stein, "In Hong Kong" A16). A defective sewage system facilitated the spread of SARS after the index patient visited his brother in the building, had diarrhea, and used the bathroom there. Soon, local residents started to "watch the disease go up each floor every day" (Greenfeld 255). With two-thirds of the patients in the complex building having diarrhea, "a very substantial virus load" was discharged into the sewerage in Block E (Hung 375). The outbreak in Amoy Gardens was taken as an indicator that the virus was now "at large in the community," and many foreigners left Hong Kong quickly (Greenfeld 264).

On April 1, a fourteen-year-old boy created a fake *Ming Pao* web page as an April Fools' prank,[4] announcing that Hong Kong had been declared "an infected port," that its "stock market had collapsed," that border checkpoints had been closed, that all citizens had been ordered to stay at home, and that the chief executive of Hong Kong, Tung Chee-hwa, would soon announce in an emergency press conference that "the outbreak is out of control" (N. Taylor, "Net-spread Panic" 2). Described as the "most dramatic online event of the years," this SARS rumor drove 7.2 million viewers to visit the DH website on the same day. In response to the mass panic created by this fake site, the Hong Kong government created the biggest cell phone spam by "sending a blanket message to about six million cell phones" to dispel the rumor (Wong A6). In late April, another bogus e-mail scam claimed that the DH "had discovered the deadly atypical pneumonia virus in air filters on Mass Transit Rail trains" (Lo 4). Denied open access to detailed risk information, the public was deeply concerned about the possibility of unknowingly contracting SARS when working or traveling near locations with recently infected cases. Sosick.org functioned as a participatory forum for local communities to concert scattered sources of risk messages and to compile a comprehensive list of infected locations.

In response to the lack of detailed official risk information about SARS, four young computer engineers in Hong Kong decided to work on and release to relatives and friends information about locations where SARS patients worked and lived in Hong Kong. On March 31, the engineers compiled the first sosick.org SARS building list. After uploading it online, they sent the URL to relatives and friends. Its information was in such high demand that in two days, sosick.org attracted over two hundred thousand accumulated hits and over one hundred e-mails a day. Only then did they realize that their circles of family and friends were not their only readers and that their website was meeting a public need. Soon, site visitors started to supply the website owners with reports and data about SARS-affected buildings. Such information was gathered through online or onsite research from news reports, news releases, or building management announcements about possible cases in communities. The four young men collected data from users who posted information on the sosick.org website and then checked the credibility of such data before adding them to the list of infected buildings. They also offered all information in both Chinese and English, which made their website bilingual and enhanced its international visibility. As a grassroots effort to list all the infected housing and commercial estates, the website soon became a major player in the extra-institutional risk communication about SARS in Hong Kong as well as in transnational risk communication processes (see fig. 3.2 for a screen capture of the website's home page).

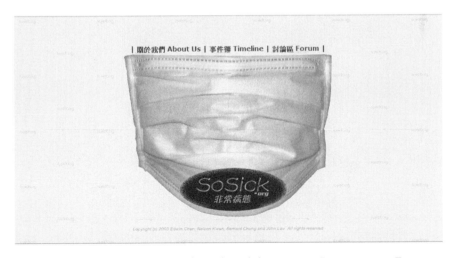

Figure 3.2. A screen capture of sosick.org's home page, June 19, 2005. From sosick.org, courtesy of Bernard Chung, Edwin Chan, Nelson Kwan, and John Lau

Building-Specific Urgent Health Notices

Building Management Official (BMO) notices are locally produced posters employed by building management offices. Building managers issue and post BMO emergency notices in commercial or residential buildings after receiving DH notifications about local infection during the SARS outbreak. Most of these urgent notices started with announcements about DH confirmatory notifications of SARS cases within the building and continued with reassuring messages about anti-infection and sterilization measures taken to disinfect public facilities. They also urged residents to stay calm, to pay attention to personal and environmental hygiene, and, in some cases, to wear masks and to seek medical treatment if any symptoms developed. Many such BMO notices also provided contact information for the DH for those who needed more information about SARS (see figs. 3.3 and 3.4).

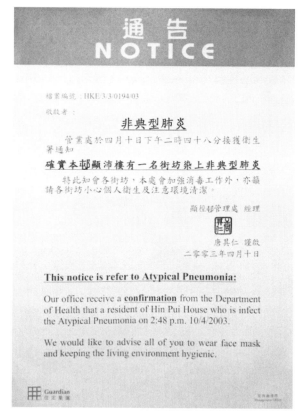

Figure 3.3. April 10, 2003, notice about identification of a SARS case in Hin Pui House, Hong Kong

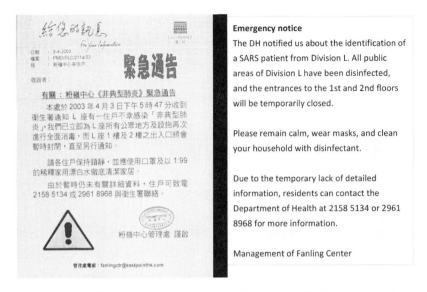

Figure 3.4. April 3, 2003, notice about identification of a SARS case in Fanling Center, Hong Kong

The DH provided limited information about SARS patients to protect their privacy. As a result, management offices did not get either the exact numbers of the infected apartments or names of the patients. Originally issued top-down by the DH to building managers, BMO notices were designed to be posted in public spaces, such as bulletin boards in the elevator lobby or outside the management offices, for limited circulation within those infected buildings. The DH centralized the production and circulation of BMO notices and restricted the access to a limited location-specific audience. The institutional channel for the production, circulation, and distribution of BMOs was featured by its well-defined routes, its limited number of contacts, and its reliance on written documents circulated in specific locations during well-defined time periods. Local residents were considered passive recipients and consumers of such risk information only when they were already within the immediate radius of infected buildings.

Bottom-Up Risk Communication in Independent Website, Public Participation

Communicative technologies, such as digital cameras and Internet forums, make it easy for users to tactically hijack texts originally designed for limited access by privileged users and to widely distribute them. Concerned citizens seized the platform offered by sosick.org, which was originally designed for private communication only, and transformed it into one for subversive bottom-up public production and civic intervention. When concerned navigators resorted to sosick.org for risk communication purposes, the site owners inventively came up with new moves to cope with the large number of risk messages submitted by navigators and created a democratic participatory model. The owners reinvented sosick.org into an open system both by encouraging public contributions and by performing rigorous quality control to ensure the validity of its risk messages.

To enhance the credibility and impacts of their risk messages, the sosick.org owners decided to offer references and external links to all buildings included in their constantly growing list. They took rigorous measures to ensure the accuracy of any new buildings they added to the website by requiring users reporting such data to obtain and include proof, such as "newspaper articles [publicizing] the names of infected buildings, or letters issued by the Department of Health to the estates' management about people on an estate being infected with SARS" (Lais 6). The sosick.org owners only accepted four types of sources: news links, website links, BMO notices, and, later, official reports from the Department of Health's website.

After users submitted the original data, the owners verified the news and performed credibility checks before posting the information online. They functioned as what Lyotard and Thebaud call "a listener, not an author" and judged the bottom-up risk messages on a case-by-case basis (72). Before uploading the newly added names to the existing list, the four engineers would first check the sources of news reports and then call estate management of infected buildings for confirmation. They spent five to six hours every night after returning home from work to complete "all steps from clearing emails to updating the address list" (Lais 6). Such caution in cross-checking the risk information ensured the accuracy of the address list of infected buildings and prevented complaints from mistakenly listed buildings (see fig. 3.5 for a visual representation of the entire risk communication process). Bernard Chung, one of sosick.org's creators and organizers, emphasized the rigorous measures they took to ensure the credibility of their list: "[W]e try to include more than one source for each [infected building]. When there is only one source, we make sure it is a reliable, mainstream source" (Taylor, "Net-spread Panic" 2).

The previously highly centralized BMO notices were profoundly changed by the active user disruption and circulation as well as the subsequent elicited

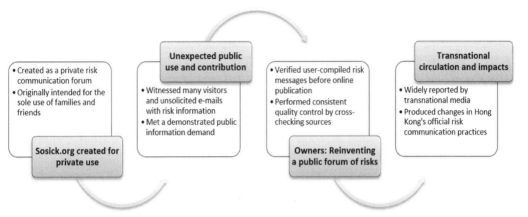

Figure 3.5. Sosick.org: changes of functions as an informal risk communication platform. From sosick.org, courtesy of Bernard Chung, Edwin Chan,
Nelson Kwan, and John Lau

confirmations from BMOs concerning local cases. In other words, the genre
of BMO notices was hijacked from the previously designed government-to-
infected-building communication route. Concerned citizens redistributed it,
transmitted it to an alternative site, and ushered it into constantly ongoing
and mobile participatory risk communication processes.

In addition, because of the rapid submissions from visitors, the website
greatly facilitated the timely circulation of urgently needed risk information
among the public. For instance, it "recorded the spread of SARS from Amoy
Gardens to the nearby Lower Ngau Tau Kok Estate *one week* before this
became generally known" (Lais 6; emphasis added).

Reaching Transnational Media, Risk Communication Channels

Sosick.org attracted so much attention that by April 9, the corresponding
e-mail address for the site received over one thousand messages reporting
infected locations every day. Altogether, 411 buildings and 18 affected air
travel flights were included in the final compiled list, and a total of 180 BMO
photos were submitted to the website as evidences of local infections. On
April 11, the website's cumulative hit count reached two million, and on April
12, sosick.org became one of the top 10 most searched words in Yahoo.com.hk,
one of the top search engines in Hong Kong ("Sosick.org Timeline"). Sosick.
org's extra-institutional risk communication efforts and its highly reliable
risk messages attracted enormous attention from transnational media. In

fact, the creators were interviewed or reported on by over twenty domestic and foreign print, televisual, and online media, including CNN and National Public Radio (NPR) in the United States. Sosick.org was listed as one of the prominent web sources for SARS information by the leading medical journal *The Lancet*, along with official websites of WHO, national health ministries, and world-renowned research institutions (Larkin 389). Such transnational media exposure demonstrates the huge impact sosick.org had on the global risk communication processes and the recognition of the important role it played in shaping official risk communication approaches.

Institutional Appropriation of Extra-institutional Risk Practices

Despite repeated public requests for location-specific risk information, health officials repeatedly denied such inquiries. They rationalized that "it would be difficult to conclude there is a need for such information" and that "[such information is] not necessarily in the public interest" (Philips 1). They also claimed that if the DH did so, "the general population might take personal hygiene for granted if they lived in other buildings" (Benitez and Lee 1). By mid-April 2003, SARS was spreading among residents of Amoy Gardens at such an alarming speed that over three hundred residents had been infected with SARS. The public fear was growing so high that "rumors of a cover-up" and "a huge volume of e-mail speculation on which buildings [had] been infected" were widely circulated in alternative media (Taylor, "Net-spread Panic" 2). In response to these developments, the DH announced on April 9 that it would soon publish a list of buildings where confirmed cases of SARS had been found. On April 11, an additional sixty-one confirmed SARS patients were reported in Hong Kong's daily SARS update, with eleven medical workers and eleven residents from Amoy Gardens (Moy 1). The government refused to disclose the location of new cases, insisting that all the new cases came from different parts of the community and showed "no sign of a new concentration of cases in any area" (Ng and Lee). However, sosick.org broke the official silence on the same day by listing new cases at eight locations, including Aberdeen, Central, Diamond Hill, Repulse Bay, and Tai Koo Shing.

On April 12, the DH's official website published for the first time a list of infected buildings where confirmed SARS cases had been found. The public believed that the move was prompted by sosick.org, "which had [been], for more than a week, providing details of SARS hot spots, including the names of buildings where infections had been confirmed" (Lais 6). The DH denied, however, that it was driven by public pressure to name infected buildings. A DH spokesperson stated that "in light of recent developments [the DH will] put the list on the Web, but the right thing [is] to maintain personal and environmental hygiene" (Benitez and Lee 1). Another official announcement reinforced the emphasis on hygiene, claiming that the information was provided to "encourage members of the public and building management offices to adopt stringent hygiene measures to prevent the spread of SARS in the community ("List of Buildings"). In addition to public hygiene, health officials stressed the importance of not discriminating against people infected by SARS or their families in the affected buildings. They cited two reasons: First, "residents in the same building [are] not be subject to any risk," and, second, only with moral support could those quarantined "stay at home with ease of mind" ("Isolation").

Alternative Media and Extra-institutional Risk Communication

This rhetorical study of the use of alternative media in tactical risk communication enhances our current understanding of extra-institutional risk communication, the use of mobile communication technologies in risk communication, and ethical decision making. Alternative media have value because they provide professionals with quickly accessible communicative channels that allow them to send out risk messages even when professional codes or official orders forbid such communication. As a cultural site less regulated by power apparatuses and more readily accessible to the public, alternative media, such as sosick.org, serve as one possible entry point into power systems for tactical intervention to challenge dominant discourses. To borrow Kimball's terms, alternative media offer tools for "tactic technical communication both within and outside the workplace" at different cultural sites (83).

Figure 3.6 presents the extra-institutional risk communication channels explored in this chapter. Chapter 2 discusses the technocratic model of risk communication, which describes the one way top-down risk communication processes that start with technical experts evaluating risk situations and end with power apparatuses employing mass media to disseminate risk messages. Chapter 3 focuses on the leakages that may take place alongside official risk communication processes. Such leakages result from participatory extra-institutional risk communication efforts made by anonymous professionals and whistle-blowers who resort to little-controlled alternative media to distribute contesting risk messages.

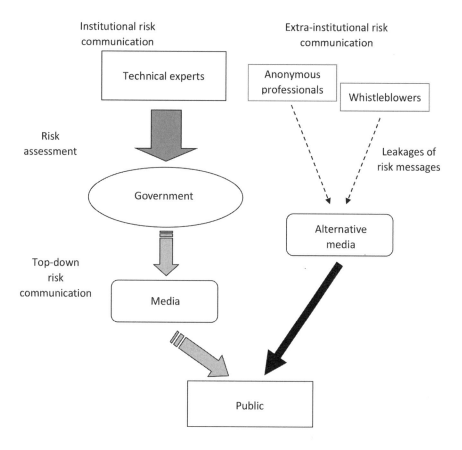

Figure 3.6. Leakages and extra-institutional risk communication

Emerging epidemics, such as SARS, provide an interactive and dynamic space for rhetorical contestation and unofficial risk communication amid uncertainty and official silence. When the official channel of risk communication gets shut down because of economic and political considerations, the tactical extra-institutional risk communication in alternative media can circumvent censorship and release risk messages to the public. Less regulated by the dominant power, alternative media function as a physical and rhetorical space for the production and circulation of unauthorized extra-institutional risk messages first by professionals with access to inside information and then by the larger public.

Like a double-edged sword, alternative media bring professional communicators as much opportunity as challenge and danger. Blurring the line between workplace and private life, alternative media empower professional communicators with the means to circumvent institutional control of risk information while exposing them to personal consequences if they choose to speak about risks as unauthorized insiders. In addition to possible personal losses, professional communicators also face the confounding difficulty of presenting risk messages to the public when they only have limited information about the actual risk and the need to defend the limited credibility of their risk messages. To speak up about the imminent risks via alternative media is not a simple task. It requires well-informed decision making and carefully calculated action. It also requires that we acknowledge and discuss alternative media, extra-institutional technical communication, and ethical decision making in professional communication classrooms, as we introduce future professional communicators to and prepare them for difficult risk communication situations.

4

Constructing SARS: The United States, China, and WHO

How did different key cultural players construct the global epidemic of SARS and the SARS-China relationship? What forces motivated and shaped such rhetorical constructions, and what impacts did they have on the global anti-SARS campaign?

In his famous treatise titled *On Guerrilla Warfare*, Chairman Zedong Mao provides detailed definitions for his notion of people's war:

> The revisionary war is a war of the masses; it can be waged only by mobilizing the masses and relying on them. [. . .] The masses, the millions upon millions of people who genuinely and sincerely support the revolution[,] is the real iron bastion which it is impossible, and absolutely impossible, for any force on earth to smash. (88)

Mao clearly lays out the approach to launch a people's war. In addition to having a strong army, "we must also organize contingents of the people's militia on a big scale. This will make it difficult for the imperialists to move a single inch in our country in the event of invasion" (89–90). Among his list of ten principles of operation for a people's war, two of them are particularly pertinent to the people's war against SARS that the Chinese top leaders launched in late April 2003: "Fight no battle unprepared. [. . .] Give full play to our style of fight—courage in battle, no fear of sacrifice, no fear of fatigue, and continuous fight" (90).

Several factors contributed to China's belated response to SARS: the country's lack of knowledge about the emerging mysterious pneumonia from November 2002 to February 2003, its backward public health facilities, and its institutional disarray and official inaction. As a result, WHO employed biopolitical measures, such as travel advisories, onsite inspections, and technical support, to intervene in March. Closely collaborating with WHO, China managed to launch an aggressive people's war against SARS through mass mobilization. China eventually managed to eradicate SARS with the operation principles that Mao articulates above, namely, full preparation, courage, sacrifice, and tireless and continuous fight. In contrast with China's long and challenging battle with SARS, the United States took a proactive approach to contain the import of the SARS virus in March 2003 and successfully prevented the spread of SARS within its borders.

Priscilla Wald defines what she calls "the outbreak narrative" as "a formulaic plot that begins with the identification of an emerging infection, includes discussion of the global networks throughout which it travels, and chronicles the epidemiological work that ends with its containment" (2). Outbreak narratives have explicit politics that "consistently register anxieties about the global village that reflexively imagined the containment of disease in national terms against its actual and threatened border crossings" (Wald 63). Circulating across media and genres, outbreak narratives "make the act of imagining the community a central feature of its preservation" (Wald 52). Wald's cases examine the outbreak narratives about AIDS and Typhoid Mary within individual countries and the rich scientific, journalistic, and fictional discourses surrounding such outbreaks.

When applied to a transnational context, the study of cross-cultural epidemic rhetoric and outbreak narratives would necessarily investigate epidemic narratives told both by epicenters and by little-affected regions. The analysis of outbreak narratives told by countries and regions both inside and outside the epicenters would yield new understanding about the differences between the ways individual countries construct emerging epidemics originating elsewhere and the ways epicenters tell their own stories about local outbreaks. For instance, the analysis in this chapter reveals that despite China's final success in eradicating SARS, SARS coverage in American media did not achieve full closure. Both WHO publications and Chinese media employed full-fledged outbreak narratives, with different focuses on technological inadequacy and infrastructural backwardness. The media coverage in the United States, however, paid close attention to China's underreporting and utter confusion about SARS throughout the outbreak but discussed very little the final containment and eradication of SARS in China. Thus, the US outbreak narrative about SARS seems to tell a story about a country failing to cope with an emerging epidemic because of ideological and political reasons. Then, mysteriously and luckily, that failing country somehow managed to get the job done.

As a comparative rhetorical study about transcultural narratives of SARS, this chapter examines the transcultural rhetorical construction of SARS in

American mass media, in Chinese mainstream media, and in WHO's public health discourse (SARS updates, travel advices, press releases, and the like). To explore the interactions among the three key players, SARS discourses in national and regional US media are analyzed before moving on to study rhetorical and biopolitical interactions between China and WHO. This analysis of the three types of SARS discourses, however, does not provide satisfactory answers to the frequently raised questions in American media: How could China prevent the spread of SARS in its hinterland and its vast rural areas with poor public health infrastructure and with densely populated towns and villages?[3] Regional media reports, particularly those from SARS-affected areas in China, are explored to look for answers to this important question.

War in Iraq Coverage and SARS in American, Chinese Media

Throughout history, wars and epidemics often go hand in hand. The 1918 Spanish flu erupted during the final stages of World War I. The infamous epidemic started in the United States in March 1918, and it lasted until June 1920. Whereas the first phase of the plague caused few deaths, when the flu surfaced again in fall of 1918, it struck viciously (Barry, "Anthrax Pranks"). With crowded troop quarters, massive troop movement across regions, and intercontinental business and missionary travelers, the Spanish flu circled the world, killing over fifty million people. The pandemic of the killer disease caused "unusually high death rates among adults," with half of the dead being people in their twenties and thirties (Crosby 12). As Kathleen Minnix describes, "World War I and the Spanish flu fed each other" in 1918.

Wars not only influence the development of epidemics but also complicate the development of and media coverage about epidemics. When violence, terror, and hunger threaten people's physical survival on a daily basis, the less visible and thus less fearsome phantoms of viruses become a more distant concern. When one surveys the international context surrounding SARS, one important event that occurred around the same period was the 2003 invasion of Iraq the United States spearheaded from March 19 to May 1, which also signified the beginning of the war against Iraq. Both the invasion and the ongoing war drew a lot of media attention. With the military involvement of the United States, the United Kingdom, and other Western countries in Iraq, the distant, emerging SARS outbreak became one of the less immediate concerns. Therefore, Western countries had different degrees of involvement in the SARS outbreak in 2003. Next is examined the reporting patterns about SARS and Iraq in American and Chinese media.

The article pattern of SARS was analyzed in two American mainstream news media, the *New York Times* and the *Washington Post*. The findings revealed consistently higher coverage of the domestic issue the US War in Iraq than that of the international situations of SARS (see fig. 4.1). The month of May witnessed the most frequent reports about SARS in both newspapers, partly because of the increasing amount of SARS information China released.

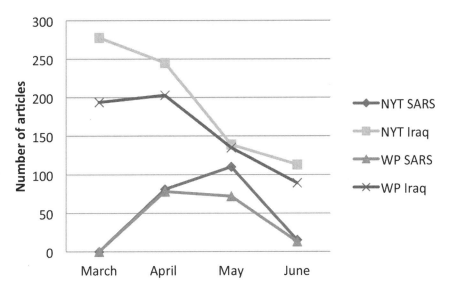

Figure 4.1. Articles about the War in Iraq and about SARS in the *New York Times* and the *Washington Post*, March–June 2003

Compared with the American media's preoccupation with the War in Iraq, *People's Daily* covered the foreign event of the Iraq invasion much more comprehensively than domestic SARS outbreaks in March and April. The reporting patterns of March and April are completely the opposite of those in the US coverage: the number of articles on the War in Iraq is hundreds more than the number of reports on the domestic issue of the SARS outbreak in China (see fig. 4.2). Whereas *People's Daily*'s coverage of SARS before April is characterized by underreporting, the coverage in May and June shows a pattern of overreporting in most of its sections, as the Communist Party's newspaper devoted over half of its space to report about the development of the anti-SARS campaign and about informative tips on SARS prevention.

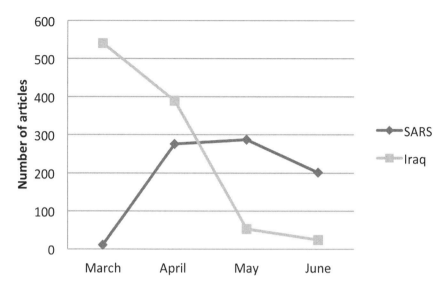

Figure 4.2. Articles about the War in Iraq and about SARS in *People's Daily*, March–June 2003

SARS as Ideological Pathologies in the US Media

The epidemic of SARS simultaneously existed at biological, political, ideological, cultural, and economic levels, mediated both by the at-first erratically attentive, then uninterested American media and by the at-first suppressed, then overreporting Chinese media. For most Americans, SARS was and remains a media reality packaged for mass consumption. The spectacle of SARS the media created refracts the entrenched cultural fantasies the media continuously revived and reinforced. My analysis of various rhetorics of SARS sheds light on ideological constructions as well as on cultural biases that shaped American SARS discourses.

In the WHO Global SARS meeting, Gao Qiang, executive vice minister of China's Ministry of Health, divided the SARS epidemic in China into three stages: onset (before March), spread (April), and decline (May and June) before WHO removed Beijing from its travel advisory on June 24 ("Speech of Mr. Gao Qiang"). As a sharp contrast to Gao's clearly divided stages, SARS coverage in the United States evolved from a narrative about the information cover-up before mid-March to information manipulation until mid-April and finally to questions about the quality of information and China's credibility before China eradicated SARS in late June. To some extent, the press portrayed a story of SARS originating in China, spreading with the help of official censorship, and growing out of control before China's official admission. Then, suddenly and mysteriously, the epidemic disappeared in June more because of pure luck than because of China's prevention and control effort. As Lynn Windt and Theodore Hinds point out in their analysis of cold-war rhetoric, the function of political rhetoric requires three essential conditions: "a raw event and/or events [. . .], a rhetoric that clarifies and assigns meanings to the events, and publicity for the rhetoric as others share it at the time" (7). The same conditions operated in the construction of the SARS-China relationship and in the wide circulation and acceptance of such interpretations in the United States.

The US media's early coverage of SARS in April focused on the underreporting and undercalculation of SARS cases in China. Some previously unreported details about China's handling of SARS were publicized in various American media, and a recurring theme dealt with the international criticism of China's slow response at the early stage of SARS. Some of the news headlines reflect this theme: "China Admits More Mystery Illness"; "China Squelches Early Alert on SARS"; "A Beijing Doctor Questions Data on Illness"; "China Getting a Black Eye for Early Secrecy on SARS"; "Virus Badly Underreported in Beijing"; "China Admits Underreporting Its SARS Cases"; and "A Reticent China Undercuts Its Milder New Image." As the reports describe, the Chinese government "ordered local reporters to play down reports of the disease," labeled early health reports about SARS in Guangdong as "top-secret documents," and forbade health officials to discuss it lest they "leak state secrets." The state-controlled press was "banned from reporting SARS" at first, then a "strict limit [was] set on what could be covered." Soon a logical leap was made by resorting to the Communist Party's traditional penchant for secrecy to explain China's early inaction. For instance, China had been accused of considering "[negative] health statistics as state secrets" and of being particularly reluctant "to release bad news occurring in Beijing, the capital"; therefore, its "slow and secretive" early response was characterized by "reticence" and "obstructionism."

China started its belated-yet-full-scale anti-SARS campaign on April 21, acknowledging its mistakes and expelling two top officials who had manipulated the SARS statistics. China quarantined suspected cases, closed down schools and public entertainment venues, and issued stringent laws to punish those who willfully spread the disease. Despite the changes in China's efforts to contain SARS, American media still resorted to the myths, logical leaps, and stereotypical ideological differences mentioned above to interpret all the changes. The US media provided very little description of China's anti-SARS measures, which was followed by the routine questioning of issues, such as early inaction, censorship, crisis of credibility, and the Communist Party's tradition of information manipulation. Such critiques existed as a consistent theme in American SARS coverage throughout the outbreak.

In addition to dwelling on China's slow response to and cover-up of SARS before April, many reports continued to question China's efforts to contain SARS and the quality of its data. Although WHO reported no systematic underreporting in Shanghai, suspicion of a continual cover-up still remains: "China is the epicenter of SARS, [so] Shanghai has no escape" (McLaughlin). The media repeatedly predicted that China could not possibly prevent SARS from reaching the economically backward hinterland (Bradsher, "Relapse" A5; Eckholm, "As Cases Mount" A10). When SARS was almost brought under control in early June, the same questions were raised about the reliability of the data, the "many imponderables about [the] SARS epidemic," and "the crackdown on the media to maintain tight control" (Altman, "SARS Enigma" A18; Pomfret, "China" A16).

Another central logical operation in the construction of the SARS-China connection employs historical analogies to attribute China's early inaction to the Communist Party's penchant of secrecy. In addition, it compares the construction of the Xiaotangshan SARS hospital near Beijing to the mass-mobilization movement in the Cultural Revolution and describes the international critique of the Chinese government as the same as that after the Tiananmen Square event. Connections were made between China's Communist Party and the cold-war stereotypes associated with communism, namely, totalitarian governments and aversion to freedom.

In *Permanence and Change*, Kenneth Burke warns that "the great danger of analogy is that a *similarity* is taken as evidence of an *identity*" (97) and explains:

> The business of interpretation is accomplished by the two processes of over-simplification and analogical extension. We oversimplify a given event when we characterize it from the standpoint of a given interest— and we attempt to invent a similar characterization for other events by analogy. (107)

He continues with his discussion of the method in the judging of historical events:

> Those who attempt to interpret history by ambitiously driven analogical extensions lay much emphasis upon the factors of history that can be called recurrent. But one can note the recurrent only by abstracting certain qualities from the given historical complexities. One must have special informing interests of his own. (107)

In historical analogies, a series of traits or premises commonly believed to be true about the prior event gets projected onto the current event. Transforming similarities into essential features of identities, analogies oversimplify the complex contexts and features of the current event and dramatically change its nature by repackaging it as another similar occurrence of the prior one. Such historical analogies help to create a sense of continuity and consistency in the understanding of the present in light of the past.

As an instance of historical analogy, Joseph Kahn claims, "China has suffered much larger natural and man-made disasters in the past, including floods, famines, earthquakes, and epidemics taking millions of lives," compared with which SARS was a much smaller disaster ("Contagion" A11). Here, Kahn compares SARS with "the famine caused by Mao Zedong's forced collectivization in the late 1950s," with both demonstrating China's routine failure to "grapple with natural or created disasters" ("Contagion" A11). He later compares SARS to the Tiananmen Square demonstration in 1989 in terms of the seriousness of leadership crisis ("China Getting" A10). Such historical analogies define the nature of the events surrounding SARS as the same as previous man-made disasters and the Tiananmen Square event. Doing this abstracts features, such as leadership crises and political maneuvers, from vastly different historical contexts surrounding those events. These analogies also create melodramatic narratives by stereotyping current events, motives, and actions against the backdrop of previous political events and add multiple layers of ideological and political meanings previously associated with China. Such comparisons oversimplify the "historical complexities" surrounding SARS (Burke 107) and allow the inflection of a long-existing linguistic and ideological epidemic about Communist China to be transferred to SARS. These comparisons revive the preexisting ideological, political, cultural, and linguistic epidemic associated with communism, the cold war, and China.

A new myth comes into existence: SARS stands for the routine failure of Communist China to deal with disasters. Whereas international risk regimes urged China into taking measures to contain SARS, the US media lumped SARS together with other perceived "Chinese sicknesses" and soon transformed it into an icon laden with political, cultural, and ideological meanings (Waldron). Examination of SARS reports and editorials reveals the construction of a SARS/China myth: SARS signifies not the way China deals with an epidemic outbreak but what China really is as a country. This logical movement quickly melts historically specific conditions and responses into routine decisions and entrenched habits. Through the use of existing stereotypes of communism, the framing helps construct an equation:

Death

↑

SARS = denial = Communist censorship = China

Diagram 4.1

The use of existing cultural biases about China reflects ideological differences and relies on long-existing binaries, such as health versus pathology, democracy versus totalitarianism, and us versus them. Such selective coverage excluded changes taking place at the second stage of the outbreak and the immense efforts China made to quell SARS. By labeling all anti-SARS efforts as Mao-style and communist regimentations, the media lumped together quarantines, strong anti-SARS decrees, and concerted medical resources as blameworthy oppressive schemes rather than measures commonly taken by other countries to contain SARS. Therefore, the American understanding of SARS is anchored in the larger picture of the cultural, political, and ideological differences between China and the United States, in the perception of communist governments as totalitarian, and in the entire linguistic and ideological package attached to the term *communist China*.

Visual Representations of SARS

Time Asia's special issue on SARS employs a visual synecdoche,[1] or the equivocation between parts and the whole, on its cover to depict China as the "SARS nation" (see fig. 4.3). The graphic on the cover superimposes the image of China's national flag on that of a radiographic photo of the pathological lung structure of a SARS patient. Equating SARS with China, the graphic suggests that China has become the epicenter of SARS, the cause of SARS, and the synonym of SARS. The title employs red letters for the acronym *SARS* and black letters for the word *nation*. The subtitle, printed in a smaller font size, suggests, "How this epidemic is transforming China." Combined, the graphic and the text suggest the convergence of the spatial and epidemiological mappings of SARS: as the origin of SARS, China became a country that exported the epidemic to the rest of the world. The visual metaphor suggests not only the equivalence between SARS and China as a nation but also the attempt to put a national and ethnic identity to the epidemic of SARS.

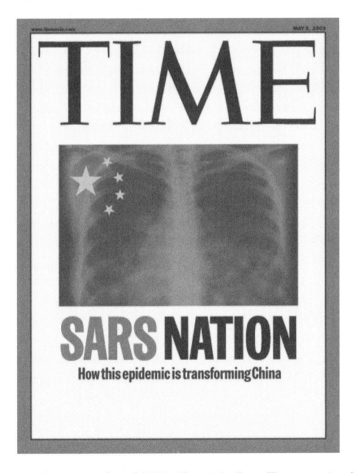

Figure 4.3. Cover story about SARS in *Time* Asia. From *Time* magazine, May 5, 2003, © 2003 Time Inc.; used under license; *Time* and Time Inc. are not affiliated with, and do not endorse products or services of, licensee

Cultural Circulations and Adaptations:
SARS in Political Posters

With SARS bringing huge economic and political impacts, wider cultural, artistic, and political forces began to appropriate the acronym of SARS for non–public health purposes. The cultural circulation of the acronym invited rhetorical and artistic transformations, adaptations, and recontextualizations of the term. It offered new and interesting outlets for the expression of ideas about contemporary cultural and political issues, which ranged from epidemic control to domestic and international politics in the United States. Transforming the original meaning of SARS into something more relevant to the contemporary issues in the United States, such rhetorical adaptations offered artists interesting ways to express their political and cultural concerns.

For instance, Clinton Fein, a comic artist, made a tourist poster for the "World Tour 2003" of SARS, in which he listed all the starting dates of local SARS outbreaks for the cities of Shanghai, Hanoi, Hong Kong, and Toronto and finished with the usual advertising line of "coming soon to a city near you" (see fig. 4.4). Adapting the traditional design of a tourist or performance poster, Fein followed the conventions of the genre closely but used language, colors, and design elements effectively to emphasize the quick pathological tour of SARS and the increasing apprehension it brought to the international communities. A closer look at the dates of arrival shows an interval of about two weeks between the beginnings of SARS outbreaks in the four cities, which almost suggests a regular schedule of shows or tourist trips. The arriving dates listed in the poster do not correspond with the actual dates on which the four cities started to have SARS cases, as they were most likely invented to better conform to the generic convention of tourist posters and to achieve dramatic effects. Considering the increasing distances between those cities, such regular intervals revealed the high speed with which the SARS virus traveled around the world and indicated the immense fear brought by the "World Tour" of SARS.

Another political poster adopted the acronym of SARS to protest against the Bush administration's policies (see figure 4.5). The poster applies the symbolic icon of the facial mask to a portrait of President George W. Bush in front of the national flag of the United States. The poster reinvents the full name of SARS as "Sardonic American Rhetoric Syndrome" and, in a yellow tag, states that "symptoms include lies, propaganda and hypocrisy." At the

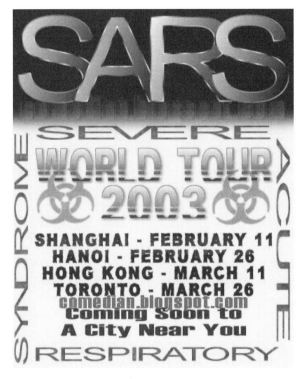

Figure 4.4. SARS world tour 2003. From Clinton Fein, SARS, 2003, Annoy.com

bottom of the poster, a different yellow, script font in italics is used in the short statements "Avoid politicians" and "Avoid media." Without looking at the visual and verbal components of the poster, the format of the message is almost identical to that of a public health educational poster about SARS: The name of the epidemic is spelled in full with its symptoms explained and possible preventive measures listed. The iconic figure of a masked man suggests SARS and the widespread fear it caused. Yet, a closer look at both the graphic and the text produces a completely different message. The post strategically juxtaposes Bush, the masked man standing in front of the national flag, with eye-catching words "lies," "hypocrisy," and "propaganda." It makes explicit connection between the reinvented acronym of SARS and Bush's faulty accusation of Iraq hoarding nuclear weapons as the rationale to launch the Iraq War in early 2003. The mask suggests the withholding of truth rather than silence in the creation of propaganda surrounding the invasion of Iraq. Its verbal messages work well to transform the poster into a politically motivated protest while its overall design still keeps the look of a public health poster about SARS prevention through the use of the mask and the acronym of SARS.

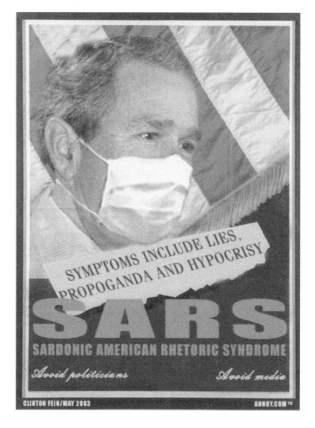

Figure 4.5. SARS: sardonic American rhetoric syndrome. Used with permission of image creator (comedian.blogspot.com)

Media Coverage in Chinatowns

The field of Asian American studies calls for the distancing from the American-centered and nation-based research paradigm and advocates instead for a community-based and immigrant-centered approach that "examines the internal dynamics of the Asian American community and their culture as a global phenomenon" (H. Liu, "Transnational" 140). Madeline Hsu, among others, refutes the dominant conception of human migration as a one-way process. Instead, she proposes to redefine the process as trans-Pacific circular

146

flows of people, money, information, and social relations across national boundaries. To analyze media reports about SARS and Chinatown with an immigrant-centered approach, it is important to survey news reports from mainstream and regional English media in the United States and from Chinese media based in Chinatowns. This section includes both mainstream and ethnic news media from Canada because of the drastic economic and psychological impact SARS had on Chinatowns in Canada.

Mainstream national news media, such as the *New York Times* and the *Washington Post,* were preoccupied with the actual scope of SARS and the ideological roots of China's belated responses. In contrast, regional newspapers focused more on local SARS situations and the ways in which fear of SARS affected local Asian communities, particularly Chinatown businesses. Relying on the quick and unsupervised technologies of mass-distributed hoax e-mails, Internet posts, and, in some cases, text messages, rumors about Chinatown businesses infected by the SARS virus were quickly circulated in big cities in the United States, Canada, Europe, and Southeast Asian countries, such as Malaysia and Indonesia. Specifically targeting businesses, such as restaurants and supermarkets, such rumors reinforced the existing fear about international travelers returning from countries with ongoing SARS infections. Moreover, these rumors indicated that Asian communities, in general, and Chinatowns, in particular, functioned as possible virus reservoirs because of the ethnic connections. Alan Kraut invents the term *medicalized nativism* to describe the association of immigrant groups with communicable disease and the subsequent justification for stigmatization of such groups (Wald 8). Medicalized nativism goes beyond scapegoating immigrant groups for an invading disease. It associates the disease with "dangerous [and primitive] practices and behaviors that allegedly mark intrinsic cultural differences" and "expresses the destructive transformative power of the group" (Wald 8). The following sections analyze how medicalized nativism operates in the discriminatory discourses about Chinatowns and other Asian communities.

According to netlore, rumors, in some cases malicious hoaxes, were "circulating via emails in cities from New York to Toronto to Sacramento and places in between," warning people to "stay away from Chinatown and other predominantly Asian neighborhood[s] due to alleged outbreaks of SARS among restaurant or grocery workers in those areas, often citing specific businesses by name" ("SARS Virus Infects"). One such e-mail explicitly urged people to "avoid going to ASIAN areas," claiming that on April 3, "the police shut down Hawaii and San Gabriel Supermarket due to the employee some-how [getting] hit by this virus" ("SARS Virus Infects").

Similar malicious rumors and Internet hoaxes were also recorded in ethnic Chinese newspapers based in North America. Jie Xiao reports the economic impact of a rumor about one cook working for a Philadelphia restaurant ("SARS"). The hoax claimed that the man travelled back to Hong Kong and became infected with SARS. It caused so much panic that it con-tributed to more than a 70 percent plummet in overall Chinatown businesses in Philadelphia. Similar SARS scares took place in Chinatowns in Las Vegas, Los Angeles, Toronto, Houston, and Dallas. They were often caused by ru-mors and Internet hoaxes that claimed that specific Chinese restaurants and supermarkets had employees returning from mainland China or Hong Kong who got infected and died soon afterward (Jiang; J. Li, "Canadian Premier"; J. Song, "SARS Fears").

By April 25, a total of 245 suspected SARS cases were reported to the CDC from thirty-seven states, with thirty-nine of them having illnesses consistent with the interim US surveillance-case definition for probable SARS cases. Among them, thirty-seven people were epidemiologically identified as having recently traveled to mainland China, Hong Kong, Singapore, Ha-noi, or Toronto. Statistics show that 49 percent of the probable cases were white, and 44 percent were Asian, and proportions for suspect cases were 54 percent and 36 percent, respectively (CDC, "Outbreaks of SARS—United States" 357). Unsubstantiated yet widespread fear occurred as a response to the transnational ethnic connections between SARS epicenters in Asia, Asian communities, and Chinatowns and concentrated Asian populations in other parts of the world. Sometimes, such anxiety resulted in the irrational fear that "going to places with concentrated Chinese populations would greatly increase the chance of contracting SARS" (Jiang). These rumors were pred-icated on the entangled links among geopolitics, ethnicity, and epidemics. They blamed the close contact between outsiders—namely, immigrants and travelers—and the epicenters in Asia, and they warned against any "intimacy with outsiders" or travelling and shopping in Asian communities, such as Chinatowns (Pernick 862).

Caucasian Americans and Canadians were not the only groups that stayed away from Chinatowns. Asian Americans and immigrants were reported to have stayed away from Chinatowns because of the perceived geographical link between epicenters in Asia and Chinatowns in North America. Christie

Blatchford coined the term *SARS neurosis* to describe the neurotic epidemic of hate and racism SARS caused. She argued that because "the substantial chunk of the [Chinatown] business" came from the Chinese, it was other Chinese who racialized SARS and punished Chinese businesses (A1). Her claim seems a little far-fetched since she ignored the reasons behind people of Asian descent's decisions to stay away not only from Chinatowns but also from other public places. Asian immigrant communities took very different risk reduction measures both because of the racial stereotyping, profiling, and shunning they encountered on a daily basis and because of their knowledge about the SARS situations in Hong Kong and China. Many cities witnessed a sharp "rise in anti-Chinese feeling" because "SARS originated in China" (Abbate A8). Antonella Artuso reported Chinese Canadians' bitter experiences with "racial slurs, hate messages," "stories of stereotyping and targeting," rejection of services in restaurants, real estate agencies, auto shops, and casinos, as well as the singling out of their children for special treatment (5). A Canadian Chinese community leader compared the stigmatization of SARS to that of AIDS: "Just as AIDS is not a gay disease, SARS is not a Chinese virus" (Artuso 5). Despite public health officials' and civic leaders' repeated emphasis on SARS as "an equal opportunity disease," SARS panic persisted, and its accompanying stigma stayed (Blatchford A1).

Adding to these experiences of racial stigmatization was the anxiety caused by underground and official reports in the transnational Chinese media about SARS outbreaks in the larger communities in Hong Kong and later in mainland China. Because of "family and business ties" with Hong Kong and China, many Asian immigrants obtained information about SARS from transnational Chinese media, online news portals, and discussion forums. Being "web savvy and bilingual," those immigrants were much more aware of the SARS outbreaks in the epicenters because of "trans-Pacific travels, calls, and emails" (Murphy A4). Chapters 2 and 3 in the current volume describe the tremendous sense of uncertainty and fear experienced by Guangdong and Hong Kong before China started to aggressively combat SARS in late April. It is very likely that such anxiety greatly influenced the risk behaviors of Asian immigrants who read print and digital reports about the SARS situation in China. Many Asian immigrants were "getting information about SARS from websites in Hong Kong, where the authorities are much more alarmed about the disease's spread" (Murphy A4). One San Francisco health official lamented about the competing risk information from Asia, which was "not under our control" (Murphy A4). Asian immigrant communities encountered on a daily basis two sets of highly contradictory risk definitions and prevention tips as well as news about more-alarming risk situations in Asia, which contributed to a "psychology of fear" of the "far-off killer" (Murphy A4).

People of Asian descent reported radical behavior changes. Many of them no longer went to restaurants or grocery stores in Chinatowns. In response to their experiences with suspicion from colleagues and with racial shunning "on transit, in schools and other public places," Asian immigrants tried to reduce their trips to run errands around the city and to "cut their ties to their own communities" to prove that they were "'clean' of SARS" (Goossen, Pay, and Go A15). They avoided not only trips to public places but also contact with other Asian people as part of their "precautions to avoid infection" (Alphonso NA9). In some radical cases, such precautions resulted not only in people's efforts to avoid "any human contact" by wearing masks and gloves in public places but also in openly acknowledged fear to go out because "it is better to be safe than sorry" (Sims A7; Murphy and Arenson A12).

Media construction of local epidemics brings not only discursive effects but also material impacts, such as economic losses, racial discrimination, and isolation on communities stigmatized by intentional or unintentional media coverage. SARS has been portrayed in mainstream media as an invading global epidemic that originated from China, a vast country with not only the competing ideology of communism but also an increasingly competitive economy. Therefore, transcultural communities (Chinese immigrants in Chinatowns), Chinese sojourners (students and travelers), and, in some cases, Asians, in general, became a convenient catch-all scapegoat during the SARS scare throughout North America.

The circulating malicious and unsubstantiated rumors heightened consumer fear, hysteria, panic, and misunderstanding of the local threat of the disease, which resulted in huge reductions in business and economic losses of up to 75 percent in Chinatowns (Swingler 2). Numerous cities with China-towns in North America and Asia (i.e., Boston, Chicago, Honolulu, Las Vegas, Los Angeles, Manila, New York, Philadelphia, San Francisco, and Toronto) witnessed huge decreases in patronage and business, which was caused by rampant Internet hoaxes and cellular phone text messages wrongly claiming that owners or staff of Chinese restaurants and grocery stores contracted and died from SARS and that businesses were shut down by state authorities (Matthews; Rosenwald B1; Surendran A1).

Chinatowns play important economic and cultural roles in the cities where they are located. As major assets for local authorities in Europe and North America, Chinatowns "are often included in initiatives to regenerate derelict areas and considered part of the tourism industry" (Christiansen 177). For instance, in Chicago, Chinatown contributed about $65 million in sales tax revenue in 2003 (Chao). As numerous scholars in Asian American studies point out, the ultimate goal of immigrants is often economic success rather than assimilation (Y. Chen, *Chinese San Francisco*; Madeline Hsu, *Dreaming*; H. Liu, "Transnational"). Immigrants rely on geographically dispersed social relations and expanded networks in both their host countries and their home countries to "explore economic opportunities beyond national boundaries and to create alternative social spaces away from home" (H. Liu, "Transnational" 141).

With unfounded rumors and fear bringing economic blows to the communities, local Chinatown businesses and political leaders made active efforts to dispel SARS rumors and to publicize the absence of any health threats in Chinatowns. Luming Mao and Morris Young define Asian American rhetoric as "systematic effective use and development of symbolic resources in social, cultural, and political contexts" (4). Asian American rhetoric is "employed to address specific occasions, whether responding to acts of racism or forming community" (6). It aims not only to "carve out new space for critical and productive engagement" but also to "resist social and economic injustice and reassert their discursive agency and authority in the dominant culture" (4). As Asian American rhetorical discourses, Chinatowns' responses to rumors about local SARS threats certainly worked to destabilize the asymmetrical power relations between the majority and minority cultures and brought material and symbolic consequences.

Let's examine how Chinatowns in New York City (NYC) and Toronto responded to SARS. NYC Chinatowns suffered tremendous economic losses from the September 11 terrorist attack in 2001. In a phone survey of 112 business owners in NYC Chinatowns, 84 percent of respondents claimed that their business plummeted after the first reports about SARS in Asia (Harrison 8). By the end of April 2003, NYC Chinatowns suffered heavy economic tolls because of hoaxes and rumors related to SARS, even though no SARS cases had been found there. The community collaborated to resist the stigmatization caused by the faulty ethnic links between SARS and Chinatowns. John Wang, president of the Asian-American Business Development Center, urged the state and municipal governments of New York to form a task force to "promote tourism and provide tax breaks to area businesses" (Harrison 8).

Similar calls for official and public support were heard from Chinatowns all over the world. Community leaders organized publicity events, public health workshops, and press conferences and sponsored advertisements in leading regional English newspapers. Functioning as community advocates and spokespersons, chambers of commerce and local leaders in various Chinatowns launched public education campaigns and placed advertisements in mainstream newspapers to denounce the rumors. Rather than staying as passive victims of malicious hoaxes, restaurants targeted by such hoaxes held press conferences and invited reporters from both ethnic Chinese newspapers and English newspapers to dispel those rumors (Emery; Jiang). At the 2003 Canadian Critical Race Conference, Victor Wong, executive director of Vancouver Association of Chinese Canadians, criticized "the racialization of SARS" in his presentation: "SARS is not an ethno-specific disease but it has become the modern day yellow peril." Wong listed various rhetorical artifacts created by his association to combat the marginalization of Chinese Canadians, including a website about SARS and Chinatown, a TV public service announcement on SARS that was aired on two Vancouver TV channels, and online daily bulletins of news articles and media commentaries on SARS. Wong also called for the adoption of the multilingual, multicultural health approach instead of relying on the existing Eurocentric and bureaucratic approaches to healthcare to better assist the anti-SARS campaign in Canada.

Rhetorical messages sent by most Chinatowns emphasized their economic contributions to local areas, dispelled SARS rumors, and rejected the alleged ethnic and geographical connections between SARS and Chinatowns. As Asian American rhetorical discourses, they brought about "changes that affect[ed] the attitudes, beliefs, and actions of their intended audiences" (Mao and Young 5). One can clearly see the rhetorical impacts of Chinatown's call for support in the New York City Department of Health and Mental Hygiene's SARS update issued on May 14. The update starts by stressing the need to promote public understanding of SARS: "SARS is not a disease that specifically targets the Asian communities or any other ethnic groups in NYC.... There is no need to avoid travelling in Asian communities in NYC" (Frieden). People were urged not to "trust any unofficial claims or rumors" (Frieden). In addition, the department's director promised in the update to "continue to meet regularly with organizations in the community so as to inform them of the SARS situation in NYC in a timely manner" (Frieden).

In many parts of the world, state and municipal health and political authorities took action to help local Chinatowns recover from the SARS scare and to attract tourists and shoppers. Public health officials held community meetings and passed out informative fliers to dispel rumors about SARS cases in local Chinatowns. The mayors of Boston and New York ate lunches in Chinatowns, and the Canadian premier visited Toronto's Chinatown to demonstrate moral support, to promote tourism, and to dispel false rumors of SARS threats in the areas (Rosenwald B1; Westfeldt). The US senators from New York, including Hillary Rodham Clinton, participated in dining in Chinatown and were part of press releases that supported local businesses. Such gestures from highly prominent officials were reported as top news in ethnic Chinese newspapers to serve as solid evidence about the absence of SARS cases in Chinatowns.

One influential piece of Asian American rhetoric, however, went beyond symbolic gestures of support from high-profile politicians and public health officials. It exposed the "systemically racist structure" that operated to stigmatize and oppress Chinese and Filipino immigrants in Toronto (Leung 142). The Chinese Canadian National Council (CCNC) issued a report titled "The Yellow Peril Revisited: The Impacts of SARS on Chinese and Southeast Asian Communities" in 2004. Carrianne Leung, one of the coauthors, later published an abridged version of the report in an academic journal, in which she criticizes the "systemic racism" embedded in "the process of the response [to SARS] everywhere on different levels of governments, health institutions, communities, [and] the public" (Chinese Canadian National Council 140; 144). She argues that the "social crisis" of SARS is "constituted through racist ideology," which is well supported by personal narratives obtained from interviews and focus groups with Southeast and East Asian communities in Toronto (137). With Chinese Canadian communities and Chinatowns constructed as "a problem of public health and national security," Chinatowns were historically connected with disease and filth and were often targeted as spaces requiring "sanitation reform" (137). The same historical discourses operated again in the context of SARS to contain and regulate Chinese and Filipino Canadians through alienation, discrimination, harassment, layoffs, and isolation of such racialized bodies. The report records people's experiences with overt targeting and stigmatization in public transport, workplaces, schools, hotels, international borders, and other public places. CCNC's recommendations to prevent racial targeting include the reduction of racial stereotyping in media portrayal, funding for antiracism advocacy groups and Chinatown businesses suffering from huge economic losses, and inclusion of minority communities in public health response plans (36–38). Leung's study goes beyond individual accounts to present a collective narrative about "the racialization of SARS and its gendered and classed effects" on Southeast and East Asian communities (147; see also Chinese Canadian National Council). Started as a political document put together by the CCNC, the report records numerous incidents of labeling, stereotyping, status losses, and individual and structural discrimination widely experienced by Asian immigrants (Ali 47–49). Leung deliberately and strategically brought more media and scholarly attention to this issue by publishing an excerpted version of the document in an academic journal in 2008, which continued to facilitate the circulation of the report as one of the studies on SARS and its racial impacts in transnational media. Leung's case attests to the importance of minority communities to rally together and to take collective action, either through community leaders or community-industry-academia partnership to maximize the cultural circulation and political impacts of their rhetorical discourses. Asian immigrants are situated in complicated trans-Pacific networks of relations. They develop complex transnational and multicultural identities as well as social networks, and they actively perform political and rhetorical acts at the intersections among local, regional, and global contexts to promote their economic vitality.

College Antipathy toward Asians: Orders of Exclusion

Efforts to put an ethnic face on SARS came not only from media discourses surrounding Asian communities, particularly Chinatowns, around the world but also from university decisions about admissions and access to various academic events. University of California (UC) Berkeley announced on May 2 that it would ban students from China, Taiwan, Hong Kong, and Singapore from taking its summer courses on campus (Murphy and Arenson A12). The university soon changed the policy on May 6 to target only Chinese students after the CDC lifted its travel advisory for Singapore.

Students from China and Taiwan represented "nearly 16% of U.S. foreign students in 2001–2002" (Marklein 1A). For the 2011–12 academic year, a total of 764,495 international students were enrolled in universities in the United States, with 194,029 (25.4 percent) of them from China (Institute of International Education). China's booming economy, reinforced by the traditional Confucian emphasis on education, drove China to surpass India for the first time as the top spot of origin for international students (Lewin 4). International students are a less privileged group in what Aihwa Ong calls flexible citizens. They travel across national boundaries in search of educational opportunities, and often they either have to pay expensive tuition and fees or have to obtain financial support to fund their study in the United States. As consumers of higher education, students travel in pursuit of better education rather than privilege or profit, and they have much more limited mobility compared with transnational business travelers. In other words, international students' access to the United States is controlled by universities that offer them both admissions and legitimate status to enter the country. My analysis here does not suggest that international students can be dismissed as powerless transnational consumers. Instead, the huge revenues they bring to American universities give international students, parents, and their countries of origin strong negotiating power over issues of access. During global epidemics, when foreigners from epicenters are often considered possible sources of health threats, universities may deny international students the access to their campuses to protect their local communities, as UC Berkeley did in May 2003.

UC Berkeley cited lack of resources as the primary reason behind its decision, arguing that the university faced "a shortage of space for isolating students who showed signs of the disease" and, thus, was incapable of coping with potential local outbreaks caused by students from epicenters (Burress and Russell). Commenting on international students' preference for "group-living arrangements" in International House on campus, Gary Penders, director of UC Berkeley Summer Sessions, said, "We could create a worldwide plague ourselves by bringing all these students together for the summer and then sending them back home" (Burress and Russell). Labeling international students as a pathological entity, the ban created an imagined geography of illness not only for international students but also for the group-living community that such students share on campus. Barring those students from campus, the university transformed them into an insidious health threat, a sick Other, who should be either controlled by structures of segregation or excluded as dangerous outsiders. As a result, UC Berkeley lost

$1 million in course income, and, by the end of the SARS epidemic, not one American university had reported any SARS cases on campus.

With international students bringing huge revenues, many US universities "wrestled with how to deal with SARS" (Locke). Some schools took drastic steps to cope with the perceived risk of incoming Asian students importing the virus to campuses. For instance, Washington University in St. Louis discouraged people from SARS-affected areas from attending graduation ceremonies, and the University of Pennsylvania decided to screen and possibly quarantine students coming from China. Other schools, including St. Joseph's University, cancelled summer programs that would have brought Chinese students on campus. In addition, other universities, such as Stanford, Duke, and Syracuse, issued advisories on their websites (Sternberg and Marklein). All these risk reduction efforts, made at the regulation site of universities, registered circulation-related anxieties about the permeable borders between communities and natures and the "containment of disease in national terms against its actual and threatened border crossings" (Wald 63).

UC Berkeley's decision targeting Asian students, however, was considered an unusual, if not extreme, "overreaction" by leading experts. It resulted in intense international criticism that the university had "overreacted to the potential health risks of SARS" (DiMassa). WHO "cautioned against 'irrational behavior' and 'the exclusion of people' coming from SARS-affected areas, such as China," for Berkeley's move could cause panic and frustration (Fagan A04). WHO also emphasized that "the best defense is not exclusion but good management of the situation in the unlikely event that someone attending a meeting were to become sick with SARS" (Fagan A04).The CDC also issued similar guidelines, urging organizations not to overreact to SARS or to "let fears of the SARS virus disrupt graduation ceremonies, conferences and other meetings open to foreigners" ("CDC Cautions" A18).

Many Asian American organizations and writers responded to UC Berkeley's ban by publishing letters of protest. They also mobilized transnational business and cultural connections in the United States to fight against what was perceived as racist and discriminatory measures against the Chinese people. Chinese for Affirmative Action, a civil rights group in San Francisco, condemned the ban as "discriminatory and too broad" (V. Wong). Similarly, Iris Chang, the author of *The Rape of Nanking*, criticizes the measure for its "blanket ban on Asians," for its "anti-Chinese sentiment," and for its "exclusion based on nationality, not sound medical diagnosis" (A31). Calling it "discrimination under a different name," Chang demanded "more careful reasoning from American institutions" (A31). She compares the decision to discriminatory measures, such as the Chinese Exclusion Act passed in 1882 and the blanket quarantine of all Chinese in Hawaii in a local bubonic plague outbreak in 1899. Chang mobilizes historical events that similarly transformed medical panic into racial prejudices to address issues of travel and mobility, containment and community, and imagined geographies (Mao and Morris 6). Ling-chi Wang, a UC Berkeley employee, published a letter of protest online, criticizing the ban for having no clear rationale for selecting "countries targeted for exclusion." He ends his letter eloquently:

> With reports of sharp declines in visits to Asian restaurants from New York to Honolulu and fewer tourists visiting Chinatowns across America, such a sweeping and arbitrary decision could not come at a worse time. On a predominately Asian campus in a multiracial state, it could be particularly divisive, contributing to hysteria and racializing and politicizing a public health issue that now affects more than three dozen countries around the globe.

Here, Wang connects the hoax e-mails and rumors about SARS outbreaks in Chinatown, which came in a bottom-up fashion from unknown sources, with UC Berkeley's ban of Chinese students, which were issued by top officials from a well-respected university. Putting the two anti-Chinese events together, Wang demonstrates the danger of racializing a medical epidemic and its repercussions at all levels throughout the American society. As Wald would argue, Berkeley's SARS policy "implicitly pathologize[s] particular human beings, human behaviors, and spaces" (268). Portrayed as potential carriers, international students from the epicenters not only crossed borders to enter the United States but also crossed the porous borders between health and sickness and those between the vulnerable campus and the group-living community of International House. Such images dramatized the "dangers of life in a global hot zone" (Wald 268) and greatly stigmatized the populations of international students.

In addition to official and unofficial protests from overseas Chinese, Hong Kong, led by Arthur Li, its secretary for education and manpower, actively intervened and negotiated with UC Berkeley to argue for the inclusion of students from Hong Kong in summer programs. Li mobilized transnational networks and affiliations, including the US Consul-General in Hong Kong and the Economic and Trade Offices in the United States in this political lobbying. These transnational efforts helped to produce a partial lift of the ban for students from Hong Kong on May 10 (Ng). UC Berkeley announced a modified policy that allowed eighty students, mostly from Hong Kong, to enroll for summer classes. The ban on five hundred other students from mainland China and Taiwan remained unchanged.

Part of the reason for the change in the policy, according to UC Berkeley Chancellor Robert M. Berdahl, was because "our decision to limit enrollment in our summer programs has created the impression here and abroad that UC Berkeley was actually banning students from studying here, or not welcoming Asian students at all." At a press conference held on May 10 to announce modifications to the campus's SARS policy, Berdahl emphasized:

> Nothing could be further from the truth. [. . .] This is a time [to express] support for our friends who have for so long entrusted us with the education of their children. We at Berkeley are proud of our long-standing relationship, and the many friends we have in East Asia, and we honor the mutual trust that has developed. ("Text")

The contention surrounding UC Berkeley's SARS policies demonstrates that international students are caught in the political and geographical space between their home country and their host country. They also suffer from the competing and asymmetrical power relations surrounding their transnational presence. Students from Hong Kong benefited from the active intervention of Hong Kong officials and organizations, which effectively pushed UC Berkeley to change its SARS policy. As a "long-standing" source of international students, Hong Kong had forged strong economic connections and historical ties with UC Berkeley, which eventually pushed the university to make a small compromise (admitting eighty students from Hong Kong) to acknowledge the mutual interests between the two parties. What needs to be emphasized here is the arbitrary nature of this compromise. Early May witnessed the rapid increase of SARS cases and the spread of SARS in the wider communities in mainland China, Hong Kong, and Taiwan. Berkeley decided, however, only to drop its discriminatory admission ban for students from Hong Kong because of the city's transnational lobbying. It could have worked equally well to implement the same risk reduction measures for students from all three parts of the Greater China, which, unfortunately, did not take place because of racial targeting.

My analysis of the contestations surrounding the cartoon on SARS world tour, hoaxes about Chinatowns, and UC Berkeley's SARS policy illustrates the micropolitics among travelers from epicenters, immigrants, and the United States. Moreover, it demonstrates "the historical, cultural, and economic moments of entanglement and contradiction" between overseas Chinese and the dominant US culture. All three of these anti-Asian events fit into what Foucault calls "biological-racist discourses," which function as "a principle of exclusion and segregation" (*Society* 61). Such discourses help to normalize society, which indicates "the appearance of a state racism" or "the internal racism of permanent purification" (62). Employing this racism for social normalization, the United States directs internal racism against itself, against its own elements (immigrants and ethnic communities), and against its own products (transnational travel, the travel industry in ethnic communities, and the educational industry catering to tuition-paying foreigners).

Rhetorical and Biopolitical Interactions between WHO and China

My study of both WHO discourses and *People's Daily* articles identifies two stages in the formation of the global biopolitical surveillance in the SARS outbreak in China, in which WHO played a prominent mediating role. The first stage of SARS (from November 2002 to the end of March 2003) has three unique features: great anxiety and uncertainty about SARS in the global community, WHO's thwarted efforts to obtain permission to investigate the SARS situations in China, and ineffective biopolitical surveillance of and risk communication about SARS in China. Witnessing positive changes in China's collaboration with WHO, the second stage (from April 1 to June 30) featured the increasingly close collaboration among China, WHO, and the global biomedical communities; effective biopolitical surveillance; transparent reporting practices; the gradual construction of the urgently needed public health infrastructure; and the eventual eradication of SARS. A variety of rhetorical tensions and points of contention marked the dividing points of these two stages. In what follows is an examination of the rhetorics employed by *People's Daily* and WHO's public discourses as well as the international media's coverage of the WHO-China interactions surrounding SARS to explore the rhetorical negotiations among the two key actors in China's anti-SARS campaign.

Before April: Uncertainty, Urgency
versus Reassurance, Certainty

WHO and *People's Daily* employed drastically different rhetorical approaches toward SARS in February and March 2003: one with anxiety and urgency and the other with reassurance and claims of victory. WHO's updates and daily summaries of reported cases featured anxiety, uncertainty, urgency, and constant action and progress. WHO's discourses during this period exemplified Foucauldian biopower in its most comprehensive form. WHO quickly assumed a leading role in both public health and scientific research in the global anti-SARS campaign. Acting as the most prominent technical supporter, WHO spoke about SARS in predominantly technical terms. It offered frequently updated SARS definitions and detailed recommendations for its surveillance and treatment as well as an evolving emergency guideline for travelers and airlines, which later developed into highly influential travel advisories. Such travel recommendations established a global, macrolevel epidemiological gaze into different nations and regions for signs of epidemics. They not only divided the world into affected and dangerous areas, vulnerable areas, and unaffected and safe areas but also disciplined outbreak areas with travel advisories. Creating "an atmosphere of heightened awareness," WHO's global travel advisories helped to achieve three significant results in the global response to SARS: the activation of a "well-designed national preparedness plan in many countries," sensitive surveillance with cases "quickly identified, [promptly reported,] and immediately isolated," and "strict protective measures in countries with imported cases" ("Severe Acute Respiratory Syndrome").

In addition to issuing technical guidelines, WHO frequently communicated with "all national authorities" while offering "laboratory and clinical support to ensure appropriate investigation, reporting, and containment of these outbreaks" ("Severe Acute Respiratory Syndrome"). In other words, WHO's emphasis on the technical aspects about SARS pushed individual countries to strengthen their national surveillance, which helped to contain the international spread of SARS by stopping any "onward transmission of the disease beyond those initially identified" ("Update 8"). Besides the global, macrolevel epidemiological surveillance, WHO also employed a microlevel gaze to study the etiological and clinical features of SARS by forming networks of leading laboratories and clinicians and by resorting to state-of-art technologies, such as daily teleconferences and restricted websites, to achieve constant data sharing and regular reporting.

In sharp contrast to the uncertainty and urgency in WHO public discourses, news reports in *People's Daily* during the same period were full of reassurance, certainty, and claims of victory. Most reports repeatedly reassured the public and the international community that the outbreak was under control and that it was safe to work and travel in China. In the eighteen SARS-related articles published in *People's Daily* in March, Chinese Minister of Health Zhang Wenkang and Foreign Ministry spokesman Kong Quan were cited several times claiming that the outbreak was "effectively under control," that "patients had recovered gradually," and that "the lives of local residents had returned to normal" ("Mystery Pneumonia"; "806 SARS Cases"). These topoi of "SARS is under control" and "China is safe" were heavily emphasized in *People's Daily* from March to April 9, 2003.

Chapter 5 examines the transnational risk negotiations between WHO and China about SARS in mid-April, which are full of institutional interactions and extra-institutional interventions from whistle-blowers and anonymous professionals. WHO employed transnational surveillance tools, such as travel advisories, which brought huge economic and political repercussions to those listed as severely SARS-affected areas. WHO's biopolitical measures, along with international criticism, forced China to provide WHO with more transparent information and with open access to affected regions, to adopt rigorous anti-SARS measures, and to mobilize governmental institutions and medical care workers in its national anti-SARS campaign. As a result of those radical changes, the topos of "SARS is under control" disappeared in the national media and was replaced by a more pragmatic focus on governmental measures taken to contain SARS.

China's Rhetoric of Infrastructural Inadequacy

To understand the rhetorical arguments China made against the international criticism of its early undercalculation and of the dramatically increased cumulative SARS cases in Beijing, one key text has to be examined, namely, the transcript of the press conference held by the Information Office of State Council, China's cabinet, on Sunday, April 20. In this unusual press conference, Gao Qiang, the executive vice health minister, announced that the mayor of Beijing, Meng Xuenong, and Minister of Health Zhang Wenkang had been dismissed from their posts because of their failure to effectively manage SARS risks in Beijing ("Press Conference").[2] Gao then introduced the latest SARS situation and anti-SARS measures taken by the Chinese government. Marking one of the most drastic tipping points in China's official responses to SARS, Gao's argument both emphasized resolute measures taken by China to combat SARS and represented the rhetorical interaction between China and its Western critics. He made several strategic rhetorical transformations and defended China's risk management of SARS against several common charges. Gao's argument works on several fronts to rhetorically transform the Western media's accusation of China's intentional cover-up into an admission of bureaucratic incompetence and infrastructural backwardness. It also attributed the dramatic increase in SARS cases to the simultaneous use of different classificatory schemes and to the miscounting of cases rather than to purposeful underreporting. As a rhetorical platform, the press conference directly engaged with foreign criticism by recontextualizing China's failure to effectively manage SARS risks and by highlighting material constraints both in its public health infrastructure and in its legislative and institutional systems.

Gao made a key rhetorical move by transforming the accusation of faulty risk definitions and an "intentional cover-up" of the SARS situation into infrastructural inadequacy, "inaccuracy of SARS statistics," and bureaucratic incompetence due to institutional disarray ("China Holds"). He blamed the weak health infrastructure as an important reason for the underreporting. He started by acknowledging the mistakes China had made in dealing with SARS. More specific, he criticized the MOH's lack of preparation for a public health emergency, its weak epidemic-control system, and the absence of a unified system for information collection and reporting. In addition, "a lack of effective communication and information exchanges among hospitals in Beijing" posed great difficulty for city health officials to collect accurate and comprehensive SARS statistics ("Official Explains"). Gao pointed out that "Beijing has 175 governmental hospitals at the municipal, district, and county levels, 14 hospitals run by the Ministry of Health and the Ministry of Education, 16 run by the military and air forces, and 14 hospitals belonging to various ministries" ("Official Explains"). Modeled after the Soviet Union's governmental structure, most ministries in China have to serve political and social functions in addition to professional ones (F. Lu, "Danwei"). They provide employees with comprehensive services covering social welfare, housing, medical care, child care and education, family planning, policing, and retirement; they function like small independent societies of their own. For instance, the Ministry of Defense has its own national and regional universities, schools, hospitals, police forces, factories, courts, and even tourism industries, which are not subject to the administration of any other institutions. The wide distribution of hospital management to various institutions and the lack of coordination among them resulted in poor communication and inadequate mechanisms for epidemic reporting and surveillance.

WHO's SARS "Update 32" supports Gao's argument about the lack of coordination among military, police, and civilian hospitals as one key reason for underreporting. Published on April 17, the update complains, "The military hospitals, which are not obliged by Chinese law to report cases to health authorities, have been the focus of considerable rumors over the past several days." It adds after a few lines: "The recent decision of military hospitals in the Guangdong Province to report SARS cases to the authorities may set an important precedent." After a North Carolina man caught SARS during his visit to Toronto in late May, David Heymann, the WHO's chief infectious-disease expert, discussed the lack of collaboration between central and provincial governments as another reason that contributed to China's underreporting of SARS. Criticizing the conflict between Canada's federal and provincial health agencies, Heymann said, "SARS has shown us that relationships between federal, or central, and provincial or state governments are very important in public health, and very difficult to establish. . . . We understand that this has been a problem in China" (Alphonso and York A1).

Rather than dwelling on the damage done by this lack of institutional coordination, Gao quickly moved on to its remedy. On April 15, the State Council sent a monitoring team to work with the Beijing municipal government and related departments. Moreover, the Beijing municipal government had set up a unified mechanism for epidemic control to mobilize all medical resources and to systematically collect and report information about SARS.

By refocusing the public attention on inadequate health infrastructure, Gao highlighted "the essential difference between inaccuracy in SARS statistics and intentional deception" and promised to come up with an effective reporting system ("Official Explains"). Although not thoroughly effective in defending China against the international criticism of information blackout, Gao's argument helped to partly repair the political damage caused by China's belated response by shifting the focus of the contention. It called attention to the impacts of local material conditions and political structures on risk management approaches, which reconstructed underreporting as unfortunate consequences of material restraints instead of ideological differences.

Epidemiologist Jeffrey McFarland, one of WHO's two experts who visited Beijing's 309 military hospital, spoke highly of some "extraordinary measures" taken by China to unblock "the previously choked bureaucratic pipeline" after "President Hu Jintao ordered 'no delay' and 'no deceit' in combating the outbreak" on April 17 (Hong and Leow). Such measures included requiring military hospitals to report directly to the MOH instead of the Ministry of Defense, "granting the WHO a meeting last week with Vice-President Wu Yi, who was in charge of public health—the first in a decade," and speeding up the issuing of visas into China for WHO experts from the usual four weeks to twenty-four hours (Hong and Leow). Measures like those mentioned above demonstrated China's resolute efforts to combat bureaucratic red tape to facilitate its anti-SARS campaign, which, in turn, supported Gao's claim about the negative impacts caused by infrastructural inadequacy.

Firing top officials for their failure to effectively cope with SARS carries significant yet different symbolic meanings for international and domestic audiences. For the international community, the dismissal suggested internal conflicts and contradictions concerning appropriate ways to cope with SARS and the power conflicts between the new general leadership of Hu and Wen and officials loyal to Jiang Zemin. It also indicated the determination of new national leaders to fight an all-out battle against SARS, which contributed to "an enlightened and open international image," according to a *People's Daily* report. The latter was further confirmed by the punishment of over "120 central and local governmental officials" who were "derelict in their duties in an unexpected calamity" ("Slack Officials"). These punishment decisions were "taken as practical measures" by top leaders to "improve the government work style" and were "applauded by Chinese people"; they were "well received by both domestic and world opinion" ("Slack Officials"). Domestically, leaders had not been appointed direct responsibilities in crises and disasters in the past, which resulted in the "sluggish and perfunctory reactions" to SARS. Therefore, such severe punishment of negligent officials functioned as "a radical campaign" launched by top leaders to fight "against stubborn diseases in the public administration" and to urge officials to "make people's health and lives a priority" ("Slack Officials").

Gao's arguments highlighted the internal problems with China's institutional structures and underfunded public health system, which created new ways through which China's responses to SARS were mediated in the transnational media. The comparison of the American media's construction of SARS as ideological pathologies and Gao's rhetoric of infrastructural inadequacy brings home the complicated construction of the epidemic-epicenter connections and the accompanying stakes of such construction.

The competing representations of China's belated responses to SARS carry not only symbolic force but also political implications. Infrastructural and material inadequacies are problems within the system, which can be improved through enhanced funding and institutional commitment. In contrast, ideological pathologies suggest the existence of two competing and incompatible systems and mark the binary between us and them. As an outsider, the other has only two options: either become one of us or be eliminated as the enemy.

After April 20: Infrastructure- versus Technology-Centered Rhetoric

China's post–April 20 coverage of SARS marked a dramatic change in focus and tone. The reassuring tone about "China is safe despite SARS" disappeared and was replaced by a pragmatic, honest, yet still predominantly positive tone. Top leaders, such as President Hu Jintao, Premier Wen Jiabao, and Vice Premier Wu Yi, repeatedly urged governmental officials to accurately report local cases, stressed the immediate dismissal of those who lied or underreported, and called for patriotism and people's war against SARS. The mandatory daily update of SARS cases offered transparent reports about the actual situation of SARS, which was rarely seen in any media before April 20. In contrast to the American media's continued preoccupation with ideological blame, *People's Daily* took a pragmatic approach, focused on the anti-SARS measures taken by governments and institutions at all levels, and provided prevention tips for communal and personal battles against SARS.

With WHO's travel advisories in place, China suffered from sharply reduced tourist bookings and domestic consumption, widespread withdrawals of foreign investments, and intensifying international criticism. In order to restore its social and economic stability, China worked hard to establish centralized and well-coordinated biopolitical surveillance to combat SARS. Some of China's major infrastructural problems were the underinvestment in the public health system in the last twenty years, the lack of adequate health care facilities in the countryside, the absence of a public health emergency system, and the outdated legislation about epidemic prevention and control.

News reports in *People's Daily* focused on measures taken to fix existing problems in the public health system, on material supports, and on unprecedented domestic collaboration among various governmental sectors. To remedy the insufficient funding for biomedical research and disease control and prevention, a special fund of 2 billion RMB (US$243 million) was created to mobilize leading clinical and basic science researchers to jointly develop effective treatments and diagnostic tools ("China Holds"; "China Creates"). The fund was also used to finance the treatment of farmers and urban residents who had no medical insurance and to upgrade diagnostic and SARS-proof equipment for county-level hospitals as well as designated SARS hospitals in central and western China ("China Creates"). In addition, 3.5 billion RMB (US$421.7 million) were set aside to establish a new nationwide public health system and a national quick-response mechanism to improve China's emergency-response capacity for epidemics ("China Sets Up; "Chronology"; "China Planning"). Over 3 billion RMB (US$363 million) was provided to central and western regions to build their state centers for disease prevention and control ("State Treasury"). To solve Beijing's institutional disarray in SARS reporting, the Beijing Municipality set up a unified mechanism for epidemic control and directed the mobilization of all medical resources after mid-April ("China Holds"). To prevent SARS from spreading to rural areas in the most severely affected regions, a fund of 812.6 million RMB (US$98.3 million) was allocated to improve the infrastructure and capacity of local health and medical facilities, including the purchases of desperately needed equipment and vehicles ("China Sheds"). Finally, a new public health emergency regulation was quickly enacted in mid-May that required "the State Council and provincial governments to establish both contingency headquarters to coordinate the efforts of all relevant departments" and the creation of "monitoring, early warning, and reporting systems" ("Legal Framework").

China's anti-SARS campaign produced several unexpected outcomes: preventing SARS from spreading to the hinterland of China; eradicating SARS without any diagnostic tool, treatment, or cure; and vanquishing SARS despite the country's inadequate public health infrastructure. Through all these reports, *People's Daily* transformed SARS from a medical epidemic to one of domestic infrastructural backwardness, which eventually was fixed both through political and economic commitment from top leaders and through concerted institutional collaboration.

In addition to focusing on infrastructural improvement, Chinese mainstream media also appealed repeatedly to nationalism and patriotism to win support from the people. Zhongping Ren's award-winning *People's Daily* commentary lauds nationalism as the "great anti-SARS spirit." Ren pays tribute to many people who contributed to "the construction of our new Great Wall" against SARS: unified and determined national leaders, heroic medical care workers and biomedical scientists, and the patriotic, self-sacrificing public (1). For Ren, Chinese nationalism has both "patriotism at the core" and "unity, peace-loving, diligence, bravery, and vitality" as its central elements (1). It has been evolving throughout history and has been continuously renewed in major disasters, such as SARS (1). Ren explains how patriotic conduct serves collective interests in SARS control work throughout China:

> As a people's war without bystanders, the anti-SARS battle closely connects individuals, families, communities, and the nation in a shared destiny. This close connection requires everyone to participate in the anti-SARS campaign by performing their duties, whether it is to fight against SARS in the frontline as medical care workers, to continue their normal life as ordinary citizens, to work hard as employees, or to stay quarantined and to cooperate with health workers as close contacts or suspected cases. (1)

Ren concludes his commentary by stressing the need to "resolutely carry out the Central CPC's calls both for serious engagement in SARS control work and for unwavering attention to the central task of economic development" (1). He announces, "With the strong leadership of Central CPC, with rich material foundation accumulated since the economic reform, with advanced science and technologies, and with our great nationalism, we have the capacity to conquer the epidemic and win a comprehensive victory" (1).

The media also put great emphasis on China's tremendous sacrifice to eradicate SARS and its role as a responsible power in the Asia-Pacific region. *People's Daily* compared China's success in quelling SARS to its performance in the 1997 Asian financial crisis, during which China took many positive measures to improve the mutual trust and cooperation between China and other Asian countries ("China Sheds"). A *Washington Times* editorial predicts, however, "[E]arning international trust back will take time," for "China will be nursing a black eye for its silence on SARS long after the last patient from this outbreak recovered" ("SARS and the Beijing Olympics" B02).

Playing a leading role in the global anti-SARS campaign, WHO negotiated the allocation of public health resources among countries and imposed global surveillance through rigorous reporting systems and travel advisories. In China, WHO functioned as the international inspector, biomedical expert, and technical supporter. It helped China to investigate the SARS situation in different areas and to combat SARS more effectively through infrastructure construction. For instance, on April 16, WHO recommended "a nationwide surveillance system and health network to report the atypical pneumonia epidemic quickly to ensure the disease is controlled effectively" ("WHO Suggests").

According to Alan Schnur, WHO's team leader of Communicable Disease Control in China, an important component of WHO's work was "to work with Ministry of Health (MOH) and other partners to establish and strengthen disease surveillance and response system[s]" (34). On April 20, Schnur proposed four strategies to curb SARS in Beijing: "surveillance and reporting, hospital management and infection control, community information and contact tracing, and good government support" ("WHO Expert: 'I Trust'"). The MOH accepted all those suggestions and worked to establish a nationwide surveillance system and health network, to report daily updates of SARS cases, and to allocate a special fund to help those who could not afford SARS treatment.

Although applauded by WHO, the dramatic changes China made had little impact on WHO's technology-centered rhetoric. As WHO added new areas to the growing list of places to be avoided in its travel advisories, the updates explained the technical criteria for assessing the nature and magnitude of SARS outbreaks. Such criteria included "the number of prevalent cases and the daily number of new cases, the extent of local chains of transmission, and evidence that travelers are becoming infected while in one area and then subsequently exporting the disease elsewhere" ("Update 37"). WHO also recommended control measures that all nations should adopt, which included "early identification and isolation of patients" and "rigorous contact tracing" ("Update 58"). As chapter 5 discusses, WHO faced international outcries and challenges concerning its ambiguous and subjective application of travel advisories both in 2003 and in 2009: when Toronto was listed in WHO's SARS travel advisory on April 23 and then taken out on April 30 after Canada's intensive political lobbying and when Asian countries protested against WHO's decision not to require epicenters in North America to implement border screening at the beginning of the H1N1 flu. These two historical controversies surrounding WHO's use of travel advisory clearly demonstrate the potential impacts of global and national political and economic interests on major public health decisions.

From April to June, WHO officials inspected the anti-SARS work in Guangdong, Shanghai, Beijing, and SARS-affected provinces in central and western China. WHO's media reports focused on anti-SARS facilities and measures, which listed among others the community-based prevention and control networks throughout the countryside, the setup of special funds, the division of fever clinics from other parts of local hospitals, and efforts of mass mobilization and mass education ("WHO Experts: No Big Risk"; "Chinese Leaders").

In late May, Beijing started to witness a steady decline in its daily new cases from over one hundred to fewer than twenty (see fig. 4.6). When discussing Beijing's SARS situations, Dr. Henk Bekedam, the WHO's representative in Beijing, still dwelled on the poor "infrastructure of the Chinese health system, which has been weakened over the last 10 to 20 years as the Chinese government has focused on economic development and invested less in public health" (Altman, "WHO Expresses" A14).

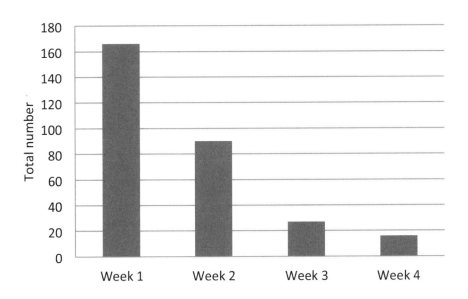

Figure 4.6. Mainland China's weekly numbers of new probable SARS cases in May

WHO's June 3 update shifted its focus from poor infrastructure to the quick mysterious drop in SARS cases in China. Heymann, WHO's executive director for communicable diseases, discussed the urgent need to "work with the [Chinese] government to determine the factors that have led to such a rapid fall in SARS cases compared to other sites where outbreaks have occurred" ("Update 72"). The update wondered whether the problematic use of technologies, that is, inadequate case-detection approaches and information gaps in China, had contributed to the decrease of SARS cases in MOH's official updates:

> Although great improvements in surveillance, reporting, infection control, and public awareness have occurred in China in recent weeks, WHO remains concerned about the sensitivity of case detection in some provinces. [. . .] A particular problem is the large number of new cases reported—approximately half—without information on the source or setting of exposure. The absence of this information makes it difficult for WHO to assess the extent of local transmission. ("Update 72")

The update continued to cite technological rigor as the reasons for China's dramatic progress and hinted at the importance of top leaders' political commitment to public health concerns:

> The daily number of reported new probable cases of SARS in mainland China has declined considerably in recent weeks [. . .] to an average of 2.5. [. . .] [T]his progress [. . .] demonstrates the decisive importance of high-level political commitment and determined application of control measures that have proven their effectiveness. ("Update 72"; see fig. 4.6)

This tone of suspicion about possible information gaps was replaced by a much more confident tone on June 6, when the *New York Times* cited Bekedam's announcement that WHO "now believed that statistics released by the Chinese government were generally reliable" (Rosenthal A10).

On June 16, a joint press conference offered by WHO and the MOH witnessed a flood of questions about the credibility of the drastically decreased SARS statistics in Beijing. Heymann again used highly technical language to explain the radical drop in China's cases, citing contact tracing and surveillance activities as reasons, along with the mass "mobilization of the whole population" and the timely identification and treatment of SARS patients ("SARS Information").

On June 24, when WHO announced the removal of travel advisories for Beijing, its official update put similar emphases on both technological rigor and political priority:

> At the peak of the outbreak, towards the end of April, Beijing was report-ing more than 100 new cases each day. Containment of an outbreak of such dimensions is a tribute to the effectiveness of centuries-old control measures, including isolation, contact tracing, and quarantine, sup-ported by government commitment at the highest levels. ("Update 87")

The update emphasized WHO's consistent use of technical criteria for the issuing of travel advisories: "the magnitude of probable SARS cases, the pattern of recent local transmission, and the last dates of export of cases." The reason for the removal of WHO's travel advisory for Beijing was based on two facts: "[N]o cases have recently been exported from Beijing," and compared to the lack of information about contact histories in early June, "[A]ll recent cases have been traced to known chains of transmission" ("Update 87").

WHO's consistent use of technology-centered rhetoric helped to sustain the credibility and authority of its risk policies, to coordinate research and public health resources across affected countries, to defend itself against accusations of ill-informed decisions, and to maintain its ethos as the lead-ing global agency in the anti-SARS campaign. In addition to the consistent focus on technology, WHO also took care to maintain the goodwill of na-tional authorities and to ensure their full cooperation. It achieved those goals through the use of highly diplomatic and politically sensitive discourses, as demonstrated in my discussion of the more subtle praise of and emphasis on top leaders' commitment to anti-SARS work. It should also be noted that WHO's credibility as the leading health authority in the global battle against SARS relied a lot on its use of technological criteria for and the scientific reasoning surrounding travel advisories. During SARS, WHO's discourses promoted travel advisories as a scientifically tested and technically rigorous tool that objectively evaluated health risks in various SARS-affected regions. Chapter 5 shows, however, that the use of travel advisories and border screen-ing measures both in Toronto's SARS outbreaks in 2003 and in the H1N1 flu in 2009 were surrounded by controversy and by high-level political and economic negotiations.

CPC's Interaction with WHO:
Party Organ's Approaches

One question yet to be addressed on the WHO-China relationship deals with the CPC's interaction with WHO during SARS. Here I use corpus-assisted discourse analysis to examine how *People's Daily*, the Party's official mouthpiece, reported WHO's activities in and negotiations with China.[4] Particular attention was paid to the construction of roles played by the CPC and governmental institutions during the outbreak. Using a recursive reading and coding process to analyze the *People's Daily* corpus, I came up with seven categories, or codes: positive interaction between WHO and China (poz interaction), facts about SARS in China (domestic facts), facts about SARS outside China (international facts), risk evaluation and risk definitions (risks), positive evaluation of SARS efforts made by China (poz evaluation), WHO-China collaboration (collaboration), and hope and/ or requests related to SARS control work (hope/requests). Since Western media reported widely about WHO's critiques of China's anti-SARS work and conflicts between WHO and China, I added an eighth category, conflict and critique, as well. Since I am interested in exploring the way the CPC interacted with WHO, I focus only on results related to this topic in this section.

A total of 195 thematically coded instances were identified, with domestic facts, ($n = 88$), being the most frequently occurring topic, followed by positive evaluation ($n = 28$), positive interaction ($n = 20$), international facts ($n = 19$), collaboration ($n = 17$), risks ($n = 19$), and hope and requests ($n = 9$) (see fig. 4.7). These findings suggest the official mouthpiece focused mostly on domestic facts about WHO experts' meetings with their Chinese counterparts as well as WHO's visits and inspection tours in Beijing, Guangdong, Shanghai, Heibei, Guangxi, Henan, Shanxi, and Inner Mongolia from April to June. Interesting, no instances of conflicts between WHO and China or WHO's critique of China were found in the corpus. This surprising finding indicates that *People's Daily*, and perhaps the CPC's Propaganda Ministry behind the scene, preferred to highlight China's willingness to fully collaborate with WHO and the subsequent progress made in its anti-SARS campaign as a part of China's health diplomacy efforts. It also indicates attempts made both by WHO and by the CPC to avoid direct confrontation and to ensure smooth collaboration during the SARS outbreak.

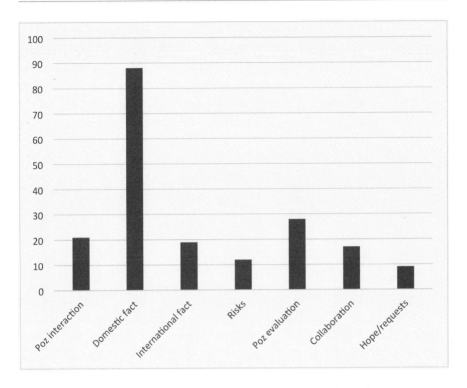

Figure 4.7. Occurrences of individual codes in the *People's Daily* corpus

When I looked at the chronological distribution of categorized instances, new insights started to emerge. One interesting pattern is the large number of instances in April's SARS discourses (77 compared to 66 in June and 37 in May), even though figure 4.2 shows a slight increase of SARS coverage in May over April (about 20) before a quick decrease in June (about 80). My readings of the corpus suggest that in May, *People's Daily* shifted its previous preoccupation with WHO's positive evaluation of China's anti-SARS campaign to the actual work that got done in China as well as progress made in SARS-related scientific research all over the world. For the entire month of May, WHO lost its prominent presence in the coverage and was replaced by a clear and pragmatic focus on frontline anti-SARS work. In contrast, many more reports in April and June fall into the epideictic mode by frequently citing WHO's praises for China's all-out eradication efforts.

The three most frequently used codes for June are domestic facts ($n = $ 30), positive evaluation ($n = 18$), and positive interaction ($n = 6$). Surprising, April witnessed a similar pattern of frequency: domestic facts ($n = 32$), collaboration ($n = 12$), positive interaction ($n = 9$), and positive evaluation ($n = 8$) (see fig. 4.8). In contrast, May witnessed frequent occurrences of domestic and international facts ($n = 18$ and $n = 9$, respectively), but little focus on any other category. Given China's official apology about its belated response to SARS on April 20, what does this surprisingly similar rhetorical focus in April and June suggest about the SARS coverage of the Party's mouthpiece?

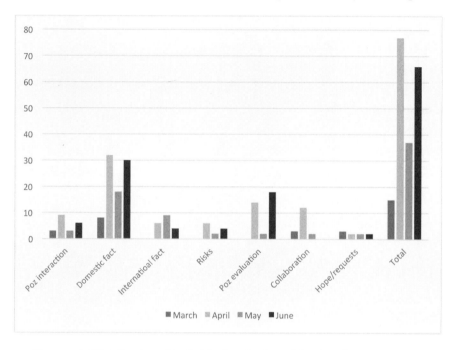

Figure 4.8. Distribution of individual codes from March to June 2003

Before I address this question, it is important to look at the distribution of all codes in April, using a ten-day interval. Two major events warrant this decision: Dr. Jiang Yanyong's April 8 open letter accusing the MOH of underreporting by providing case numbers obtained through personal investigations, as discussed in chapter 3, and China's official apology on April 20, as discussed earlier in this chapter. Figure 4.9 demonstrates a clear cluster of coded instances (46 out of 77 for the entire month) from April 1 to April 10, when little was known about the SARS outbreak in Beijing. The top four categories for the first ten days of April are domestic fact ($n = 23$), international fact ($n = 6$), positive evaluation ($n = 6$, of Guangdong's anti-SARS work), and collaboration ($n = 6$). As a sharp contrast to the abundance of instances in the first ten days of April, the last ten days were much quieter. It witnessed the presence of only five out of the seven categories ($n = 19$): positive interaction ($n = 5$), risks ($n = 4$), positive evaluation ($n = 6$, of Shanghai's anti-SARS work), collaboration ($n = 3$), and domestic facts ($n = 3$).

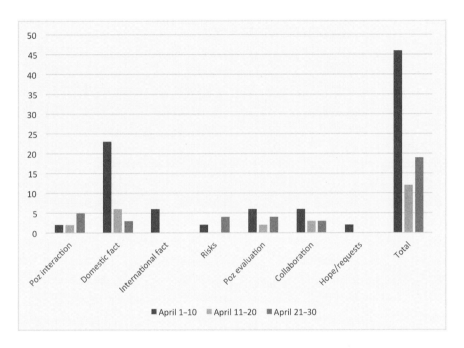

Figure 4.9. Distribution of individual codes from April 1 to April 30, 2003

The corpus analysis results show that in early April, the Party organ often cited WHO's responses in its Guangdong inspection to defend China's anti-SARS approaches, to praise the effectiveness of Guangdong's work, and to demonstrate China's willingness to cooperate with international communities. This epideictic discourse disappeared in late April and May. A highly pragmatic discourse on actual anti-SARS work emerged when the CPC and governmental institutions devoted full attention to the national anti-SARS battle. When SARS showed a clear pattern of decline in June, the CPC returned to ceremonial discourses to celebrate the hard-won victory. For instance, Beijing's acting mayor, Wang Qishan, officially attributed the success to "the strong and correct leadership of the party center and the State Council" and "the strong support of the People's Liberation Army, the armed forces and the central ministries" (Pomfret, "WHO Lifts" A12).

These findings also corroborate my previous discussion about WHO's and China's respective focus on technological inadequacy and infrastructural backwardness in their SARS discourses. Over half of the extensive reports on domestic facts deal with WHO's inspection trips from April to June 2003. In their inspection tours of SARS-hit areas, WHO paid great attention to technical details in local work, that is, diagnostic criteria, reporting mechanisms, and practices of record keeping, physical checkups, and quarantines and isolation. It should be stressed that WHO's technology-centered rhetoric and China's rhetoric of infrastructural backwardness are not mutually exclusive. Instead, they are often overlapping and mutually complementary. From time to time, the international agency would strategically direct conversation about local, short-term anti-SARS measures to suggestions about long-term infrastructural improvements. For instance, WHO suggested that China should build both a nationwide "SARS observation network" and "epidemiology and public health laboratory facilities" to effectively control SARS ("WHO Suggested"; "WHO Initiates"). In addition, Dr. Jong-wook Lee, WHO's director general, stated that SARS "exposes fundamental weaknesses in global health infrastructure" and highlighted "the need for local and national surveillance and response mechanisms" ("WHO Initiates").

Similarly, *People's Daily*'s coverage of WHO's inspection trips often emphasized local prevention techniques at all levels. Such techniques ranged from the transportation sector's use of health forms and temperature monitoring of all passengers to "patriotic public health campaigns" that emphasized daily practices, such as personal hygiene, good exercise, hand washing, no spitting, and regular sterilization of businesses and residences ("Humankind Is Able"; "SARS—an Opportunity"). The close connections between technology and infrastructure make sense because short-term technical measures helped to contain local SARS outbreaks. The eradication of SARS, however, required large-scale and long-term infrastructural improvements. In other words, driven by shared goals, WHO and the CPC quickly became strategic partners despite competing political and economic priorities. They took different approaches and made different arguments in their shared journey to combat and eventually eradicate SARS.

Case Study: Construction of Xiaotangshan Hospital

The construction of Xiaotangshan Hospital was taken as a radical measure to help relieve the heavy burden on the public health system and to treat the increasing number of SARS patients in Beijing. It took only eight days in late April for China to construct a one-thousand-bed field hospital complex in Xiaotangshan, on the outskirts of Beijing. Applauded as one of the key anti-SARS measures in China, this event went through highly contradictory rhetorical constructions in the media discourses in the United States, China, and WHO. This section examines the way different cultures discussed the construction of Xiaotangshan Hospital. It also explores the cultural, ideological, and political forces driving such vastly different rhetorical transformations.

Faulty Historical Analogies, Ideological Turn in US Coverage

As discussed earlier, preoccupied with ideological and political differences, the majority of American media discourses about SARS focused on the Chinese government's early slow responses and turned a blind eye to the pragmatic effort taken to fight against SARS. The few reports about Xiaotangshan Hospital again resorted to ideological transformation and inappropriate historical analogies to interpret the project. A *New York Times* editorial compares SARS in China to the Chernobyl accident in the Soviet Union, which served as "graphic evidence" of the failure of "the ossified political system" ("Diagnosing SARS" A20). It describes China's anti-SARS reports as "depressingly familiar communist methods of exhortation and regimentation," including "a Mao-style order to build a hospital from scratch in barely a week" (A20). Joseph Kahn makes a similar comparison between the effort and "Mao's mass mobilization campaign," the construction workers and an army, and the hospital complex and a military encampment ("Beijing Hurries").

The order to construct Xiaotangshan Hospital mobilized not only the army to build the hospital complex in eight days but also volunteering medical workers to run its infectious wards and to treat severe SARS patients. In epidemics, mass education and mass mobilization are essential to severing transmission chains and to containing the epidemic. However, the historical analogy makes a sweeping comparison and transforms mass mobilization from a practical public health tool into one employed exclusively by totalitarian governments for political purposes. It uproots the construction of Xiaotangshan Hospital from an all-out anti-SARS campaign and recontextualizes it in the civil war and the ideology-driven event of the Cultural Revolution, both led by Mao. The use of faulty historical analogies helps to insert certain common traits (dictatorship) or premises (totalitarianism) to bind different events together. In this case, the construction of the new SARS hospital is transformed from an important anti-SARS measure into either a violent civil war or an ideologically driven and violent political event like the Cultural Revolution.

Infrastructural Improvement, Rhetoric of Quantification in China's Coverage

Numerous reports were published about the construction of Xiaotangshan Hospital in China, stressing it as a symbol of vital infrastructural improvement, resolute governmental determination, close institutional collaboration, intense biopolitical efforts, and great personal sacrifice made by medical care workers. One dominant theme is the China-style efficiency or the "lightning-quick" Xiaotangshan speed ("Miracle"). Media attention was paid to both the enormous challenges Xiaotangshan encountered and the surprising miracles it achieved in May. In late April, major hospitals, such as You'an, Ditan, and China-Japan Friendship Hospitals, were all "running in excess of their abilities, without enough beds to admit more patients for treatment," which was the catalyst for the construction of Xiaotangshan as "Beijing's dedicated SARS facility" (H. Li, "Emergency Construction"). Medical personnel working at Xiaotangshan greatly outperformed the initial goal of using it as a "pressure reducer." The field hospital functioned as "a Noah's Ark made to brave the storm of SARS" and was later lauded by WHO as "a miracle in the world's medical history" (H. Li, "Emergency Construction"). To some extent, Xiaotangshan stands for China's aggressive post–April 20 measures to strengthen its poor health infrastructure. It becomes a symbol of biopolitical and political successes that China achieved during the SARS outbreak.

Rhetoric of quantification is constantly used to indicate both the magnitude of the problem and the efficient construction of the facility (Petersen and Lupton). According to Alan Petersen and Deborah Lupton, the rhetoric of quantification argues that statistical figures, not subject to doubt or ambiguity, hold immense symbolic power. Statistics have rhetorical and political dimensions in addition to scientific ones. Many reports about Xiaotangshan Hospital often start with numbers to introduce its construction and function:

> Xiaotangshan hospital was constructed as a specialized SARS hospital with 1000 beds. It mobilized and recruited 1383 medical workers from military hospitals all over the country. However, it was built in only eight

days (April 23–30) around the clock by 7000 construction workers and started to function at its full capacity with all medical supplies in place upon completion. (F. Mu 15)

Calling the Xiaotangshan hospital a "miracle," China's Central Television Station (CCTV) stressed that as the largest SARS hospital built in one week in China, Xiaotangshan had over five hundred wards and was equipped with medical facilities costing over 13 million RMB (US$1.6 million) and with medicine costing 90 million RMB (US$10.9 million). By stressing the size, complexity, and importance of the hospital and the quick speed with which it was constructed, such use of numbers calls attention to Beijing's urgent need for health infrastructure to cope with SARS. It also emphasizes the immense investment of funds and manpower, official commitment, and the incredible efficiency of workers.

With a large number of severe SARS patients admitted into the hospital, the rhetoric of quantification worked to highlight the magnitude of local outbreaks and to praise the medical successes achieved there. Rather than relying on the use of numbers alone, it employs another rhetorical tool, or what Rebecca de Souza calls "statistical relativity," to "put the numbers in perspective by providing a broader context within which to read them" (260). Using statistical relativity, the media discourses compared the number of patients and infection, death, and curing rates in Xiaotangshan with those of other SARS-affected countries, which helped to put the figures in perspective. Applauded as one of the key transformational biopolitical measures, Xiaotangshan Hospital treated and cured 680 confirmed patients, which were one-tenth of the world's total and one-seventh of China's total number of patients. The fractions one-tenth and one-seventh show the large proportion of patients that Xiaotangshan treated, the magnitude of medical challenges it met, and the key role it played in the global and national anti-SARS campaigns.

News reports also compare SARS statistics across cultures to highlight the achievements that Chinese doctors made in treating and curing SARS patients. Xiaotangshan achieved the best medical records during the global SARS outbreak: 0 percent medical worker infection and only a low 1.2 percent death rate compared with the 5 percent average all over the world. By relativizing the numbers, such reports call attention to the medical successes achieved by Xiaotangshan in terms of its control of in-hospital infection, a prevalent issue plaguing many hospitals treating SARS patients, and of its extremely successful regimen of treatments for severe and diagnosed SARS patients.

All this rhetorical use of statistics highlights China's reliance on the ideology of heroism, patriotism, and unified efforts in its post–April 20 official narratives about SARS. In late April, state-run mass media were urged to promote a "national spirit" to help to "unite the people and boost public morale" in the fight against SARS ("Chinese Media"). Chinese media at all levels devoted great attention to successes achieved by medical care workers and reported intensively about self-sacrifice and altruism demonstrated by those working on the frontline against SARS. Stories about heroic doctors and nurses humanized the tremendous efforts made by medical care workers, which helped to produce impressively high recovery rates and low death rates of SARS patients in China.

WHO's Focus on Technological and Technical Aspects

WHO welcomed the construction of Xiaotangshan Hospital as a biopolitical measure to relieve the burden on Beijing's medical system. On June 3, the WHO team inspected and evaluated the facilities, operation, and anti-infection measures in Xiaotangshan Hospital. The team spoke highly of the great efficiency in constructing the hospital and staffing and providing supplies for it, of the large number of patients being treated, of the extremely low death rate, and of the zero-infection rate among medical care workers. As positive validation of the Xiaotangshan project, WHO's comments were widely reported in Chinese media. As the technical support and coordinator of the global anti-SARS campaign, WHO provided recommendations to improve the technological and technical aspects of the hospital, such as possible ways to improve the ventilation and air conditioning systems. WHO also suggested that Xiaotangshan could simplify its excessively rigorous measures, which had protected medical care workers from in-hospital infection.

Putting the Puzzle Together: Narrow Escape of the Countryside

In early May, Beijing witnessed a huge increase in its SARS cases. From April 26 to May 12, altogether eighty-five towns reported SARS cases, and over fifty agricultural towns reported a total of 155 diagnosed SARS cases. From March to May 15, in a replay of contagion-induced flights commonly seen in plague outbreaks, eight million migrant workers returned home to the countryside, and altogether twenty-six provinces reported the identification of local SARS cases on May 28 ("155 Confirmed SARS Cases"). Ji Yunshi, the provincial chief of Hebei, a neighboring province of Beijing, succinctly summarized the intimidating difficulty that all provinces in the hinterland encountered:

> Hebei has 67 million residents. Our densely populated cities are located in big plains and are connected by well-developed transportation networks. The medical infrastructure in many parts is rather backward. [. . .] Therefore, if SARS goes out of control in Hebei, it will cause more complication and damage than the outbreak in Beijing. The effective prevention of the spread of SARS from Hebei to neighboring provinces and municipal cities will directly influence the health of Beijing and of the entire nation. It will partly determine the outcome of the entire anti-SARS war in China. ("Hebei Province Chief Ji Yunshi")

Premier Wen Jiabao stressed in a national video conference in Beijing that "the prevention work in rural China is the key to the nation's ongoing SARS battle" and that governments at all levels must "be on top alert to guard against the killer disease in the countryside" ("Premier"). This focus on SARS prevention in the countryside illustrates the immense national fear of massive SARS outbreaks in the countryside. The mass migration of farmworkers from big cities back home only exacerbated the risk of importing the SARS virus with them. To many people's surprise, by the end of July 2003, when WHO announced that SARS had been eradicated throughout the world, China had reported no large-scale SARS outbreaks in its rural areas. How did China manage to prevent the spread of SARS to its vast countryside, one of the most feared risks, when no diagnostic kits, vaccines, or cures for SARS existed? How did transnational media interpret this surprising success achieved by China?

My analysis of SARS discourses as employed by the mainstream American and Chinese media as well as by WHO publications offers little clue. Neither can the rhetorics of infrastructural inadequacy or technological backwardness provide a satisfactory answer. Indeed, those two rhetorics employed by China and WHO pinpoint the fatal weaknesses in the anti-SARS battle in the countryside that could have resulted in rampant outbreaks. Moreover, after examining transnational coverage in leading international news publications, I realized that the same question perplexed many Western journalists and readers. To put the puzzle together, I went beyond English publications, including the English versions of Chinese national newspapers that considered Western readers and overseas Chinese as their primary audiences. I turned to national and regional news reports published in Chinese, particularly those in newspapers published in provinces with large numbers of SARS cases, to look for locally invented strategies and grassroots tactics that helped to prevent returning migrant workers from importing the SARS virus to small, rural towns and villages.

Gao Qiang, China's executive vice health minister, summarized the five top lessons China learned from SARS as: having a strong command system to organize all forces, improving legislation to ensure the fulfillment of obligations, relying on science and technology, mobilizing the broad masses of the people, and increasing international cooperation. Whereas my analysis of China's SARS control work in other parts of the book has addressed most of the five points Gao mentions above, here the focus is mainly on two of the five lessons Gao discussed above, namely, government leadership and mass mobilization. Leaders at all levels had to play exemplary roles and stood up to daunting challenges. In addition, the anti-SARS campaign had to rely on the masses and to mobilize every citizen for "mass prevention and mass control" ("Behind Beijing's Sustained Decrease"). This call for mass participation provided the panicked public not only with mechanisms for individual contribution but also with tips and tools for everyday practices.

As discussed in chapter 1, maintaining stability and economic development has been the top priority in China in the past few decades. It was particularly emphasized in mainstream media in the 2003 SARS epidemic, which reported President Hu Jintao's repeated calls for the entire nation "to unite as one to defeat SARS and to pursue continuous economic development" ("Chinese President"). China paid a high price for SARS, as the epidemic caused a total loss of US$28.2 billion (Hai, Zhou, Wang, and Hou 57). Meanwhile, the Chinese government gave full support to its anti-SARS campaign by providing massive investments in public health infrastructure. In addition to the 2 billion RMB (US$242 million) fund provided by the State Council, more than 5 billion RMB (US$602 million) was allocated by regional governments for SARS control work. China also offered preferential tax exemptions and special subsidiaries for industries and individuals affected by SARS, particularly small- and medium-sized enterprises, which were major employers of low-income earners.

Considering China's dramatic financial investment in the anti-SARS campaign and its tremendous economic losses, it is understandable why top leaders put so much emphasis on economic development and growth. One *People's Daily* report explains: "The true picture of the SARS epidemic had not been made available to the public until April 20 *exactly because of a fear of instability*. The political and economic stakes were especially high, given the broad consensus that this country cannot afford to lose its hard-won economic fruit" ("Chinese New Leadership"; emphasis added). Economic concerns also drove national media to call repeatedly for the patriotic action of every citizen to "firmly implement governmental measures to focus on economic development while doing good work in preventing and treating SARS" ("Editorial"). The broad masses of workers were urged to "implement the proactive financial policy, [to] maintain normal orders of production, study, and writing," and to ensure China's sustainable economic development ("Editorial"; "President Hu").

Containment and People's War
against SARS in Beijing

Launching people's wars against SARS functioned as an integral part of China's all-out battle against SARS. SARS task forces were established in every constituency, both in cities and in rural areas, with CPC members, medical staff, and military reserve forces functioning as the mobilizing forces to contain SARS at all fronts. Andrew Ross describes two types of containment in American, political, post–cold war thought, with the first focusing on a "threat outside of the social body," which should be "excluded, or isolated in quarantine, and keep at bay from the domestic body" (42). The second meaning of containment refers to the "domestic contents of the social body," or an "enemy in our midst," which must be "neutralized by being fully absorbed" (64). Interesting but perhaps not surprising, neither of the two types of containment exists in regional news reports about SARS control work. The official SARS discourses focused solely on the mobilization of the broad masses to eradicate the epidemic and demonstrated great support for those quarantined or treated for SARS. Considering the high infection rate among medical care workers in China, the authorities' careful avoidance of stigmatizing individual SARS patients helped to direct the public attention to the larger issues of personal hygiene, community sterilization, and social responsibilities to avoid contracting or spreading SARS. Focusing on the epidemic itself, government at all levels emphasized the anti-SARS battle at the personal and communal levels and avoided victimizing any individual patients, including patients with high viral loads who infected many close contacts and medical care workers.

In late April, SARS cases in Beijing increased exponentially. All hospitals in Beijing were overwhelmed, and medical staff overworked. To make things worse, of Beijing's thirty-two thousand registered physicians and thirty-four thousand certified nurses, fewer than three thousand were familiar with respiratory diseases. Hospitals that did not specialize in infectious diseases were not prepared to deal with the epidemic because of their inadequate physical layouts and the shortage of trained staff. Neither were they familiar with rigorous disinfection measures that specialized hospitals routinely use. As a result, noninfectious disease hospitals became "one of the most important sources of infection" because of clusters of SARS cases in medical workers and outpatients ("April 30 News Press").

To relieve the medical burden on the civilian hospitals, the Beijing municipal government started the construction of Xiaotangshan Hospital, and the Defense Ministry recruited twelve hundred military doctors and nurses from all over the country to help treat Beijing's severe SARS patients in the new hospital. In addition, a couple of top comprehensive hospitals were temporarily converted into specialized infectious-disease hospitals, and measures were taken to transfer doctors and nurses with expertise in respiratory diseases from all over the country to Beijing. Meanwhile, Beijing's comprehensive hospitals, like hospitals in other parts of China, set up over 150 fever clinics, which functioned as isolation areas and had separate facilities such as testing, pharmacy, and fee-charging centers from their main buildings. This arrangement helped both to diagnose possible SARS patients with fever symptoms and to reduce in-hospital cross-infection to a minimum ("April 30 News Press").

Despite all these anti-SARS measures, the virus ran rampant in the larger community, and fear of the epidemic was heightened both in Beijing and in neighboring regions. On April 29, the Beijing municipal government issued "Guideline for the Strengthening of SARS Control Work in the Communities," which describes a typical approach of SARS control work adopted by governments at all levels throughout China. Starting with the claim that "SARS control work directly influences people's health and survival as well as the stability and development of the capital," the guideline calls for the "full participation and support from all businesses, organizations, and residents at the levels of streets, residential areas, towns, and villages." The guideline states that it is absolutely necessary to mobilize all forces and integrate all resources in the communities so that all residents will participate in the "mass prevention and mass control work" as "owners of communities" to "win this people's war against SARS" ("Beijing Municipal Guideline"). As a part of the mass-mobilization mechanism, grassroots CPC organizations and volunteers functioned as the four-level, coordinated information monitoring network in Beijing. Building administrators, neighborhood committees, street-level committees, and district-level directing centers worked together in the information network to screen possible SARS cases and close contacts at all levels. Community volunteers worked with local quarantine officers both to monitor the temperatures of those under home quarantine through daily phone calls and to deliver food, medicine, and other needed commodities to them. Meanwhile, Beijing municipal government stipulated that any company with employees under quarantine should keep their positions and pay their normal salaries during the quarantine, which protected the economic interests of those who cooperated with official quarantine orders.

As a result of this mass prevention and mass control campaign, approximately thirty thousand Beijing residents were quarantined in their homes or in quarantine sites from March to July 2003. The Chinese Field Epidemiology Training Program of the Chinese Center for Disease Control and Prevention (China CDC) conducted a survey at the end of SARS to evaluate the efficacy of quarantine as a risk reduction measure. The China CDC's findings suggested that even though quarantine criteria were unclear and their application inconsistent at the beginning of the outbreak, quarantine did work for the close contacts of symptomatic SARS patients. For people who had contact with SARS patients during their incubation period, however, none of those close contacts developed SARS because of the lack of infectivity of SARS at its early stage. A total of 6.3 percent of the sample of quarantined close contacts of symptomatic patients developed SARS. The contraction rate was 31.1 percent for those who cared for SARS patients, 8.8 percent for visitors, and 4.6 percent for those who lived in the same buildings. The survey authors conclude, "The use of quarantine, in combination with enhanced surveillance, isolation of SARS patients, and comprehensive use of personal protective equipment by health-care workers, appears to have been effective in controlling the recent epidemic of SARS in Beijing" (Ou, Li, Zeng, Dun, Qin, and Fontaine 1040). They also suggest that to improve the efficiency of quarantine and to allow for better focus of resources in future outbreaks, quarantine should be limited to "persons who have contact with an actively ill SARS patient" (Ou, Li, Zeng, Dun, Qin, and Fontaine 1040).

People's War against SARS in the Rest of China

Beijing helped with the anti-SARS work in neighboring agricultural towns by mobilizing individual villages to take charge of disinfection, to distribute thermometers to each household for daily temperature monitoring, and to cancel any mass gathering, including weddings and funerals ("April 30 News Press"). All villages kept rigorous track of individuals entering their communities by monitoring visitors' temperatures.

Henan Province exported over six million migrant workers, with over half of them working in the worst-affected areas, such as Beijing, Guangdong, and Shanxi. To combat the mass return of migrant workers, the province set up a rigorous accountability system, with CPC leaders at all levels taking charge of local SARS control work. The eighteen prefecture-level cities in the province formed a preventive network with all counties, villages, and households functioning as dynamic and independent combat units in the mass prevention and mass control of SARS. In addition, clinics and small-town health centers coordinated the use of all medical resources and developed medical surveillance networks for all communities. Communal residents were mobilized to improve their own personal hygiene and self-protection as well as to contribute actively to local SARS control work. After WHO's visit to Henan in late May, James Maguire from WHO's team of experts spoke highly of Henan's proactive monitoring system that mobilized the entire society in its anti-SARS campaign.

Other agricultural provinces with large numbers of migrant workers, that is, Sichuan, Shanxi, and Guizhou, resorted to the military reserve forces to build multilevel, cooperative SARS surveillance networks. These civilian soldiers actively took charge of tasks, such as educating the public about SARS prevention, disinfecting local communities, supporting medical workers, and taking the temperature of and registering returnees and floating people (Gao and Wang). The civilian soldiers also formed "spring planting and harvesting teams" to help families whose members worked in the cities with laborious agricultural work ("Guizhou's").

Like many other SARS-affected countries and regions, China designated the diagnosis and treatment of SARS cases to medical care workers and the production of epidemiological data to epidemiologists. However, it took a more rigorous approach in finding and quarantining close contacts, which became the new duties of the so-called neighborhood committees that consist of retired volunteers directed by communist party members. As a CPC-sponsored, grassroots force, neighborhood committees penetrated all residential communities throughout the country, and they played significant roles in many communal things, including supervising migrant populations and monitoring residents' birth-control practices. Lisa Movius, an American freelance writer living in Shanghai, describes the grassroots SARS control work conducted by her neighborhood committee members in Shanghai's southern Xujiahui District who were "assisted by about 100 'official helpers,' retired volunteers who patrol specific streets and buildings." To a great extent, neighborhood committees helped to ensure the success of people's wars against SARS and the mobilization of all residents to practice temperature monitoring and home quarantine whenever necessary.

Containment rhetoric at the local level seems to function within the mechanism of mass prevention and mass control of SARS. President Hu's call for people's war against SARS mobilized all individuals to actively participate in the national anti-SARS campaign. Therefore, communities at all levels, including households, dormitories, buildings, villages, streets, business units, and companies, should all vigilantly protect themselves against risks posed by visitors and travelers, who might be asymptomatic SARS carriers. This containment rhetoric, like its counterpart in official SARS discourses, differs from the two types of containment described by Andrew Ross. For Chinese people during the SARS outbreak, the threat comes both within ourselves (the nation as a whole) and from outside (of local communities). For communities outside the SARS-affected regions, to contain SARS often meant to identify, monitor health conditions of, and quarantine, if necessary, travelers and/or returnees from other parts of the country. With each community fighting a local battle to keep SARS out, the binary between us and them and the healthy and the sick got redefined on a case-by-case, village-by-village basis. The goal was no longer to discriminate and segregate but to defend us, a community unaffected by SARS, against all possible outside sources of infection. This practice of localized containment was exactly what China's mass prevention and mass control mechanism attempted to achieve: recruiting all citizens to participate in the anti-SARS battle and casting a wide net by catching anyone with fever and by treating him/her as a possible SARS case instead of missing one real SARS patient. The weapons in this extremely localized anti-SARS battle were very old-fashioned low technologies: thermometers, health registration forms, and quarantines.

To Floating People in SARS-Affected Cities: Stay Put, Don't Leave

One risk factor that had been frequently discussed in the global media about China's anti-SARS campaign was the potential import of the SARS virus to China's hinterland and poor countryside by panicked floating people, or migrant workers and college students from small agricultural towns and rural areas. High levels of fear during emerging epidemics are associated with uncertainty, lack of information, and a widespread perception of loss of control (Eichelberger 1285). People resorted to whatever little information was available to them to respond psychologically and to take risk reduction action. In early May, SARS spread quickly in metropolitan cities, such as Guangzhou, Hong Kong, and Beijing, and caused enormous social and economic disruption. Fleeing from severely affected cities to avoid contracting SARS, migrant workers and college students traveled across the country via trains or long-distance buses to return to their hometowns, often in poor provinces with few SARS cases reported. This massive trend of emigration of farmworkers and students from epicenters caused great concerns at all levels of governments, which soon came up with strategies to prevent the much-feared spread of SARS to all parts of China.

Beijing's experiences with SARS again demonstrate the interconnectedness between mass panic and official risk management approaches. Before the end of April, the guerrilla media overflowed with rumors and sensational killer-disease stories amid official denial and resulted in panic shopping and price hikes. With political commitment from top leaders and with open communication about SARS situations in late April, mass panic disappeared and was replaced with creative grassroots risk tactics and mass prevention and mass control campaigns even though SARS cases in Beijing continued to increase rapidly in the first half of May.

Liu Jian, vice agricultural minister in charge of SARS control work in the countryside, talked about China's strategies at a State Council press conference in mid-May. Describing the guideline as "urban-rural coordination and multi-sector collaboration," Liu listed five strategies: control the return of migrant workers to the countryside; for those who did return, report early, quarantine early, and provide treatment early, if necessary; strengthen the case-reporting mechanism at the levels of counties, towns, and villages; improve the capacity of medical treatment in the countryside; and enhance mass education (Zeng and Shen). Putting governmental officials and hospital administrators in charge of their local anti-SARS work, governments at all levels implemented rigorous accountability mechanisms, and those who failed to carry out their duties were punished. For instance, in Shanxi Province, one of the worst SARS-affected provinces in China, altogether 117 officials and hospital directors received disciplinary punishments ranging from written warning to dismissal from their positions (Gao).

Resorting to the trope of responsibility taking during crises, both Beijing and Guangzhou issued numerous directives and policies requesting companies hiring migrant workers to seal off their construction sites and work units to assist in the national anti-SARS campaign. Both cities warned companies against irresponsible practices, such as the closing of businesses, the dismissal of migrant workers, and the firing of employees infected with SARS. To help to provide better onsite surveillance of migrant workers, the Beijing Bureau of Labor and Bureau of Social Security employed six criteria for the evaluation of construction companies, which included housing no more than fifteen workers per dormitory, improving ventilation, and disinfecting dining halls, dormitories, and restrooms (Yang Liu, "Beijing Bureau"). In addition, all companies were required to comply with anti-SARS guidelines and to report about the SARS control work among their own employees to Beijing's monitoring networks. Many construction sites that did not meet the requirements were either fined or forced to stop their operations to improve their working conditions ("Beijing's Rigorous Examination"). Punished for its failure to comply with official risk reduction measures, an interior-decoration company was expelled from Beijing after one of its employees was hospitalized for medical observation, four put in quarantine, and 101 left Beijing for home ("Interior Decoration Company").

After suspected SARS cases were found in two universities in Beijing, universities in Beijing and the neighboring Hebei Province sealed off their campuses. They implemented rigorous registration and monitoring of anyone leaving or entering the campus and monitored students' temperatures on a regular basis. Many universities issued guidelines for student behavior in late April, which urged students not to leave campus. When large numbers of students fled back to their hometowns in the hinterland, policies were issued to punish those who left or returned to campus without approval from college SARS control groups, those who failed to report their onset of SARS symptoms in a timely manner, and those who did not comply with quarantine arrangements.

Sheldon Ungar identifies both talk radio and the Internet as the two alternative media for the voice amplification of public concerns and recommends the search of both media to "locate a signature of public concern" in global risks ("Moral Panic" 280). When government authorities moved away from false "no-risk" assurances to transparent risk communication and calls for mass mobilization, students quickly responded to such official calls, using the Internet as their deliberative forums. Soon the topic of whether college students should leave their universities for home became the most discussed topic in bulletin board systems (BBS) run by universities in Beijing, which provided traces of "personal worries and agitated conversations" during SARS (Ungar, "Moral Panic" 278). One student post appealed to the traditional Confucian value of putting "nation before community and society above self": "One of the most valued Chinese virtues is the fearless attitude toward death. . . . During SARS, this virtue of 'dare to die' indicates a life attitude that would sacrifice one's own interest for the larger interests of other people, communities, and the nation" (Lou, "History of SARS Attacks" 12). Another post elaborated on the relationship between individual survival and community interests:

> The fact that the affected areas are still not sealed off does not mean we can leave freely. . . . We choose not to leave not because of outside forces, but because of our sense of duty to the society. Each 'one ten thousandth' [chances of us developing SARS would] quickly develop into countless 'ten thousands' [of infected SARS cases], which [would] throw us into greater danger. (A. Liu, "College Students")

At Chinese Agricultural University, the CPC committees of two colleges jointly issued a letter of advocacy for the entire campus, urging students "not to return home for the interests of the society, families, and oneself" (Liu, "College Students"). They cited as rationales the high risk of contracting SARS when traveling home via public transport and of becoming sources of cross-infection to families and local communities. One post on the Beijing University BBS said,

> Social responsibility sounds huge and general, but now everyone of us is confronted with its most concrete and ordinary side. . . . Each of us is a fighter, and our way of fighting is to stay in the affected area—despite

its accompanying danger, we do this for ourselves as well as for others. ("We Worked Together")

These calls for self-restraint and personal sacrifice for communal interests remind one of Confucius's definitions of ren, the cardinal virtue, in the *Analects*: "Be the first to undertake difficult tasks and the last to think about reward" (6.22). As Confucius preaches, a true gentleman is willing to "sacrifice his life to preserve ren rather than to survive at the cost of compromising ren" (15.9). The online posts urging students not to return home reflect some of the key components of ren, that is, gravity, modesty, diligence, generosity, self-restraint, and perseverance in adversity (Ding, "Confucius' Virtue-Centered Rhetoric" 149). As a limited, regional risk reduction effort, online debates on going home or not witness the metamorphosis of individuals into social beings as college students pondered their personal responsibility to the larger groups of families, communities, and the nation. It helped students to put forth small initiatives that helped to facilitate official attempts to compartmentalize and control a wide variety of high-risk space in Beijing. These discussions clearly demonstrate students' sense of interdependence and interconnectedness that "interfused biological, social, and political belongings," which foregrounds responsible citizens as their master trope of identity (Wald 79). These discussions also suggest the influence of emotions and values in people's experiences of and responses to health risks, as Steven Katz and Carolyn Miller stress in their affective-value model of risk communication.

To Floating People in Little-Affected Provinces: Don't Enter or Return

Agricultural provinces exporting large numbers of migrant workers to SARS-affected areas encountered numerous challenges in their efforts to first prevent the import of the SARS virus and then to control local outbreaks. Such provinces took all kinds of measures both to dissuade migrant workers holding jobs outside the province from returning home and to monitor the health conditions of all returnees. With all their SARS cases being travelers or migrant workers returning from outbreak areas, agricultural provinces mobilized all forces, including local officials, medical workers, civilian soldiers, neighborhood committees, families with members in SARS-affected areas, and migrant workers themselves to build a comprehensive defense line against the epidemic.

One SARS-control strategy commonly employed by all provinces was to set up health monitoring stations in all ports, long-distance bus stations, highway checkpoints, and railway stations to supervise health conditions of inbound travelers. All floating people were required to register their names, identity numbers, and contact information. To prevent the repeated import of SARS cases, provinces like Hunan and Zejiang and transportation hubs, such as Wuhan in Hubei Province, took the radical measure of either imposing two-week quarantines on or forbidding the entry of any travelers or returnees from severely SARS-affected regions (X. Wu, "Hunan's Stipulation"; "Zejiang Province"). All these health-monitoring measures, mild or extreme, attempted to maintain the boundary between the healthy and the sick by creating closely guarded biopolitical and geographical defense lines for provinces, cities, and towns that still had few SARS cases.

Provincial governments of Henan, Anhui, Jiangsu, the Autonomous Region of Ningxia, and the Autonomous Region of Inner Mongolia issued urgent directives asking local officials to ensure that local migrant workers working in epicenters would refrain from returning to their rural homes. Jiangsu's urgent notification required that governmental officials of all towns and districts "take full responsibility for persuading migrant workers with local hukou from returning" and for monitoring health conditions of all returnees from SARS-affected regions (Shen and Jiang). Henan's directive states that all means should be used, including "reasoning and emotional appeals" to persuade migrant workers with Henan hukou to "stay where they were instead of returning home, to follow the directions of their working units, and to continue their life routines" (Han and Pan).

Other provinces, such as Shandong, Henan, and Guizhou, directly appealed to their migrant workers by issuing open letters or friendly announcements to them. Many agricultural towns and villages started cooperative arrangements, including civilian soldiers and multifamily agricultural teams, to cope with the shortage of labor in the spring planting and summer harvesting seasons. The Provincial Government of Henan states in its open letter,

> If you are a Henan farmer working in SARS-affected areas, please do not worry about agricultural work at home. Keep your job there. Don't return home. Local government will help your family with wheat harvesting and fall planting. (Han and Pan)

Governmental officials and village leaders mobilized all families with members working in epicenters to either call or write to those family members, asking them not to return home to "help sever the transmission channel of SARS" (Fuming Lu, "Shandong Initiated"). Shandong initiated a "Green-Love Mail Channel" that, with the help of the Communist Youth Leagues throughout the province, arranged the delivery of three hundred thousand "green-love envelops" with paid postage and thousands of "green-love prepared phone cards" to all families with members working in outbreak areas (Fuming Lu, "Shandong Initiated").

Management of Travelers from SARS-Affected Areas: People's War

Despite numerous official strategies to dissuade migrant workers from returning home in the hinterland, millions of panicked floating people still travelled back to the rural areas. In late April, many migrant workers resorted to public transportation systems and took trains or long-distance buses to go home. To track down all close contacts who shared the same vehicles with suspected or confirmed SARS cases, travel alerts were widely publicized in newspapers, online news services, and radio and TV broadcasts. The travel alerts aimed to inform those passengers of the health threats they had confronted and to urge them to seek medical treatment if any symptoms appeared. Regional institutions, such as local health bureaus, public transportation bureaus, and mainstream media, took charge of the entire process of initiating and disseminating such national or regional travel alerts.

Deterred by the rigorous health monitoring measures at highway checkpoints, bus stations, and railway stations, migrant workers soon chose to travel by rented vans, motor tricycles, tricycles, or bicycles. Imagined by the public as ambiguous bodies with possible infection, many migrant workers rejected such perceptions and considered it safer for them to travel home than to continue living and working in Beijing. A small town in Hebei witnessed over eight hundred man-powered tricycles traveling on a major expressway south from Beijing on the single night of April 25 ("Hebei Province").

In addition, unlicensed "black buses" recruited passengers outside long-distance bus stations, and licensed buses picked up and dropped off passengers along their way in suburban areas, which often resulted in excessively overloaded buses and at-will travel of passengers outside officially appointed stops. Such illegitimate practices also turned those "black buses" into blind zones for local SARS control work since many passengers who got on "black buses" outside bus stations were migrant workers who did not go through regular temperature monitoring or health registration (Y. Cai). In mid-May, a highway supervision division caught a bus between Ningbo, a rich coastal city, and a rural town in Anhui Province that illegally picked up passengers outside the bus station. With over one hundred people on a bus with only thirty-one seats, the "air quality inside the bus was extremely poor" (Y. Cai). The reporter commented on the threats caused by such "black buses": "If there were any confirmed or suspected SARS patients on this bus, the infectivity would be very strong. Anyone who got infected on such buses would then produce large outbreaks in the rural areas" (Y. Cai). Black buses posed great challenges to official efforts to convert all physical space and mobile space, such as public transport, into strictly partitioned and constantly monitored social space. Similar efforts to circumvent official health checkpoints and surveillance networks brought huge pressure to SARS control work.

With the ever-tightening anti-SARS networks cast for rural areas, some migrant workers chose to walk back home via back roads, mountain trails, or village lanes. To cope with migrant workers who evaded all official SARS monitoring measures, many rural towns set up local, rigorous mass-prevention networks. Barefoot doctors working in individual villages took charge of monitoring the health conditions of returning floating people. In addition, directors of village committees were required to monitor the entrance points of their villages, and family with recent returnees were required both to supervise their temperatures and to ensure seven- to fourteen-day quarantine for all returnees ("Migrant Farm Workers").

In addition to top-down measures to control the movement of floating people, SARS-affected cities and panicked villages also employed locally improvised tactics to protect their borders and to reduce local SARS risks in early May. Most villages "built makeshift barricades and posted sentinels to keep out strangers" (Eckholm, "With Virus at Gate" A14). Many of them blocked most entrances to their communities and set up checkpoints in the few open ones to monitor visitors' temperatures, to spray disinfection on car tires, and to direct returning migrant workers to quarantine sites outside the villages. Some cities blocked the highway entrances and forbade all cars from epicenters from entering. Small agricultural towns and desperate villages located near major expressways with heavy traffic from epicenters took extreme measures, such as setting up roadblocks or digging up sections of the expressways to keep travelers and vehicles from epicenters, such as Beijing, Shanxi, and Inner Mongolia, from passing by. These blockades in the highways stopped all traffic from and to epicenters without authorization and greatly impeded the transportation of much-needed medical supplies and everyday commodities to SARS-affected areas. The blockades soon brought intensive media coverage as well as official countermeasures. Both the Ministry of Construction and the Ministry of Public Security issued emergency circulars requiring public transportation departments and police to "take all-out measures to maintain the regular flow of traffic" ("Premier"; "Ministry of Public Security").These measures soon brought highway traffic into order and ensured the smooth transportation of much-needed SARS materials to the epicenters.

On June 13, WHO removed its travel advisory against nonessential travel to Hebei, Inner Mongolia, Shanxi, and Tianjin. Dr. Heymann in the update complimented the efficiency of China's anti-SARS measures, particularly its mass mobilization efforts:

> We've seen that there has been a massive effort to mobilize the population both in urban and rural areas across the country, encouraging people to monitor themselves for fever and to ensure that SARS cases are quickly identified, isolated and treated. . . . China has made huge strides in its effort to contain the outbreak of SARS. (WHO, "Update 80")

In its efficient and much shorter battle against SARS, Singapore also mobilized both Confucian values of personal sacrifice and governmental paternalism as well as self-restraint and cooperation to put similar emphases on individual responsibility and mass mobilization (Weber, Yang, and Shien 154). A ministerial panel announced on May 3, "While all ministries are involved in the war against SARS, every individual has to play his part, whether in obeying regulations to stay home or changing what was previously accepted social behaviour, such as working while sick" (Henson). As part of the mass-mobilization efforts, Prime Minister Goh Chok Tong emphasized,

> There is no excuse for anyone in Singapore not to know the part he has to play and that when he has a fever, he may be a potential infector. So the message is a simple one. All of us as ordinary citizens, you and I, have a part to fight SARS and keep Singapore cool. (Henson)

The sole message repeated in all Singaporean media was, "Do the right thing." Only when everyone carried out his/her own duty as a citizen fighting in the national battle against SARS could affected countries and regions effectively contain and eradicate SARS.

As a comparative study of the cultural and institutional rhetorics about SARS, this chapter demonstrates the intricate interconnectedness among rhetoric, culture, ideology, politics, and economic interests. It focuses not only on the different narratives told by cultures and institutions about the same epidemic and the rhetorical strategies employed in such storytelling events but also on factors motivating the construction of such narratives and their impact on the actual stories being told. Preoccupied with ideological and political differences, the American mainstream media rhetorically transformed SARS from a medical epidemic into one of ideology. Changing its contour and shape in its circulation in regional media and other cultural sites of the United States, the rhetoric surrounding SARS encountered attempts to put an ethnic face to the epidemic as well as the appropriation of the term *SARS* as another venue for political criticism and dissenting voices. In contrast, WHO was restrained by its function as a global institution of public health and by the limits on its power to prescribe actions that member states should take. To ensure the fullest and quickest cooperation of China, the origin and epicenter of SARS, WHO rhetorically transformed the medical epidemic of SARS into one of technological inadequacy to achieve minimal conflicts of interest and to focus all attention and efforts on the urgent task to contain and eradicate the global epidemic. Meanwhile, WHO's SARS discourses also emphasized the essential role played by national authorities' political and financial commitment in their anti-SARS campaigns.

The Chinese media focused on material conditions and constraints rather than on ideology or politics and transformed the medical epidemic of SARS into one of infrastructural backwardness. My analysis of the discourses to mobilize the nation to contain SARS in the hinterland and countryside, however, reveals the use of ideological tools, particularly the promotion of patriotism and the mobilization of nationalistic identities and united efforts in its anti-SARS campaign. It also calls attention to the importance of providing both emotional and valuative support and participatory mechanisms so that affected communities and ordinary citizens can participate in the overall campaign against emerging epidemics.

SARS is a highly infectious disease that threatens to come back with full speed with one missing case, as demonstrated by Toronto's brief encounter in late May with a second SARS outbreak and an exported SARS case in North Carolina. One selfish act or one missed or misdiagnosed case "is all it takes to undo the Government's efforts to fight the SARS scourge" (Henson). Considering the Singaporean government's exemplary performance in its anti-SARS work and its aggressive use of home-quarantine orders, the world has much to learn from what the city-state concludes about lessons learned in its battle against SARS: "Even with the Government responding as *one Government*, that was just 'half the shop.' The other half? *The people*" (Henson; emphasis added).

5
Transnational Risk Management
of SARS and H1N1 Flu
via Travel Advisories

*How did transnational risk analysis and risk communication op-
erate among intergovernmental bodies and affected countries with
competing interests and agendas during the global epidemics of
SARS and the swine flu? What tools were employed to mediate
such transnational interactions and negotiations? What forces were
involved, and how were various knowledges produced, legitimated,
and disqualified?*

To address the questions raised above, this study investigates the transnational risk policies surrounding SARS and the H1N1 flu in 2003 and
2009, respectively. Both risk management processes biopolitically monitored
global flows of people from and to outbreak areas through the transnational
use of travel alerts, advices, and advisories.[1] This chapter begins by examining
the dramatically different risk negotiation approaches taken by China and
Canada, two of the countries most affected by SARS, to influence WHO's
response to local outbreaks. Then the chapter investigates WHO's risk management of the 2009 H1N1 flu epidemic and the agency's reluctance to employ
any exit screening or travel advisories because of economic and political
considerations. In conclusion is a discussion of theoretical implications for
transnational rhetorical and risk communication studies.

Travel Alerts, Impact of Local SARS Situations
As a biopolitical genre, travel advisories are adapted as rhetorical responses to
possible health threats posed by outbreak areas to travelers. This section considers the use of travel alerts as transcultural risk management tools during
global epidemics. Travel advice has been used by national governments and
intergovernmental organizations to inform the public of geographically specific health or terrorist threats. For instance, since 1958 WHO has "issued
weekly lists of areas infected with quarantinable diseases so that national
authorities can decide whether to apply public health measures to arriving

travelers" ("Update 19"). However, WHO had never issued "an emergency global travel advisory" before the SARS outbreak (Altman and Bradsher A7).

During the first six months of 2003, WHO employed global travel advisories to exert biopolitical surveillance on SARS-affected areas. The transnational risk management of SARS, however, was in no way a unidirectional or top-down process. In fact, my analysis shows that risk analyses surrounding SARS were constantly shaped, negotiated, and transformed by competing networks of rhetorical-material forces distributed across national and institutional boundaries. Two countries, namely, China and Canada, were most profoundly influenced by WHO's global travel advisories. For this reason, this chapter examines the ways that China, Canada, and WHO negotiated about possible transnational risk management approaches in light of the vast economic and political repercussions brought by travel advisories. My study of transnational risk management reveals strikingly different contours, approaches, and strategies that brought unpredictable results. To fully understand the implications of these differences, one needs to comprehend the impact of the severity and scope of local outbreaks on the local use of travel alerts.

Mainland China launched the most prolonged and challenging anti-SARS campaign to combat local outbreaks that began in November 2002 and were eradicated in June 2003. Exacerbated by early inaction and China's severely underfunded public health system, SARS infection spread to multiple regions as early as late March. WHO's travel advisories recommending against elective travel to parts of China yielded tremendous economic and political damage, which, in turn, forced China to fight SARS more cooperatively and aggressively in April.

Canada's story proceeded differently. With small clusters of SARS cases occurring in hospitals and communities in Toronto from March to June, WHO listed Toronto as one of the affected areas with ongoing SARS infection. WHO also recommended against elective travel in Toronto from April 23 to April 30. However, Health Canada, Canada's federal department in charge of national public health, issued domestic travel advice from late April to mid-May to endorse traveling in the Greater Toronto area, which directly contradicted WHO's risk definitions. With few cases in the United States, the CDC in Atlanta exerted all its surveillance efforts on international travelers arriving in the United States. When WHO listed Toronto in its April 23 travel advisory, the CDC issued only a contradictory, downgraded health alert for Toronto.

WHO's Mediation of Transnational
Risk Conflicts via Travel Alerts

WHO issued its first global health alert on March 12 to warn national health authorities about spreading outbreaks of mysterious pneumonia in various parts of the world. To manage the global risks posed by SARS, WHO adopted the disciplinary technology of ranking, or defining "the place one occupies in a [hierarchical] classification" to "transform confused multitudes into ordered multiplicities" (Foucault, *Discipline* 47–48). It developed classificatory schemes to divide and rate various parts of the world in terms of the types and severity of their health threats, which helped to distinguish high-risk areas from low-risk ones. On March 24, WHO listed for the first time in its travel alert three areas severely affected by SARS: Hong Kong, Singapore, and Vietnam. On March 27, WHO expanded the list of affected areas to include Canada and China ("Update 11"). WHO defined "affected areas" as areas where "local chains of transmission . . . are occurring as reported by national authorities" and the severely affected areas as those with both local and onward transmission ("Update 9"). On April 2, WHO issued the first travel advisory in its history to contain the spread of an infectious disease (SARS) by reducing travel to high-risk areas. Two areas in China were listed in WHO's April 2 advisory, the Guangdong Province and the Special Administrative Region of Hong Kong, because of evidence of the spread of SARS in wider communities ("Update 18").

In addition to ranking, WHO employed meticulous individualizing partitioning, another disciplinary tactic that "organize[s] an analytical space" to establish presences and absences that "supervise[s] the conduct of each individual [country and area]" (Foucault, *Discipline* 143). Such measures of differentiation help to "project subtle segmentations of discipline onto the confused space of internment" (Foucault, *Discipline* 199). WHO achieved partitioning by recommending different hierarchized surveillance measures for travelers from and to affected regions. For countries and areas with limited clusters of SARS outbreaks in hospitals and households, for instance, the United States, WHO recommended no travel restriction because of the little health risk to inbound and outbound travelers. On March 27, WHO recommended the exit screening of outbound air passengers for a small number of severely SARS-affected areas to prevent travel-related spread of SARS (see table 5.1 for a complete list of WHO's travel advisories).

Table 5.1. WHO travel advisories timeline, March 15–July 5, 2003

Date of advisory	Travel advisories to postpone nonessential trips	Areas with recent local transmission
March 15	WHO issued a rare global emergency travel advisory for international travelers and airlines to warn them of the emerging global epidemic	Toronto, China, Hong Kong Special Administrative Region of China, Indonesia, Philippines, Singapore, Thailand, and Viet Nam added
March 18		Taiwan (China) added
March 27	Screening measures recommended for international airports	
April 2	Hong Kong and Guangdong Province, China, added	
April 23	Beijing and Shanxi Province in China, and Toronto, Canada, added	
April 28		*Vietnam removed*
April 30	*Toronto removed*	
May 8	Tianjin, Inner Mongolia and Taipei in China added	
May 14		*Toronto removed for the second time*
May 17	Hebei Province, China, added	
May 21	Taiwan added	*Philippines removed*
May 23	*Hong Kong and Guangdong removed*	
May 26		Toronto returned
May 31		*Singapore removed*
June 13	*Hebei, Inner Mongolia, Shanxi, and Tianjin regions in China removed*	*Guangdong, Hebei, Hubei, Inner Mongolia, Jilin, Jiangsu, Shaanxi, Shanxi, and Tianjin provinces removed*
June 17	*Taiwan removed*	
June 23		*Hong Kong removed*
June 24	*Beijing removed*	*Beijing removed*
July 2		*Toronto removed*
July 5		*Taiwan removed*

Political and Economic Impacts of WHO's Travel Advisories

WHO's travel advisories called attention to potential global health risks posed by outbreak areas and brought immense political, social, cultural, and economic impacts. As Michel Foucault points out, medicine is always "embedded in social, economic, and political variables" (*Birth of the Clinic* 43). WHO employed epidemiological surveillance techniques, such as notifications, travel advices, and contact tracing, to visualize "the presence and location of disease" in the world from a "central and comprehensive vantage point" (Waldby 96). Given the interconnectedness of global economy and global health, national health authorities closely collaborated with WHO to contain the increasingly spreading epidemic of SARS. Meanwhile, SARS-affected countries challenged WHO's authority and competed for the right to participate in defining risks within their national borders. More important, countries listed on WHO's travel advisories negotiated with WHO to help shape transnational risk policies concerning their local SARS outbreaks and to minimize the subsequent economic and social disruptions.

Before mid-April, Chinese media featured few discussions about WHO travel advisories against elective trips to Guangdong, Hong Kong, or Beijing due to early censorship directives (Ding, "Rhetorics"). In contrast, Canadian media were full of reports and commentaries about the negative economic, political, and cultural impacts caused by WHO's April 23 travel advisory for Toronto. Numerous metaphors associated this advisory with the consequences of contagious and fatal epidemics, as well as the stigmatization caused by political failures or rejections. WHO's travel advisory labeled Toronto as a host of plague (Granatstein 4). "Blacklisted" and "stigmatized," Toronto suffered from its "international pariah status" (Granatstein 4) and had "a black mark" attached to its name (Blackwell A2). The impacts on tourism in Toronto were compared to those of the September 11 terrorist attacks in the United States and to those of "failed Olympic bids," in which a world organization evaluated Toronto as failing to be "good enough to bring visitors from around the world" (Granatstein 4). In addition to cultural and social disruptions, WHO's travel advisory singling out Canada brought huge economic losses. The economic damage in Toronto alone was estimated at over $1 billion, nearly half of the estimated $2.1 billion in damages that SARS caused to the entire Canadian economy (Blackwell A2).

Since WHO's travel advisory for Toronto lasted only seven days, the economic and political impacts that SARS had on Canada were much smaller compared to those on mainland China, Hong Kong, or Taiwan. Therefore, analysis of the Canadian media coverage of WHO's travel advisory can shed new light on the impacts of global travel advisories on outbreak areas outside Asia. The following section examines the drastically different rhetorical strategies taken by China and Canada in their efforts to influence WHO's transnational risk management approaches. Challenged by Canadian authorities about its use of global travel advisories, WHO stressed its use of objective technical criteria and denied the influence of any political considerations on its decision-making processes. By investigating the transnational negotiations about the use of travel alerts, we can better understand global power dynamics, knowledge production and legitimation processes, and biopolitical negotiations surrounding the transnational risk analysis of SARS.

Transnational Risk Negotiations between WHO and China

Epidemiological data play a vital role in risk calculations and policy-making processes during epidemics. Such data serve as the foundation for the knowledge production of epidemics and help to determine appropriate measures to contain them. As discussed earlier, disciplinary tactics, such as classification, ranking, segmentation, and partition, require the establishment of analytical space and detailed knowledge about the target population. The transnational risk management of SARS also required technical details and epidemiological data for experts to calculate SARS risks. However, in the world risk society, "the social mechanics of risk situations disregard the nation-state and its alliance systems" because of the increasingly mobile political and economic constellations (Beck 65). The knowledge legitimation processes surrounding global risks are constantly mediated by dense cultural-political networks, interconnected rhetorical-material forces, and global and local actors with competing interests. As a result, risk constructions are continuously shaped, regulated, and recast, "often in unpredictable ways, by shifting power networks and through contradictory processes and structures that span and move across local and global boundaries" (Scott, "Kairos" 137). As demonstrated by the analysis below, China's and WHO's early risk negotiations were centered on the access to clinical resources and epidemiological data. In addition, the negotiations were shaped and transformed not only by biopolitical measures and international criticism but also by dissenting actors actively participating in such transnational risk negotiation processes.

Utter Confusion, Lack of Knowledge before Mid-March

As discussed in my 2009 article "Rhetorics of Alternative Media," the domestic and transnational risk management of SARS before late March were characterized by uncertainty, a lack of knowledge about atypical pneumonia, and confusion caused by Hong Kong's avian flu cases. On February 9, WHO learned through Internet reports about Roche's press release claiming that Guangdong's outbreak was avian flu and that Tamiflu was the only effective cure ("Drug Firm"). On February 10, WHO formally requested more information about the pneumonia outbreak in Guangdong, and on February 11, it sent another request for more details about the cases. The Ministry of Health (MOH) on February 11 reported 305 cases and 5 deaths in Guangdong and offered more description about symptoms of the atypical pneumonia on February 14, but it denied any flu outbreak in Guangdong. On February 19, WHO received another report about the death of an avian flu patient in Hong Kong, which further fueled the fear that an avian flu outbreak might have taken place in Guangdong. The next day, WHO asked Chinese authorities for permission to send an expert team to Guangdong to investigate the local outbreak, which was granted. When the team arrived in Beijing, they received official updates and briefings; however, they were never allowed access to Guangdong and left in frustration after their two-week stay in Beijing.

Taking the politically safe approach of patient diplomacy, the WHO office in Beijing tried to build a cooperative relationship with the MOH and politely and patiently urged them for more data and better collaboration. As early as March 13, international medical communities were speculating about the possible connections among the "flu-like mysterious outbreak[s]" in Hong Kong, Guangdong, and Hanoi (Lo 4). In response, WHO officials stressed the need to obtain tissue samples for analysis from Chinese authorities before establishing any link between those outbreaks. On March 19, Henk Bekedam, head of the WHO office in Beijing, met with Health Minister Zhang Wenkang and asked for close cooperation. On March 22, Bekedam said it was "likely" that the outbreaks in Guangdong and Hong Kong were linked and that the outbreak actually had originated in Guangdong (Yeung and Benitez 9). On the same day, the Guangdong municipal government released its first update since its February 11 press conference, claiming that the outbreak had been brought under control and that the only location in which new patients were reported was the capital city, Guangzhou (Ying, "Illness" 9). Pressed by WHO's repeated requests, the MOH issued new figures on March 26. This update listed a total of 792 cases and 31 deaths in Guangdong by the end of February, including 487 new cases reported from February 10 to February 28 ("Update 10"). Compared with Guangdong's repeated official claims that no new cases were seen in the province since February 10, this update sent a highly contradictory message: it suggested the continual growth and spread of the epidemic and confirmed growing international suspicions.

WHO initiated direct biopolitical and rhetorical interaction with China when a five-member team arrived in Beijing on March 23 at the MOH's request for technical support. This team brought "additional expertise and equipment . . . to bolster" the investigation of SARS in Guangdong ("Update 11"). They also came with many pressing questions, the most urgent of which asked whether the atypical pneumonia in Guangdong was connected with SARS outbreaks in other parts of the world and, if so, whether they were actually the same disease.

Risk contestations between WHO and China were intensified when WHO listed China as one of the infected areas on March 27. Concerned with the spread of SARS through international air travel, WHO issued a travel alert on the same day recommending "the screening of departing passengers" at airports in the four affected areas of Canada, Singapore, China, and Vietnam ("Update 11"). Facing huge economic losses, China complied with WHO's global anti-SARS technical guidelines. It "issued the first reports of cases and deaths in ongoing outbreaks of SARS" in Beijing and Shanxi Province on March 27 and joined the WHO collaborative network on March 28 (WHO, "Update 12," "Update 13").

Political Economy of Transnational
Risk Conflicts in Guangdong

Early April witnessed heightened WHO-China biopolitical interactions to manage local and transnational risks SARS posed. Even after one week in China, WHO's request for permission to investigate the SARS situation in Guangdong was still pending and being processed on April 1. Although WHO had no access to SARS facilities and data in Guangdong, it responded quickly with risk definitions based on whatever limited information it had obtained from Chinese authorities, stressing that "many questions about the outbreak in the Guangdong Province . . . have yet to be answered" (WHO, "Update 19"). On April 2, WHO issued its first global travel advisory recommending that "persons traveling to Hong Kong and Guangdong [should] consider postponing all but essential travel" ("Update 18"). The recommendation against elective travel in Hong Kong was based on the "continuing and significant increase in cases with indication that SARS has spread beyond the initial focus in hospitals" ("Update 18"). In contrast, the decision about Guangdong resulted from "new information provided today by provincial authorities of more than 300 new cases in March alone," which indicated the continuous spread of SARS in the wider community ("Update 18"). Originally issued as a health-related recommendation, WHO's travel advisory changed its contour as it circulated globally and encountered different, and sometimes competing, interests. Citing medical evidence as its rationale, WHO used technical data obtained from the affected areas to define levels of local health risks. It announced that "the new travel advice is intended to limit further international spread of SARS by restricting travel to areas where the transmission patterns of SARS are not fully understood" ("Update 19"). WHO stressed the need to make risk decisions despite the lack of sufficient access to and knowledge about local outbreaks. It also emphasized that it would reconsider its current risk definition once more information became available ("Update 19").

The political economy surrounding the travel advisory for Guangdong vividly illustrates the medico-politico-penal dynamics and economic functions of WHO's global travel advice. Again citing the lack of access to key data and facilities as the basis for its April 2 travel advisory, WHO employed medical and political rationales to justify its risk definitions for Guangdong. Accentuating the presence of SARS in both medical and political space, WHO successfully turned the power contestation surrounding SARS from a less visible medical issue into one with immediate social and material impacts. The sudden shift in negotiation tactics suggested that WHO changed its approaches in its biopolitical encounters with China. Therefore, China had to adopt the same negotiating language, namely, up-to-date SARS data and technical criteria, to be able to participate in transnational risk negotiations again.

WHO's global travel alerts further reduced international travel, tourism, and trade in China. With its immediate economic interests affected, China started to release its tight control of access to SARS facilities in outbreak areas.

On April 2, the same day that WHO issued the travel advice, China finally granted the WHO expert team access to investigate the SARS situation in Guangdong from April 3 to April 8. Also in early April, China conformed with WHO's repeated requests by setting up a nationwide reporting system for daily SARS updates and began taking more-rigorous anti-SARS measures.

Beijing's Outbreak: Extra-institutional Forces

In contrast to the international awareness of the SARS outbreak in Guangdong, little was known about the scope of Beijing's SARS outbreak. Top officials from the MOH and the Foreign Ministry repeatedly claimed that SARS cases in Beijing did not spread outside the hospital. At a State Council press conference on April 3 and in several other occasions, Health Minister Zhang announced that it was safe to work, live, and travel in China, that SARS had been brought under control since the beginning of March, and that only twelve imported SARS cases were found in Beijing on March 31 ("State Council"; "China Safe"). As one node in the transnational risk network, China constantly encountered contending risk messages from international institutions, other countries, and dissenting whistle-blowers. When a question was raised about the contradiction between his claim and WHO's April 2 travel advisory, Zhang employed the rhetorical strategy of "argument from authority" to justify his claim (Perelman and Olbrechts-Tyteca 135). According to him, WHO issued the travel advisory because of its lack of knowledge about the situation of the Guangdong outbreak, not because of the actual danger to live or work there. Announcing that SARS had "been gradually brought under control since the beginning of March," Zhang attempted to contradict WHO's risk definitions for Guangdong and Beijing and suggested much-smaller-scale local outbreaks. He also predicted that WHO officials would consider changing their travel advisory for Guangdong after their on-site investigation there ("China's Efforts"). As the access to affected areas had been the focal point of negotiations between China and WHO, Zhang's rhetorical claim of authoritative inside knowledge to predict future changes temporarily boosted the credibility of his risk messages. It also vividly illustrates the fierce contestation of knowledge claims in global risk conflicts and the difficulty to determine what can count as sufficient proof in such situations.

In the world risk society, no nation-states or expert groups are capable of fully controlling knowledge production or of excluding alternative forms of knowledge about global risks. Dissenting networks of key players and ad hoc individual participation may shape society from below by "chang[ing] [the] rules and boundaries" of risk politics through the use of communication networks and the creation of new linkages (Beck 39–40). The "rhetorical lives of risk constructions" are constantly circulated in and transformed by a wide, interconnected, and diffuse "network of rhetorical-material forces" and by the larger political, social, and economic dynamics (Scott, "Kairos" 137). My analysis of transnational risk politics surrounding SARS reveals the impact of a contending network of institutions, experts, and authorized and unauthorized professionals as well as the subsequent creation and circulation of conflicting and colliding knowledge claims.

An underground economy of unverified risk messages from Beijing hospitals and anonymous medical workers kept circulating in unofficial channels, particularly in guerrilla media, such as text messages and word-of-mouth communication. As early as late March, masks and disinfectants were sold out in Beijing's supermarkets and grocery stores. Widely circulated rumors claimed that SARS patients had been treated in major Beijing hospitals and that some hospitals had been so full that they ran out of beds. Such rumors were actually a mix of facts and speculations, as would later be proven by official narratives about many heroic health care workers who fought against SARS in the frontline and were infected by SARS.

In the midst of this rumormongering, whistle-blowers, such as Dr. Jiang Yanyong, drew on their personal connections in civilian and military hospitals to compile and release data about the number of SARS cases. As discussed in chapter 3, Dr. Jiang managed to circumvent official censorship and to publish his findings in contending foreign media, which sent out urgently needed risk messages to the transnational risk network (see Ding, "Rhetorics"). In response, WHO issued an unusual statement criticizing MOH's lack of cooperation and the exclusion of cases in military hospitals in MOH's SARS updates, citing "conflicting reports from health workers" and "only a minority of hospitals [offering] daily reports of SARS cases" (WHO, "Update 25"). WHO listed Beijing as a SARS-affected area on April 11 and urged for permission to conduct its own investigation in Beijing hospitals. As a result, WHO was granted access to designated SARS hospitals in Beijing from April 11 to April 15, and on April 15, WHO was given permission to visit military hospitals.

After mid-April, rumors ran rampant in Internet forums and guerrilla media. It was claimed that extreme measures would be taken to contain SARS in Beijing, including city closure, mass quarantine, curfews, and the use of airplanes to spray disinfectant. Meanwhile, mounting international criticism of China's belated response appeared in foreign media, with some urging for efforts to "isolate China" (Schiller). On April 16, WHO declared that Chinese authorities had underreported SARS cases by 160 patients in Beijing after investigating the SARS situation in two military hospitals (Lakshmanan).

Mounting international pressures and domestic grassroots risk communication efforts greatly challenged risk definitions China provided in the first half of April. However, China soon sought to repair its damaged credibility by mobilizing rhetorical and material resources to justify and transform its much-criticized risk management approaches. China did not directly respond to Dr. Jiang's data or international critiques until April 20, when officials took the unusual act of firing both Zhang and mayor of Beijing Meng Xuenong for failing to respond effectively to Beijing's SARS outbreak. The dismissal of two top officials functioned as a symbolic gesture suggesting the central government's determination to fight against underreporting and to provide transparent risk information. Starting on April 20, China issued SARS updates on a daily basis instead of once every five days. The total number of SARS cases in Beijing witnessed a huge increase from 339 confirmed cases and 402 suspect cases on April 20 to an accumulative of 692 confirmed cases and 782 suspect cases on April 23. This drastic increase further fueled international suspicion of underreporting in Beijing. The MOH explained that part of the increase was caused by the confirmatory diagnosis of those placed under medical observation as suspect or probable cases. Because WHO only required the mandatory reporting of suspect or probable cases, those under medical observation or quarantine were not included in official data until they were reclassified as suspected or probable cases. Because of the huge increase in Beijing's SARS cases, WHO "slapped a travel advisory" on Beijing and Shanxi Province on April 23 (Beech). Toronto, another major city undergoing a smaller-scale SARS crisis, was listed on the same advisory.

Economic and political factors played a key role in shaping China's responses to the SARS outbreak. Chinese media indicated significant anxiety about financescapes, or the withdrawal of global capital during the outbreak. For instance, *People's Daily* compared the economic impact of SARS to that of the Asian financial crisis of 1997 and expressed grave concern over the loss of "export and foreign direct investment" ("SARS Virus"). On May 1, International Labor Day, *People's Daily* published an editorial to mobilize dominant ideological beliefs, such as patriotism and economic stability. It called on "the broad masses of the workers to firmly implement government measures to focus on economic development," to "implement the pro-active financial policy, maintain normal orders of production to fulfill the planned [GDP] objectives for this year" ("Editorial Calls"). However, both China and WHO remained silent about those issues and relied mostly on technical language in the negotiating processes, as discussed in chapter 4. In contrast, Canada brought its economic and political concerns to the negotiating table, which helped to speed up the removal of the travel advisory for Toronto. What follows examines the ways Canada employed economic, political, and technical arguments in its transnational negotiations with WHO and the different impacts these arguments had on the outcomes of those negotiations.

Transnational Rhetorical Networks of WHO's Travel Advisories for Toronto

SARS was imported to Toronto on February 23, 2003, from the Metropole Hotel in Hong Kong, where an elderly woman stayed for three nights and contracted SARS during her ten-day trip to the city. Phase 1 of the Toronto SARS outbreak started on March 13 when the elderly woman's son died of SARS and spread the virus to family members and health care workers. The Province of Ontario issued a health alert on March 14 regarding four cases of atypical pneumonia in Toronto hospitals and declared SARS a Provincial emergency on March 26. WHO extended its travel advisory by adding Toronto to the list of areas where elective travel should be postponed on April 23 and removed the city from its list on April 30. The local SARS outbreak was brought under control in early May, and WHO removed Toronto from the list of areas with recent local transmissions on May 14.

Analysis of the risk politics surrounding WHO's travel advisory for Toronto demonstrates transnational rhetorical links, interarticulation, and negotiations and accompanying political, economic, and material impacts on outbreak areas. WHO reviewed and defined the magnitude of the SARS outbreak in various countries and areas, using criteria based on clinical and epidemiological evidence. Such criteria included "the number of prevalent cases and the daily number of new cases, the extent of local chains of transmission, and evidence that travellers are becoming infected while in one area and then subsequently exporting the disease elsewhere" (WHO, "Update 37"). On April 23, when WHO added Toronto to its growing list of outbreak areas, it cited as its rationale the continual growth of the local outbreak in magnitude, the infection of not only the initial risk group of medical care workers but also other close contacts, and the infection of international travelers during their stay in Toronto, who, in turn, exported the disease to other countries ("Update 37").

WHO's travel advisories usually last for at least three weeks, or twice the maximal incubation period of SARS, before the agency reexamines them. Ontario Health Minister Tony Clement and Public Health Commissioner Dr. Colin D'Cunha led a delegation of medical experts and top health officials to Geneva, Switzerland, to argue against the need for such severe warnings for Toronto. Under immense pressure from active public-relations campaigns in Canada, WHO took Toronto off its travel advisory on April 30, only one week after the travel advisory had been announced. The following section outlines these events in greater detail.

Nontechnical Contestation in Risk Definitions for Toronto

WHO's April 23 travel advisory for Toronto was met by bitter fury and criticism from Canadian politicians, the mainstream media, and the general public. Top officials and medical experts characterized the decision as disappointing, troubling, scapegoating, wrong, alarmist, unnecessary, unwarranted, inappropriate, unquestionably irresponsible, a bunch of bullshit, a gross misrepresentation of the facts, and bad science based on outdated information. Canadian authorities made aggressive efforts to dispute WHO's risk definitions for Toronto.

Health Canada started to issue international travel advice on March 28, which it updated on a daily basis until the end of April. In response to domestic fears the WHO travel advisory caused, the Canadian agency took the unusual measure of issuing four domestic travel health alerts on April 24, April 28, May 2, and May 13. All four stressed that existing SARS cases in Toronto occurred only in specific transmission settings and in a few defined locations. They consistently defined the risk of acquiring SARS from traveling to Toronto as being low and claimed that only travel to affected countries in Asia and close contact with SARS patients would cause SARS infection. Directly contradicting WHO's travel advisory, these domestic documents aimed to maintain the economic stability of Toronto, which accounted for "a fifth of total economic activity in Canada" (van Rijn A1).

Canada participated in the risk conflicts surrounding WHO's travel advisory with media campaigns and collaboration between political and scientific communities. As a part of the "widespread condemnation" and rejection of WHO's travel advisory, politicians focused on potential economic disasters and international stigmatization. Driven by political and economic concerns, Health Canada filed a letter of protest with WHO upon learning about the travel advisory for Toronto. Toronto Mayor Mel Lastman spoke about his outrage with WHO's decision at a press conference on April 23:

> I can tell you definitely we are in better shape today than we have been in a month. . . . Where did [WHO] come from? Who did they see? Did they go to our hospitals; did they go to our clinics; did they go anywhere? They sit [in] Geneva or someplace and they make decisions. (*Learning from SARS* 38)

On April 24, several political and personal attempts were made on the part of Canada to expedite the information flow. Canadian Ambassador Sergio Marchi was dispatched to lobby WHO on a personal level; federal Health Minister Anne McLellan called Dr. Gro Harlem Brundtland, the WHO director-general, and urged her to lift the travel alert for Toronto. In addition, top Canadian health officials held a telephone conference with WHO experts to discuss the latest SARS developments. However, all of these appeals to revoke the WHO travel alert were rejected. WHO officials cited three technical reasons for issuing the travel alert: the magnitude of Toronto's outbreak, the spread of SARS cases in the community at large, and the export of SARS cases to several other countries. Stressing the centrality of public health risks in the decision-making processes, WHO officials dismissed Canada's political and economic arguments. Rejecting the need for "court-level proof," WHO stated that it had to act on the local and available data provided by Canada, which offered "*clear and undoubtable information* that the likelihood of cases coming from Canada exist" (Thompson A4; emphasis added).

In addition to efforts made by politicians, Canada's leading health officials and scientists accused WHO of bringing political considerations into public health decisions and protested against WHO's use of confusing standards, faulty analysis, and bad science. They complained that WHO experts put the travel advisory in place based on outdated and inaccurate information without consultation with their Canadian counterparts or onsite investigations. As Toronto was listed in the same travel advisory with Beijing and the

Shaanxi Province of China, top Toronto health officers suggested that WHO was presenting "a gross misrepresentation" of facts by associating Toronto with China and other SARS hot spots in Asia (van Rijn A1). In response, Dr. David Heymann, WHO's executive director of communicable diseases, stressed the use of the same criteria for the travel advisory, for "on a lesser magnitude, but still a high magnitude, Canada has met the same criteria that those other places are meeting" (van Rijn A1). Moreover, he pointed out that Beijing and Toronto were not and could not be compared, as they were "each different situations" (van Rijn A1).

The political and practical arguments that Canada made against WHO's travel advisory were built on probable knowledge, or rhetorical invention. In other words, Canada tried to make a case by drawing evidence from contingent situations and by producing probable knowledge that supported its appeals. WHO rejected Canada's political and economic arguments, however, because Canada failed to prove either the absence of public health risks or the possibility that Canada had not actually exported SARS cases. This round of rhetorical confrontations between WHO and Canada demonstrates the conflicting interests and responsibilities between national authorities and international organizations. It seems to suggest that global health authorities focused more on objective knowledge claims related to science, technology, and public health, whereas nontechnical actors, such as politicians and the mainstream media, relied more on political and economic arguments. Although these political and economic arguments may occupy a much lower, if not peripheral, status in the hierarchy of knowledge for global health authorities, they call attention to the political and economic consequences brought by global risk policies and bring "legitimate concerns to the table" (Finlay 14).

Toronto's Arguments, Successes, and Unpredictable Repercussion

Despite the numerous failed political, economic, and personal appeals top Canadian officials made, Canada did not give up its transnational risk negotiations with WHO. Realizing that "the impassionate case to overturn the advisory must be made on the scientific facts," Canadian authorities took a different route by resorting to science, statistics, and medical evidence in addition to political concerns to make the argument (Owens and Vincent A1). With concentrated efforts from health officials and medical experts, Clement started another round of negotiations by gathering evidence and by putting together arguments to demonstrate that none of the three criteria WHO used to issue the travel advisory applied to Toronto. On April 29, Clement led a six-person delegation to WHO headquarters in Geneva to meet with the WHO director. They aimed both to deliver the most up-to-date SARS statistics and to request the removal of the advisory.

The very act of sending a delegation of senior health officials directly to WHO headquarters was unprecedented. In fact, of all the SARS-afflicted countries and regions, Canada was the first and only outside group meeting with Brundtland to argue for the removal of travel advisories. In addition to stressing scientific evidences, Clement created a spotlight for transnational media by publicizing his delegation and by hiring a public-relations firm from Brussels, Belgium, to cope with requests from domestic and international media. Canada mobilized forces from multiple sources in its second round of systematic attempts to appeal for the removal of the Toronto travel advisory. The federal government, public health and medicine authorities, and transnational media all participated in the negotiations about WHO's travel advisory for Toronto.

Ulrich Beck, scholar in risk communication, stresses the importance of examining "the colliding claims of various expert groups" and "the battle-grounds of pluralistic rationality claims" (119) to answer question of "who knows and on what basis" (120). The transnational risk conflicts surrounding WHO's travel advice for Toronto provide a rich site to investigate the way various expert groups negotiated about contending knowledge claims and their use of scientific and nonscientific arguments to support those claims. As WHO's travel advisory was based on standard technical criteria, the Canadian delegation employed scientific and epidemiological evidence to undercut those criteria. The criterion of community transmission is based on statistics and epidemiological data gathered through contact tracing and clinical records about onset dates. As a result, it was comparatively straightforward for both WHO and Canada to investigate the scope of community transmission in Toronto once they had access to updated data. The delegation claimed that "there was no evidence of community transmission in Toronto since April 9" and that all cases could be traced back to the original case at Scarborough Grace Hospital (Owens and Vincent A1). Whereas the first claim proved that no new community infection took place in the past twenty days, or twice the longest incubation period, the second claim showed that all cases were transmitted in hospital or family settings or through close contact instead of being released in the community.

The evidence for Toronto's exportation of six SARS cases to the Philippines, the United States, Austria, and Bulgaria was tricky and hotly contested. In fact, this issue was the last straw before WHO added Toronto to its travel advisory. Exported cases were considered as "indicators of how an outbreak has been managed," that is, through contact tracing and health screening at airports (Owens and Vincent A1). On March 27, WHO recommended the screening of air passengers departing from affected areas to other countries. However, Canada did not adopt any pre-embarkation screening measures until May. Canadian authorities rejected the charge of exporting cases by insisting that WHO used outdated information and that its calculation of the export of cases had been "overblown" (Owens and Vincent A1).

Several factors further exacerbated the disagreement surrounding Toronto's exported cases: the use of different SARS case definitions by individual countries, the lack of diagnostic tools, and the difficulty of conducting contact tracing and of obtaining updates and clinical diagnosis for international travelers. For example, a Finnish man traveled to Toronto in April, returned home, and developed symptoms similar to SARS. Although Finland reported positive tests for coronavirus, the SARS pathogen, in May, Ontario officials concluded that the Finnish case "could not have come into contact with the disease" after exhaustively tracing his movements in Toronto (Blackwell). Given the difficulty in reaching an absolutely definite conclusion about the case, it is difficult to determine which side neglected key evidences and whose conclusion was more credible.

When one looks beyond the immediate rhetorical networks surrounding the exported cases from Toronto, more contradictory evidence can be traced. Criticizing Canada for exerting political pressure on WHO, Heymann argued, "The political lobbying of Canada was very inappropriate. [. . .] [P]ublic health cannot be interfered with by political lobbying" (Cohn A01). The atmosphere had "become so poisoned by Canadian pressure tactics that Brundtland [for the first and only time] personally took on the task of announcing when and whether the advisory would be lifted," which distracted her and other top scientists from "the crucial battle against SARS" (Cohn A01). In addition, Dr. James G. Young, the comanager of Ontario's SARS emergency, delivered a lecture at Queen's University in 2004. He claimed that since one case from each of Toronto's two SARS outbreaks spread to the United States, "those events were sufficient to trigger the WHO travel advisory" (24).

The "closed-door negotiation" between Canadian and WHO officials eventually led to the repeal of the Toronto travel advisory (Blackwell). On April 30, WHO reviewed the latest SARS data Canadian authorities offered and removed its weeklong travel advisory. In return, Canada made a compromise: it finally agreed to implement proactive SARS screening measures at Pearson International Airport in Toronto by interviewing passengers and by installing temperature-monitoring devices at the airport check-in points (Brown).

CDC's Responses to Toronto

In the world risk society, no forces can maintain absolute control of transnational risk conflicts, and decision-making processes always operate amid uncertainty. Claims of different expert groups collide with one another, and ordinary knowledge developed by experts outside their institutional positions may also participate in the knowledge contests. When combined, these claims "open up a battle field of pluralistic rationality claims" (Beck 120). Accordingly, in analyses of the power-knowledge relations of transnational risk conflicts, one should always ask not only who creates what knowledge and on what basis but also what other knowledges and groups are excluded from such knowledge-making processes and how, if ever, they make themselves heard in the exclusive and hostile power settings.

The transnational contestation surrounding Toronto's risk definitions extended beyond WHO and Canada. In fact, the CDC of the United States adopted a much lower risk category for Toronto by issuing a downgraded travel alert, which advised travelers to Toronto to take appropriate precautions rather than avoiding nonessential travel there. Producing contesting knowledge about spatialized, travel-associated SARS risks, the three national and international authorities—Health Canada, the CDC in Atlanta, and WHO—vividly demonstrate the paradoxical economy of risk classifications when epidemics quickly unfold on a planetary scale.

The CDC employed travel advisories quite proactively for affected areas in Asia. For instance, it advised against elective travel to Hong Kong, Guangdong, and Hanoi as early as March 15 when WHO released the same suggestion for the first two areas on April 2. In the case of the Toronto outbreak, however, the CDC took a much milder approach. When phase 1 of Toronto's SARS outbreak started in early March, the CDC was invited to provide technical assistance in investigating the outbreak. On April 23, the CDC responded to WHO's travel advisory for Toronto with a less stringent, lower-level travel alert "recommending [that] U.S. travelers to Toronto observe precaution to safeguard their health" ("Interim Travel Alert").

In the CDC's telebriefing on April 24, journalists questioned why the CDC's risk evaluation for Toronto differed from that of WHO. CDC officials emphasized Toronto's well-understood patterns of transmission and its complete epidemiological picture, claiming that the vast majority of the problem in Canada had been the "hospital spread of the infection." One technical criterion WHO used for travel advisories was the exportation of SARS cases, which applied to Toronto because one of the exported cases was diagnosed as a probable case in Pennsylvania in mid-April. According to a *Morbidity and Mortality Weekly Report* (*MMWR*) article, in late March, this Pennsylvania case traveled to Toronto for a religious retreat that was later linked to the subsequent spread of SARS among that group. The CDC did not consider the person from Pennsylvania as a significant health risk because of the CDC's ability to account for the epidemiological pattern in the religious group and the Pennsylvania person as well as the lack of any subsequent transmission from the Pennsylvania person. The agency further claimed that traveling to Toronto posed no health threat to US citizens because of the CDC's capacity both to predict where the health risk was in Toronto and to help travelers to assess their risks and to predict potential exposure in any situation. Therefore, the CDC concluded that a traveler going to Toronto would not be "inadvertently coming into contact with a SARS patient" ("CDC's Response"). Although the CDC never stated explicitly the criteria for its travel alert for Toronto, its explanation during the April 24 telebriefing clearly shows a greater emphasis on the overall picture of local transmissions and less attention to the actual SARS figures. It also suggested that the close political and economic connectedness and the geographical proximity of the United States and Canada might have helped to shape their transnational risk management approaches.

The CDC openly acknowledged the confusion caused by definitional issues surrounding SARS cases and criteria for travel alerts. To address the problem, the CDC called for the development of "a consistent set of criteria for different levels of travel advisories and alerts" and for "a more global agreement about what the criteria are" ("CDC's Response"). Only with such consensuses can everyone understand the health authorities' decisions and the rationales for those decisions, the CDC said. Health Canada made similar comments in its official publication *Learning from SARS*. The book complains about the inconsistent criteria for travel advisories, the weak evidence for travel advisory criteria, and the limited warning about the decision. It also stresses that "processes for developing evidence-based criteria and giving notice to affected countries *must be developed by agreement among member states*" (*Learning from SARS* 11; emphasis added).

The transnational comparison of criteria for travel advice suggests the contingent, ambiguous, and shifting nature of such technical criteria, which may cross the border of medical arena to those of cultural, political, and economic ones. The different risk categories employed by WHO and the CDC for Toronto clearly illustrate the ambiguous, uncertain, and indeterminable nature of global risks and the fierce contestation surrounding the knowledge-production processes about such risks. With contradictory risk messages coming from two of the most prestigious public health institutions in the world, individual countries responded to the Toronto outbreak differently, and Canadian authorities focused their resources to argue against the WHO travel advisory.

This study of global risk negotiations suggests that WHO considered the use of travel advisories as a strictly technical decision about global health that should not be interfered with or influenced by economic or political considerations. The rhetorical networks surrounding the use of travel advisories extended beyond the 2003 SARS outbreak, though, as demonstrated by WHO's abrupt change in its use of travel advisories and by the confusion and contention about the use of travel advisories and border screening in 2009. During the H1N1 flu pandemic, WHO openly acknowledged economic and political concerns as legitimate and important factors. This radical difference in WHO's risk management approaches suggests impacts of global power contestation on the transnational health risk policies.

Power Struggles Surrounding Travel Advisories in H1N1 Flu

As an emerging global epidemic, H1N1 flu started in Mexico in March 2009. On April 25, 2009, WHO called the outbreaks in Mexico and the United States a "public health emergency of international concern" ("Swine Flu Illness"). The new epidemic quickly spread to nine countries in North America and Europe in late April and led to widespread outbreaks and the closedown of over a thousand schools and kindergartens in Japan after May 18, 2009 ("Japan's Radically Increased H1N1 Flu Cases"; McNeil A9).

The global epidemic of H1N1 flu fully demonstrates all features of global risks as Beck defined. At its beginning, H1N1 flu was considered highly unpredictable, incalculable, and, thus, uncontrollable because of its quick spread via intercontinental traffic, the uncertainty about its consequences, and the constantly mutating influenza viruses (M. Chen, "Concern," "Statement"). Having successfully led the world to eradicate SARS, WHO quickly assumed a leading role in the global anti–H1N1 flu campaign. Margret Chen, director-general of WHO, stressed in several United Nations assemblies that the behavior of influenza viruses are "notoriously unpredictable" ("Concern," "Statement"). In addition, no one knew how H1N1's interactions with other viruses circulating in humans would influence its behavior or whether the second wave of H1N1 flu would be much more lethal (Jordans and Cheng). Chen emphasized the need to make decisions and take actions "at a time of great scientific uncertainty" ("Concern"). Similarly, editorials published in *The Lancet* and *Nature*, two leading biomedical journals, called all existing recommendations "provisional" and stressed the need to reiterate the uncertainties associated with the outbreak ("Between a Virus" 9; "Swine Influenza").

Despite the rapid global spread of the H1N1 flu virus, WHO advised no travel restriction or border screening. Instead, after April 27, WHO only recommended prudent measures and urged sick people to "delay international travel" and international travelers with flu symptoms "to seek medical attention" ("Swine Influenza"). Emphasizing economic disruption and little public health utility, WHO announced that "scientific research based on mathematical modeling" indicated that limiting travel and imposing travel restrictions would do little to stop the spread of the disease but would be "highly disruptive to the global community" ("No Rationale"). It also claimed that historical records of previous flu pandemics, "*as well as experiences with SARS*, have validated this point" ("No Rationale"; emphasis added). Similarly, Dr. Richard Besser, CDC's acting director, cited Hong Kong's experience with SARS as an example illustrating the ineffectiveness of border screening to identify cases or to prevent transmission and used it as the rationale for not adopting such measures in the United States (cited in Grady A1). These statements indicate that despite WHO's insistence of using strictly technical criteria for SARS travel advisories in 2003, the measure may have brought marginal public health benefits and was not as objective or technical as WHO had claimed.

Having the largest number of confirmed and probable H1N1 flu cases in May 2009, the United States stressed repeatedly that H1N1 flu is curable with Tamiflu and Relenza, that its federal government had large stockpiles of Tamiflu, and that there was no need to panic (Centers for Disease Control, "CDC Briefing"). The United States closed schools with H1N1 flu outbreaks in early May 2009 and put a travel advisory in effect from April 27 to May 15 recommending the postponement of nonessential travel to Mexico. However, as an epicenter itself, the United Stated never employed exit screening for outbound travelers during the H1N1 flu outbreaks. Both WHO and the United States argued that the influenza virus can be transmitted from person to person before the onset of symptoms; therefore, health screening of travelers would be of limited use in reducing the spread of the virus.

The disputes surrounding the use of travel advisories and health screening in the H1N1 flu pandemic fully illustrate the impacts of scientific uncertainty and political considerations on the global risk management of quickly spreading epidemics. During the SARS outbreak, WHO recommended exit screening from SARS-affected areas to reduce "the risk of further international spread of SARS" ("Update 11"). On April 3, 2003, WHO issued a travel ban for Hong Kong and Guangdong Province in China based on evidence showing that SARS had been exported to other countries ("Update 17"). WHO set up a working group to examine the prevention of international community transmission of SARS, with travel advisories as one of the measures being evaluated. In its 2004 article in the journal *Emerging Infectious Disease*, the working group stated that exit screening might "have helped dissuade ill persons from traveling by air" and that "preventing passengers with SARS from boarding aircraft *would likely* have reduced transmission of infection, but the most cost-effective way to accomplish this is *uncertain*" (Bell and World Health Organization Working Group; emphasis added). The careful use of hedges in those statements indicates the lack of solid empirical evidence to support the public health benefits of travel advisories and shows the ambiguity surrounding WHO's wide use of economically disruptive travel bans during SARS.

WHO's position changed, however, in the H1N1 flu epidemic. On numerous occasions, senior WHO officials stressed the need to refrain from introducing economically or socially disruptive measures that had "no clear public health benefits [...] in a time of economic downturn" ("WHO: China"; "WHO Prescribes" A01). These arguments put much more emphasis on economic considerations than rigorous surveillance measures and tried to protect global economy at a time of uncertainty.

Asia's Official Protests against Politically Inflected Decisions

Noticing the "stark differences in [WHO's] handling of the human swine flu [and] the SARS outbreak," Asian media and leading virologists questioned "whether 'a double standard' was being applied" because "WHO dare not pressure the U.S. to [implement exit screening]"(E. Lee, "WHO's Handling" 2; Schiller A03). Up until mid-May 2009, most middle-income and low-income countries in South America and Asia (with the exception of Japan) had been little influenced by H1N1flu. In sharp contrast with the calm governmental and media responses in the United States and Canada, however, many developing countries employed far more rigorous risk management measures because of fear of huge economic disruption. Asian countries were particularly vulnerable to global epidemics because of their reliance on international trade and tourism for economic growth, their limited medical resources, their densely populated cities, and their uneven regional development (H. Song, "Economies of Asian Countries"). As all the confirmed cases in Asia during the month of May had a travel history linked to the United States and Canada, Asian countries protested against the lack of border screening in the United States and criticized WHO's sharply different risk management approaches for SARS and H1N1 flu. WHO refuted requests for exit measures "because the virus had already spread to too many countries" (E. Lee, "Health Chief" 4). In response to the lack of exit measures in the epicenters, most Asian countries adopted rigorous entry screening and contact tracing to prevent the H1N1 flu virus from getting into the community in late April and early May 2009. It should be stressed that even though most Asian countries reported about early H1N1 cases after late June, the rigorous use of official measures and social-distancing practices helped to buy precious time for vaccine development and production. Concerned about possible future outbreaks, Asian media challenged WHO's recommendation against the use of border screening and questioned the politics driving such decisions, pointing out that when WHO faces "the U.S.A., they have difficulty in making a decision at all kinds of levels" (Schiller A03). Such rhetorical contestations in the global anti–H1N1 flu discourses suggest the political, cultural, and economic repercussions brought by international public health policies and the fierce conflicts of interests among countries and regions with radically different economic and public health conditions.

According to an editorial from *South China Morning Post*, an influential Hong Kong newspaper, the "two-tier entry screening" (health declarations and temperature scans) was proved effective in blocking the H1N1 flu virus in early May ("Exit Screening" 10). With most of Hong Kong's confirmed cases coming from the United States, York Chow Yat-ngok, the Hong Kong health minister, argued for the necessity for departure ports to adopt health screening measures to deter sick people from travelling and to "stop the United States from exporting more swine flu cases" (E. Lee, "Health Chief" 4; E. Lee, "WHO's Handling" 2). Hoping to reduce the one-way flow of dangerous viral carriers from North America to Asia, he also called for "Asian countries to unite in making their concerns known, as western nations would have done if Asia had been exporting swine flu among aircraft passengers" ("Exit Screening" 10). Even though Asian authorities challenged WHO's risk management policies and repeatedly argued for the need of health-screening measures, the global risk policies remained unchanged. Hong Kong and other Asian countries suffered from their lack of rhetorical and political efficacy to influence global risk policies, which forms a stark contrast with Canada's effective efforts to overturn WHO's travel advisory for Toronto in 2003.

The contentions surrounding WHO's decisions about travel advice and border screening clearly demonstrate the contingent nature of medical knowledge on which decisions are made in global risk conflicts. It also highlights the political contestations surrounding such global decisions and knowledge legitimation processes. Paul Farmer criticizes the unidirectional nature of international concerns about emerging epidemics, arguing that only epidemics emerging from a poor population to threaten a wealthy one are considered important. In contrast, diseases, such as tuberculosis, have been "allowed to persist among the world's marginalized, contributing to these pathogens' mutation and drug resistance" (Eichelberger 1293). My analysis confirms the unidirectional nature of international risk policies of H1N1 flu. Despite Asian countries' official protests and criticism, global-risk regimes seemed to better serve the interests of developed countries while paying little attention to those of developing countries. Further, this analysis finds that despite their far-reaching impacts, international agencies and national governments and institutions are not the only forces in global-risk conflicts. Communities and individuals participate in risk management activities and influence local risk policies in a bottom-up manner, as suggested by the transnational, grassroots discussions about responsibility taking during the epidemic.

Disciplinary Rhetoric at Work: Responsibility Taking at All Levels

The word *responsibility* appears repeatedly in reports, commentaries, and Internet discussions about imported swine flu cases in Asian countries, particularly China. As Chen, WHO's director-general since 2006, points out, "radically increased interdependence" amplifies the potential for economic disruption and makes financial crises and epidemics "highly contagious and moving rapidly from one country to another" ("Concern"). A *Lancet* editorial suggests that developing countries and displaced populations, such as refugees, "are disproportionately affected by an influenza pandemic" ("Swine Influenza" 1495). The editorial cited Christopher J. L. Murray and colleagues' study of the 1918–20 Spanish flu pandemic and predicted that "the next global influenza pandemic would kill 62 million people, with 96% of those deaths occurring in low-income and middle-income settings" (1495). Stressing inequities in access to health care, Chen considered an influenza outbreak "an extreme expression of the need for [global] solidity before a shared threat"; accordingly, she urged that worldwide actors work together to "protect developing countries from bearing the brunt of a global contagion" ("Concern").

Within their own borders, individual countries shoulder the responsibility to build an inclusive health system and "to offer universal coverage right down to the community level" (Chen, "Concern"). Globally speaking, every country has the responsibility to collaborate with international agencies and other countries and to share resources and information to contain global epidemics. Part of this responsibility requires all parties to acknowledge the incalculability and uncertainty of pandemics and inconsistencies in risk definitions. It highlights the need for countries with vastly different material contexts to take different and locally appropriate risk management approaches. Therefore, serious efforts should be made to negotiate solutions mutually acceptable to all parties involved.

When threatened with contagion and deaths, communities seek to contain epidemics either by blocking health threats that come "outside of the social body" through the use of quarantines or isolations or by neutralizing or fully absorbing "threat[s] internal to the host" (Ross 46). Thus, "shared responsibility" is needed not only at national and international levels but also at local and individual levels (Centers for Disease Control, "CDC Briefing"). *The Lancet* emphasized "the vital role and responsibility of the individual" and urged those with flu-like symptoms to take home isolation and other measures of social distancing, which "are most likely to stop the spread" of H1N1 flu ("Swine Influenza" 1495). Similarly, a *Nature* editorial pointed out, "[D]uring a severe pandemic, there is only so much [governments and public health authorities] can do" ("Between a Virus"). Therefore, "much of the response will depend in local communities taking action for themselves" ("Between a Virus"). Both editorials employed what Priscilla Wald calls "social responsibility," which is "fashioned by a medicalized understanding of social being and social control" (98). Highlighting "citizen judgment and action," such social responsibility requires self-care, that is, risk reduction practices, such as hand washing and social distancing, compliance with quarantine orders, and tolerance of various degrees of personal inconvenience for the communal well-being (Schoch-Spana, Franco, Nuzzo, and Usenza 10). Social responsibility also puts equal emphasis on care for others, that is, volunteering efforts, community support, and grassroots surveillance. Monica Schoch-Spana, Crystal Franco, Jennifer B. Nuzzo, and Christiana Usenza employ the term *civic infrastructure* to describe the "dynamic assembly of interdependent people, voluntary associations, and social service organizations who can pool their collective wisdom, practical experience, specialized skills, social expectations, and material assets to work on behalf of constituent members and, in many cases, for a larger public good" (11). Their study points to the unique capacities of civic-based networks to remedy disasters and epidemics if institutions and authorities can effectively catalyze and integrate them into the risk management processes. Public health officials, communities, and individual citizens should equally shoulder this public responsibility and collaborate in mobilizing civic infrastructure to ensure better surveillance, to implement good risk reduction measures, to take better care of affected communities and individuals, and to take viral bodies out of circulation.

These discussions about individual responsibilities emphasize the important role that the individual plays in the risk management of global epidemics, and possible ways professional communicators can intervene to help to better cope with global risks. Such interventions may cause unique problems, such as privacy breaching, racial discrimination, coercion, and the risks of objectifying sick individuals. Numerous studies point out the moral quandaries and challenges associated with the delicate line between meeting public health needs and protecting individual rights (Gostin, Bayer, and Fairchild; Applegate). With restraint, caution, and collaborative problem solving, however, concerned citizens can participate in managing local risks and protecting local communities from huge losses. What follows investigates a transcultural grassroots risk management movement in which Chinese mainlanders and overseas Chinese employed global digital networks to negotiate appropriate risk measures to prevent the import of the H1N1 flu virus into China. These competing bottom-up travel advices eventually made their way into regional and national public health policies to contain H1N1 flu outbreak in China.

The First Imported Case: Netizens Activated

Amid the confusion surrounding the global risk conflicts about H1N1 flu epidemic, China witnessed a massive wave of tactical, transcultural risk management initiated by both mainlanders and overseas Chinese in affected countries in North America, South America, and Japan. Angry Internet users, or netizens, in mainland China, launched so-called human flesh searches to dig up identities of the early imported H1N1 flu cases and published thousands of Internet posts accusing them of being "selfish" (Lai 04). A type of crowd sourcing, or inviting contributions from online communities to solve local problems, human flesh searches rely on collaboration among roughly four hundred million Internet users in China who use blogs and forums to gather and share information. This practice is sometimes described as "witch hunts for a digital age" conducted by "lynch mobs" (Fletcher) or "Internet-powered manhunts" in which "thousands of cybervigilantes write to expose the personal traits of perceived evildoers and publish them" online (O'Brien). As Tania Branigan suggests, the Internet plays a very important role in China because of official media control. The term *netizens* captures this "sense of the Internet as a space for social and political discussion" as well as civic intervention (Branigan).

Transnational Bodies Encounter the Human Flesh Search Engine

At the beginning of the H1N1 flu outbreak in China, tremendous human and financial resources were spent in tracking down all close contracts of early cases and putting them in quarantine to control the spread of the virus. Because of the immense epidemiological efforts and widespread fear that the epidemic generated, the first few imported H1N1 flu cases attracted a lot of

225

attention from both official media and alternative media. Stories about the transnational chains of imported cases were dramatized and widely circulated in Chinese media. This section focuses on both official and unofficial media responses to the first imported case in China.

Official Risk Measures

On May 12, 2009, the first anniversary of the tragic Wenchuan Earthquake in the Sichuan Province, many rebuilding efforts and memorial activities took place. Media attention was redirected to another major event on May 11: the first imported H1N1 flu case hospitalized in Chengdu, the capital of Sichuan, and the mass contact tracing efforts taking place both throughout the region and in Beijing.

Bao Xueyang was an otherwise ordinary thirty-year-old graduate student returning from University of Missouri (MU) in Columbia to his home town in Sichuan. He left the United States from St. Louis on May 7, transferred in Tokyo and Beijing on May 8 and May 9, respectively, and flew from Beijing to Chengdu, Sichuan, on May 10. He developed a sore throat on May 8 and began running a fever on May 9 on his flight back to Sichuan. After his arrival on the afternoon of May 9, he took a taxi to a local hospital and was quickly diagnosed as a suspect case by the local CDC.

The municipal government of Chengdu held a rather unusual press conference at 3 A.M. on May 10, announcing the diagnosis of a suspect case, the activation of its emergency mechanism, and the search for Bao's close contacts on his flight back to Chengdu. On the same evening, the Ministry of Health (MOH) announced that China's first confirmed H1N1 flu case was found in Sichuan, and Beijing's Health Bureau convened its meeting to activate Beijing's emergency system. Over thirty institutions, including the CDC, the emergency center, the department of tourism, foreign affair office, and police forces, launched an intensive campaign to track down Bao's 144 close contacts on his flight from Tokyo to Beijing (Li, Ye, Wang, and Yang). In all, 383 close contacts from twenty-one provinces on those flights, including 59 foreign travelers, had to be tracked down and isolated. Meanwhile, all travelers and staff from the Beijing Air Travel Hotel that Bao stayed in were put on intensive medical observation for seven days, which caused "a lot of anxiety among foreigners with next-day travel plans" ("Beijing Air Travel Hotel"). Local government officials "won the understanding and cooperation from most travelers" by helping to rearrange their travel schedules ("Beijing Air Travel Hotel"). The first imported case also attracted intense attention from national leaders. On May 11, President Hu Jintao issued a directive requiring all-out efforts to prevent the spread of H1N1 flu in China. Vice Premier Li Keqiang visited Bao, medical workers, and quarantined individuals in the hospital and encouraged them to collaborate closely to cure the disease (Huo, Ma, and Yan).

Institutional Risk Responses

Whereas the official epidemiological responses focused on prevention and control through contact tracing, quarantine, and thorough disinfection, news media turned to various sources to find out more about Bao. Journalists contacted the news office of MU and returning MU students to learn about the outbreak in Missouri and at MU. An infectious disease specialist in Beijing revealed that "Bao's roommate at [the University of Missouri] had fever and Bao had close contact with his roommate without taking any preventive measures. Bao also went to local supermarkets before flying home" (Huo, Ma, and Yan). The reporters did online searches and found a blog posted by someone who claimed to be Bao's roommate at MU. In a post titled "My roommate became famous," the blogger claimed to "feel feverish" on May 7, but his physician provided no special treatment. The blogger also revealed that his roommate, Bao, went back to China to get married (Huo, Ma, and Yan).

The spokesman of Sichuan Infectious Disease Hospital provided detailed updates about Bao's situation, including that Bao did not cooperate well with his caretakers at the beginning of his treatment and often took off his mask without approval from medical workers (Li, Ye, Wang, and Yang). Another journalist interviewed doctors in charge of Bao's treatment and found out that Bao's biggest wish was to obtain access to a computer and Internet in his ward. His doctor said, "Our hospital is working hard to make this possible. We will try our best to meet his needs" (Li, Ye, Wang, and Yang). Both the news media and hospital authorities tried to personalize Bao as the first H1N1 flu case in China by exploring contexts surrounding his onset of disease and his experiences as a patient under treatment. Whereas these personal details were reported to provide a human face to the first case, they were soon put under close scrutiny by the larger online communities and evaluated through the lens of traditional values, such as collectivism, patriotism, and social responsibility.

In addition, responses from national leaders and local hospitals suggest the privileges that flexible citizens enjoy in China. In light of traditional Confucian emphasis on education, students pursuing advanced degrees abroad are often considered by the public as aspiring models for younger children at home and by officials as potential specialists and investors, or global intellectual citizens who may return to work for China (Ong, "Urban Assemblages"). Bao received special treatment in his stay in the hospital and enjoyed media exposure at regional and national levels. His experiences, however, were complicated by his additional identity as a transnational virus carrier who introduced an unknown disease to a country only six years ago recovering from its anti-SARS campaign. When questions about intentions and motivations worked along with the epidemiological needs to contain the health threats posed by his transnational travel, Bao began to encounter widespread criticism, charges of selfishness and lying, and stigmatization.

Operating via the Human Flesh Search Engine

Although the government never blamed Bao for creating a public health crisis, Chinese netizens criticized him for violating cultural virtues and shirking individual responsibilities. Concerned Chinese netizens quickly started human flesh searches and worked together to dig out personal information about Bao. His national identity number, name, age, home address, education history, and flight numbers were soon found out and published online. Also published were critiques of his intention, his requests for special treatment, and the privilege he enjoyed as indicated by the visit from top officials. Enraged by his decision to travel home despite his close contact with suspect cases, Chinese netizens nicknamed him "Bao Manman," which can be translated as "Bao Hide-hide" or "Bao Lie-lie." The online critiques of Bao soon transformed the combination of random factors surrounding his infection into a narrative of intention and behavior: coming from the epicenter and having close contact with people with flu, Bao lied about his symptoms when entering China and brought "disasters" home. To make things worse, he travelled home and "polluted" the community at large because of "personal affairs [to get married]," yet he claimed that he travelled home because of his noble goal to "assist the post-earthquake rebuilding efforts" ("Bao Manman"). One indignant poster asked, "As a piece of trash refusing to effectively isolate yourself even in the hospital, what can you offer to rebuilding efforts? To rebuild with a swarm of viruses" ("Extremely Despise").

One interesting and widely reprinted post urged netizens to push Bao to offer public apologies and to end the "heroic treatment" he enjoyed from central and local governments ("Call for Action"). The post's entire argument was based on traditional Confucian values, such as *zhi* (wisdom), *ren* (benevolence), *zhong* (loyalty), and *xiao* (fidelity) (Ding, "Confucius"). It employed a series of parallel structures focusing on the four virtues to launch its criticism:

> Bao manman is *unwise* because he neither thought about nor took preventive measures despite massive outbreaks in his region; he *acted against benevolence* because he did not report about his symptoms and neglected the well-being of fellow citizens when entering China; he is *disloyal* because he imported the virus to his motherland, wasted enormous public resources, and caused damages to the society; he *is infidel* because, instead of declaring his disease or imposing self-quarantine after the onset of symptoms, he had close contact with his family members. ("Call for Action"; emphasis added)

This post aroused a lot of interest and support because of its heavy emphasis on traditional Chinese values, its focus on nationalism and patriotism, and its reliance on collectivist values (i.e., putting communal interests above personal ones) to create the exigence for Bao's public apology. Another force that drove the rhetorical transformation of Bao's identity came from online "isolation journals" posted by Bao's close contacts who shared the same flights with him. Such bloggers were put to home quarantines or mandatory medical observation in infectious disease hospitals. While some bloggers wrote about their "imposed paid holidays" with a humorous tone, others, including overseas students returning home, were enraged about the inconveniences inflicted upon them and the interruption of their short trips back home (Yue Liu, "Bao Manman").

The online discussions quickly transformed Bao from an unfortunate transnational traveler infected with H1N1 flu into an intentional and irresponsible virus carrier, clearly demonstrating the interarticulation of people, ideas, and ideologies via the Internet. The "cybercirculation and mediation of representations" of the first imported case also reveal the intersecting ideological, cultural, historical, and geopolitical forces that help to rhetorically transform Bao's identities both as a flexible citizen and as the first imported case in China (Hesford and Schell 467).

Stigmatized

As stated earlier, culturally and ethnically speaking, mainland China and overseas Chinese are closely interconnected. In official discourses, overseas Chinese are always depicted as a patriotic group that comprises an integral part of China. One widely circulated popular song illustrates this view by describing overseas Chinese, both longtime immigrants and temporary sojourners, as "those of *us* who live abroad but still maintain an authentic Chinese heart" ("My Chinese Heart"). In addition to sharing cultural and language heritages, upon their return to China, overseas Chinese look like one of "us" and become indistinguishable from mainlanders. The fear of healthy-looking H1N1 flu carriers returning from the epicenter radically changed the transnational Chinese travelers' status as a privileged group passing as one of "us." Their ability to cross national boundaries allows them to not only temporarily become one of "us" but also bring their dangerous viral luggage and spread the virus in China. This ability to pass, in times of global epidemics, brings the fear of the implosion of the boundaries of insiders versus outsiders, inclusion versus exclusion, and finally, us versus them.

Overseas Chinese were transformed from privileged flexible citizens into suspicious virus carriers who got shunned and stigmatized exactly because of their ability to move across national borders. One returning student reported a stigmatizing experience. When he walked out of the temperature checkpoint in the Shanghai Pudong International Airport, he overheard a floor cleaner saying to her coworker in the local dialect, "Look at these people—the financial crisis drives them bankrupt and the swine makes them sick. Now they come back to exploit and infect us" (S. Chen, "Mainland Net Users" 4). Such comments clearly reflect impacts of global inequalities and the bitterness experienced by less-privileged groups who watch the emerging global elite accumulate wealth and power while being themselves left out of such transnational activities. Similar discrimination against returning overseas Chinese was widespread online and offline both because of fear about the further spread of H1N1 flu and because of the tensions at work between the global mobile elite and territory-bound populations. With three of the earliest confirmed swine flu patients being students studying in American universities who flew home for the summer, many mainland netizens suggested that the government ban overseas Chinese, particularly students studying abroad, from returning home. Having recently eradicated SARS, most Chinese people still vividly remembered the nightmarish, nationwide fear that SARS would reach the poor countryside and get out of control. Reflecting such fear, some netizens asked for self-imposed voluntary quarantines and suggested that overseas returnees should "stop talking about American criteria [in dealing with H1N1 flu]; if you like the U.S. that much, then stay there" ("Bao Manman"). Others recommended suing transnational Chinese travelers who imported H1N1 flu virus, claiming "their trips could lead to the *deaths of millions of people*" (S. Chen, "Mainland Net Users" 4; emphasis added).

The global flow of electronic and print discourses mediates "the production of cultural identity, locality, and the 'virtual neighborhood' in a transnational era" (Ong 10). Quickly and widely circulated in the global media networks, local discourses can influence discourses produced in other local or global contexts and result in what Doreen Starke-Meyerring calls "transcontextualizing" impacts (493). The trend of accusations and anger of mainland netizens stigmatized and thus alienated overseas Chinese. Xing Lu points out that the anti-SARS rhetoric employed by Chinese authorities constituted "a renewed sense of patriotism" that was "characterized by patriotism and sacrifice for the party and the country" and "reinforced the traditional Chinese cultural value of collectivism" (109). The cultural values of patriotism, sacrifice, and collectivism are shared by mainlanders as well as overseas Chinese. In fact, these values become one of the binding cultural forces that unite Chinese all over the world in times of crises and disasters.

Rhetoric of Patriotism and Restraint

Independent overseas Chinese websites and bulletin board systems (BBSs) witnessed heated discussions about the widespread criticism of irresponsible overseas Chinese spreading H1N1 flu virus in mainland China. Overseas Chinese students faced a difficult decision concerning returning home during their summer break.

Self-Restraint for Collective Interests

In response to the widespread critiques about returning students as virus carriers, a student studying at Columbia University, a Mr. Sheng, issued a public letter online on May 13, 2009, urging those with travel plans to postpone their trips to avoid introducing the H1N1 flu virus into China and possibly starting massive outbreaks (Lu and Liu 3; Wang, "About a Love"; "Love"). For those who had to travel back to China, the letter urged that they "act responsibly and impose home quarantine for at least one week before going out to public places." He also suggested that returning travelers should keep the tickets of all public transportation vehicles they took in case they fell sick with H1N1 flu and the health authorities had to track down their close contacts.

Advocating caution and restraint, the letter functioned as a transcultural, bottom-up travel advisory asking overseas Chinese in epicenters to act responsibly and postpone nonessential travel (Lu and Liu 3). It exerted huge influence on China's unofficial, transnational risk management tactics because of its effective use of ethos (showing good will) and pathos (deep care for the country and for its people). The proposal also came at a kairotic moment, when online criticism of "those selfish overseas Chinese" accumulated so exponentially that it ran the risk of alienating China's privileged flexible citizens distributed all over the world. It redirected the energy away from negative finger-pointing. Indeed, with the help of transnational networks, it tipped another social epidemic of responsibility taking and created a viral discourse on self-restraint and caution for those travelling from the epicenter.

Quick Dissemination, Rhetorical Repercussions of the Open Letter

Communication technologies, particularly the Internet, facilitate transcultural flows of public discourses. In this case, the transnational digital networks enabled the transcultural negotiations about possible ways to reduce the risk of flexible citizens importing the H1N1 flu virus to mainland China. Sheng's letter was originally published via university-sponsored listservs and his QQ groups (the most popular instant-messaging application in China) (Lu and Liu 3). It attracted so much attention from overseas students that they forwarded it to friends using instant-messaging tools, such as MSN or QQ groups. Very quickly, the letter was reposted in popular discussion forums for overseas students as well as students intending to study abroad. Most of its readers endorsed the suggestion by replying with positive comments, such as "admire," "serious agreement," "strong support," and "very practical" (Lu and Liu 3).

Guangzhou Daily published the first report about Mr. Sheng's open letter on May 14, only one day after Sheng posted his letter online. This report soon "attracted widespread attention and debates and was reprinted repeatedly in the top headlines of famous Chinese websites such as Xinhua, Sina, and Tenxun" on the same day (Lu and Liu 3). By 9 P.M. that day, the Sina report had over four thousand comments from its users. Meanwhile, Sheng's letter attracted not only major domestic media, such as China Central TV, Beijing TV, and Shangdong TV, but also thousands of visitors to his Facebook account, all within one day (Lu and Liu 3).

Sheng's suggestion functioned as a hybrid exit (from the epicenters) and entry (into China) screening measure. It urged returning Chinese to consider themselves as potential virus carriers and to voluntarily employ home quarantine and temperature checks in the incubation period, which minimized the chance of unknowingly spreading the virus in the larger community. This hybrid exit-and-entry measure was particularly effective because it facilitated a surveillance gaze coming from everyone leaving epicenters for China, rather than from official health registration forms or temperature-screening devices. It embodied the collectivist value of sacrificing individual convenience for the sake of the larger interests of the motherland and local communities.

In their rhetorical model of risk communication, Steven Katz and Carolyn Miller see "influencing," not informing, "as the fundamental communicative relationship," and they acknowledge "the important role that values and affect play in all aspects of a decision" (132). As a grassroots risk communication effort, the open letter embodies what Katz and Miller advocate: the use of both knowledge and emotion to move people into action (131). Through strong appeals to shared values (self-sacrifice and patriotism) and emotions (fear of infection and anxiety of importing the virus), the letter effectively employs ethos and pathos "to achieve consensus and cooperation" (Katz and Miller 132). It not only led to heated discussions in virtual Chinese communities but, more important, produced voluntary and significant changes of action in the high-risk group of overseas Chinese, particularly among overseas students. Because of these events, many overseas students cancelled their trips back to China, citing the following reasons for their decisions: to avoid infecting beloved ones, to sacrifice personal convenience and to show loyalty to the country, to discipline oneself in epidemics, and to act responsibly for the sake of the motherland and families ("Love"; "Student Studying in the U.S.A."; "To Return or Not"). Of those who did return home, most employed home isolation to watch for flu symptoms after their arrivals. This was true for not only of about ten thousand of study-abroad students returning to the Jiangsu Province but also of many of the early confirmed cases, who imposed home quarantines upon their return and avoided spreading the virus in crowded public places ("About 10,000").

Official Rhetoric of Solidarity

Starting as a grassroots risk management tool, the bottom-up travel advice for overseas Chinese was widely circulated in transnational networks. It attracted so much heated discussion both in national media and among netizens that the Chinese government started to intervene to avoid stigmatizing its flexible citizens studying, working, or living abroad. *China Daily* published an interview on May 15, 2009, with Zeng Guang, the chief epidemiologist at the Chinese Center for Disease Control and Prevention, who recommended that overseas students avoid close contact with high-risk populations before returning to China and report to health authorities if any flu symptom appeared (Wang, "About a Love").

On May 16, one day after his interview with *China Daily*, Zeng issued a public letter for overseas students via the Xinhua News Agency. He began by asking students to take good care and to stay away from crowded public places in outbreak areas if they had no travel plans that summer. For those who would travel back to China, he recommended self-quarantine for several days after arriving home and cooperation with public health officials if flu symptoms appeared. He also wrote, "One thing is for sure: China will open its door wide for all overseas students no matter what happens. We welcome you to return to your motherland. We also have the ability to ensure your health and safety here" (Zeng). His letter soon acquired visibility online and was widely circulated in domestic and overseas Chinese websites.

On May 17, 2009, Premier Wen Jiabao visited the first confirmed case in Beijing, a student returning from New York. During his visit, Wen said,

> Our motherland is the home for all overseas students and we care deeply about your health. . . . Those of you studying in countries affected by the swine flu should learn about preventive measures and I hope you understand the prevention and control measures taken by the government if you travel home. (cited in "To Return or Not")

During the 2003 SARS outbreak, top leaders, such as President Hu Jintao and Wen, made numerous visits to medical research centers, hospitals, and universities (Xing Lu, "Construction of Nationalism"; Lin).These official visits demonstrated top leaders' passion for the people, their all-out support for the anti-SARS campaign, as well as their benevolence (ren), the most emphasized Confucian virtue, as national leaders (Ding, "Confucius"). Premier Wen's visit of the confirmed case in Beijing in 2009 sent a clear message about top leaders' moral support for infected overseas Chinese. These official gestures of care and support indicated the determination of the Chinese central government both to ensure domestic and overseas collaboration in its anti–H1N1 flu campaign and to build solidity among mainlanders and overseas Chinese.

Official Appropriation of Local Risk Management Tools

As discussed earlier, local tactical suggestions of limited or no travel interacted with discourses from other contexts and for other purposes. These risk tactics eventually became co-opted by national and regional authorities as a strategic official travel advisory to better control transnational travelers (see fig. 5.1 for an overview of the timeline surrounding the risk management processes). With H1N1 flu cases mounting throughout the world, regional and national authorities quickly appropriated the bottom-up travel advisory and issued suggestions and policies targeting overseas Chinese. For instance, on May 20, Beijing health authorities released an open letter requiring returning overseas Chinese to "stay away from parties and relatives as well as any other activities that involved a lot of people" (S. Chen, "Italian Quarantined" 5). They issued another health alert suggesting that overseas returnees avoid taking public transportation if they developed symptoms and had to seek medical assistance ("Beijing Health Bureau").

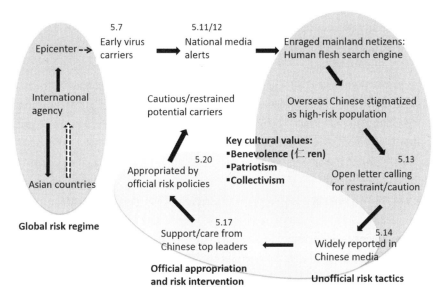

Figure 5.1. Overview of the risk management processes

This fairly quick upward movement of risk management tactics illustrates the impact of cultural values on transcultural unofficial risk tactics, official risk regime, and transnational networks. Facilitated by grassroots risk intervention and negotiations, China successfully implemented a mix of entry-and-exit screening measures, with every returning Chinese functioning as the epidemiological gaze that looked for possible symptoms to ensure compliance and self-quarantine. This co-opted risk measure helped to push many suspected cases to implement home isolation and to seek timely medical attention, which, in turn, prevented widespread infection caused by returning travelers in May and June 2009.

My analysis of the global risk management of SARS and H1N1 flu reveals several important findings for global risk communication theories. First, emotions, attitudes, and cultural values play significant roles in transcultural risk communication processes. In new and ambiguous risk situations, epistemic communities may produce contradictory and competing knowledge claims, which, in turn, confuse the public and damage the credibility of scientific authorities. Amidst such heightened fear and uncertainty, risk communicators must provide not only objective scientific narratives about the risks but also moral support based on empathy, cultural values, and concerns for humanity and equity. As demonstrated by several studies in John H. Powers and Xiao Xiaosui's edited collection on the social construction of SARS, in anti-SARS campaigns undertaken in Singapore, China, and Hong Kong, appeals to patriotism, heroism, and cultural values are as important as, if not more important than, the scattered and competing scientific findings about the unknown epidemic (Weber, Tan, and Law; Xiang Lu, "Construction"; Chin-Chuan Lee, "Liberalization"). At the beginning of new and emerging epidemics, it is far from enough to tell the public that scientists still know very little about the new epidemic, but the public should not panic anyhow because experts will get things under control. Instead, risk experts should respond both from scientific perspectives *and* the people's point of view, since *we*, not *us* the experts and *them* the ignorant public, will have to work together to contain the emerging epidemics. In fact, the public may play an equally important role whenever mass mobilization is needed to ensure that individuals shoulder their social responsibility in observing travel restrictions and social-distancing practices. Effective consideration of emotional needs and cultural values of affected communities can help experts to make better risk policies, to communicate more effectively about risk measures, and to produce more desirable outcomes.

In global risk crises, local intervention and public involvement may play different, yet equally important roles in scientific calculation and official decision making. Whenever public participation is needed for risk control purposes, grassroots risk communicators enjoy unique advantages over the experts. Instead of relying solely on rational knowledge claims, grassroots risk activists have a unique capacity to generate empathy, moral appeals, and a sense of communal needs. Both to create sticky messages and to tip an epidemic of discourses, grassroots risk efforts must strategically employ emotional and cultural appeals, kairotic intervention, and coordinated rhetorical efforts across a variety of media platforms. Accordingly, to prepare students as competent transcultural risk communicators, we must teach students global literacies, new media literacies, and rhetorical calculation, as well as the ability to analyze the cultural instead of focusing on culture as substance and empirically verifiable traits.

Transcultural communities may play an important role in global risk management and exert great impacts on transnational risk policies. Existing risk communication theories have yet to offer good analytical tools to investigate impacts of transcultural forces on global risk negotiations because of the nation-centric focuses. Concepts such as flexible citizens, transcultural connectivities, and global flows enable an in-depth investigation of how transnational communities participate in the risk management of global epidemics through the use of digital networks and grassroots movements. These transcultural forces and communication practices would remain invisible to risk communication theories that view nation-states as the unit of analysis.

My study also demonstrates the blurring line between risk issues and economic and political ones, the contingent nature of risk knowledge, and the interaction and intimate connections between global risk policies and local material conditions. The risks posed by new global epidemics are highly indeterminable and incontrollable because of the lack of knowledge about diseases, constantly mutating viruses, and global flows of people and goods that greatly facilitate the spread of viruses. In addition, such risk conflicts are further complicated by the vastly different responses from individual countries, intergovernmental organizations, and transcultural communities as well as by the challenges to coordinate responses from various players participating in the risk negotiation processes. Compared with the more relaxed responses taken by the United States, Canada, and other European countries to H1N1 flu outbreak, middle-income and low-income countries employed more-rigorous biopolitical measures because of their limited medical resources, their crowded populations that greatly facilitate the spread of the virus, and the urgent need to block the virus out of their borders. Analysis of transnational risk conflicts requires unwavering and constant attention to the unique local material contexts, political and ideological structures and priorities, communication practices, economic interests, and cultural differences surrounding all involved individual cultures and transnational key players. To better understand the cause of such drastic differences in transnational risk management approaches, one has to look beyond the discourse networks surrounding risk conflicts and investigate the material conditions and historical contexts that helped to shape and determine local responses. Only with such deep and localized knowledge can one find out ways to participate in the analysis and intervention processes and to negotiate mutually acceptable solutions to transnational risk conflicts.

Conclusion: Transcultural Communication and Rhetoric about Global Epidemics

This book contributes to studies of transcultural communication and the rhetoric of global epidemics through nuanced investigation of discourses about SARS, the first emerging epidemic in the new millennium. It proposes and applies a theoretical framework of transcultural communication to study communication about global events in their full complexity. Through thick description and analysis, I explore vastly different cultural sites where international, national, institutional, extra-institutional, and transcultural actors communicated about SARS and negotiated about possible ways to manage its accompanying risks. As viral discourses circulated in global media, SARS was rhetorically transformed from a medical epidemic into epidemics of anti-communist and anti-immigration ideologies, infrastructural inadequacy, and technological backwardness. With different magnitudes of local outbreaks, countries and regions, such as the United States, China, Canada, Singapore, and Hong Kong, took unique and radically localized approaches to manage local SARS risks. Whereas some resorted to Confucian values and patriotism for mass mobilization purposes, others turned to modern technologies and economic rationality to reduce both local transmission and economic losses. This concluding chapter elaborates on my contributions to transcultural communication, to the study of global risks, to professional communication and pedagogies, and to the rhetoric of global epidemics.

Building a Theory of Transcultural Risk Analysis

With health risks, such as SARS, developing on a global scale, the risk analysis of global epidemics poses a great challenge to existing risk communication theories, whose explanatory power is severely limited by a narrow focus on industrial practices and institutional issues within single cultures in the North American context. This study of transcultural risk management of SARS shows the indeterminable and uncontrollable nature of global risks and the contestation surrounding risk definitions among national, international, institutional, and extra-institutional actors. My proposed theoretical framework of transcultural communication serves as a useful tool for global risk analysis because of its attention to transcultural forces, global flows, power dynamics, knowledge production and negotiations and impacts of local contexts on risk communication practices.

Besides the theoretical framework of transcultural risk analysis, this project also offers insight for the study of risk communication in non-Western cultures with a critical contextualized approach. A critical contextualized approach considers the investigation of power relations, knowledge-making practices, and local cultures and contexts essential for the study of transcultural risk communication practices in non-Western cultures. Through critical contextualized analysis, my study of the 2009 H1N1 flu explains not only why Asian countries took extremely rigorous preventive measures but also what contributed to the different risk management approaches taken by the United States and by China.

Further, my investigation of informal participatory risk communication analyzes the roles that alternative media can play amid official silence, as in the case of SARS, or in confusing global risk politics, as in the case of H1N1 flu. Extra-institutional risk communication processes operated differently in relation to SARS and the H1N1 flu, with the former relying more on guerrilla media and the latter operating mainly via the Internet. In 2003, transcultural alternative media served as the platform for practitioners with access to insider information to send out unauthorized and unverified risk messages to the general public that, in turn, challenged the official containment narrative. In 2009, transnational virtual communities of mainlanders and overseas Chinese negotiated about best risk management approaches to prevent the import of the H1N1 flu virus by overseas returnees. Enraged mainlanders activated human flesh searches to dig out the identities of the first few cases and to explore ways to discipline transnational bodies as potential virus carriers. In response, overseas Chinese responded to online discrimination and stigmatization by proposing a bottom-up, self-imposed travel advisory that urged all overseas Chinese either to postpone their travel plans or to quarantine themselves at home upon their return to China. In both epidemics, concerned citizens' tactical use of alternative media produced profound changes in global risk management processes and greatly influenced the contours of global risk politics surrounding SARS and H1N1 flu.

Pedagogical Implications for Professional Communication

As demonstrated by this book, many boundaries currently taught in professional communication pedagogy no longer hold true in our contemporary globalized and digitally connected world. The three boundaries discussed below separate industry and academia, mainstream media and alternative media, and nation-states and transnational connectivities.

Dismantling the Boundary between Industry, Academia

The field has witnessed an ongoing argument concerning whether we should base our teaching approaches solely on industrial needs (Krestas, Fisher, and Hackos; Rainey, Turner, and Dayton; see fig. c.1) or whether academic research should serve as another driving force (Miller, "Humanistic Rationale"; Miller, "What's Practical"; Johnson-Eilola; see fig. c.2).

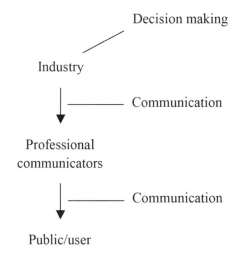

Figure c.1. Model of professional communication as service to industry

Preoccupied with the industry-academia divide, professional communicators tend to fall into alliance with one or the other. My study shows, however, that we pay relatively little attention to the third force, the public, who are often viewed as passive consumers of professional communication products, such as user manuals or risk messages. Citizens are often excluded from decision-making processes because they, unlike industry, do not usually hire professional communicators to serve as user advocates in information design processes (Salvo; Johnson; Johnson-Eilola) or in risk communication processes (Grabill and Simmons).

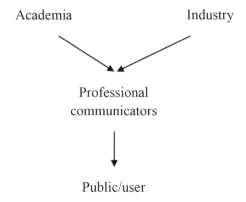

Figure c.2. Forces shaping professional communication pedagogy

The same argument can be extended to areas where no formal mechanism exists to allow professional communicators to participate in usability testing or in research on user needs. In other words, professional communicators have a civic responsibility to intervene in high-stakes communication processes, despite the fact that no institutions sponsor such advocacy for the public. Meeting the responsibility helps to protect the public's right to survival and to promote sustainable community development. We must help students understand the need to go beyond industrial service by viewing the community and the wider public as one of the key stakeholders in professional communication processes (see fig. c.3).

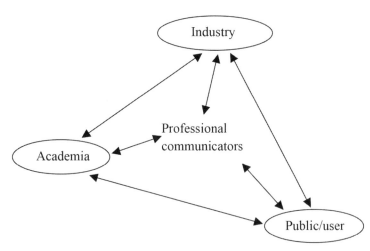

Figure c.3. Ideal model of open communication among three key stakeholders in professional communication

———

To achieve this goal, we must change the way we talk about professional communication research and practices. I argue that we must reintroduce the public as an integral part of any professional communication event that we discuss in the classroom. Raising awareness precedes planning and taking action. Only by breaking down the existing boundary, if not binary, between industry and academia can we help establish the public as an equally important stakeholder, which, in turn, helps to promote open communication concerning issues that influence the public's economic, environmental, health, and technological well-being. Figure c.3 presents an ideal model of open communication among the three stakeholders—industry (including institutions and other power apparatuses), academia, and the public—in professional communication processes. The professional communicator should function as researcher, mediator, negotiator, and facilitator in processes of communication and decision making among the three stakeholders.

Of course, it will require tremendous effort and long-term commitment to public interest to put this proposed model into practice. Here, Johndan Johnson-Eilola's revolutionary reconceptualization of professional communicators into symbolic analysts can help the field cultivate the ability to reintroduce the public as an essential stakeholder in professional communication processes. Students need the four skills of experimentation, collaboration, abstraction, and systems thinking to "develop tactics for avoiding the nearly automatic subordination of communication to technological values" (Johnson-Eilola 260). Only by helping them develop these skills can we succeed in promoting and accomplishing open communication. In addition, service learning should be incorporated as an essential component of professional communication curricula to provide students with real-world experience in working with publics to investigate local needs and to solve existing problems (Bowdon and Scott; Coogan; Sapp and Crabtree; Scott, "Practice of Usability").

Breaking Down the Boundary between Mainstream, Alternative Media

But what media outlets can professional communicators employ to access and evaluate public needs in the proposed model of open professional communication? Industries and institutions have strategic control of corporate, commercial, and mainstream media, which they employ for top-down communication to disseminate official messages and to shape public opinions.

However, thanks to technological advances, particularly open access to the Internet, the public can tactically employ alternative media and guerrilla media for bottom-up communication. Such practices of communication from below, if employed effectively, have transformative potential and can effectively influence official decision-making processes—an ability that has been demonstrated by numerous studies (Ding, "Rhetorics"; Ding and Zhang; Rheingold; Sun). Accordingly, professional communication classrooms can and should teach students media literacy and help them to cultivate rhetorical savvy to gain tactical access to media to reach desired audiences. Doing so helps students not only to know about the existence and potential of such media but, more important, to tactically employ such media to promote public interests.

Dismantling the Boundary between Nations, Transnational Connectivities

Earlier, this chapter discussed the importance of my proposed theoretical framework of transcultural professional communication and critical contextualized methodology. Both tools can function well in the teaching of intercultural communication. It is important to emphasize the limitation of using nation-states as the unit of analysis and to explore transcultural connectivities in intercultural communication practices. One way to make transcultural forces accessible to undergraduate students is to examine how communication technologies, particularly the Internet, function to mediate transnational negotiations about global risk, health, and technological issues. Well-designed cases and scenarios can be extremely useful in teaching roles played by transcultural connectivities in global events, which is discussed in more detail in the next section.

Challenges, Issues in Professional, Risk Communication

Situated in a global context, this book highlights challenges posed by professional communication and risk communication. First, those who enjoy privileged access to risk information and those who take charge of the production of high-risk health documents are often professionals, such as epidemiological researchers, physicians, or scientists, who do not perceive themselves as technical writers. In other words, we must acknowledge and cope with the fact that professionals rather than professional communicators with formal training in technical writing are more likely to serve as risk communicators in health crises.

To reduce this gap between training and job duties, we must renew our commitment to service courses in professional communication and business, technical, and scientific writing so as to reach future professionals. Only by moving away from the perception of technical writing as service to industry can we adequately address and effectively teach ethical decision making and civic action. Moreover, by reaching out to and influencing future professionals, we can help educate and produce more critical and conscientious professionals with the knowledge and skills to act ethically in difficult communicative situations.

Second, this study of alternative media in risk communication raises questions about ethical practices and possible ways to teach ethical decision making, including: When public health is seriously threatened, should professional communicators take some personal or professional risks to communicate threats to the public through formal or alternative media, or should they passively abide by top-down orders for the sake of job security? This is by no means an easy question. As Donna Kienzler points out, the teaching of critical thinking skills and ethical practices should be accompanied by explicit discussion of the dangers and consequences that such decisions may bring to students. Sam Dragga stresses the value of using narrative details in cases and scenarios to teach ethics in technical communication classrooms. Agreeing with his position, I believe that as part of teaching ethical practices, we should point out to our students possible choices and existing channels of communication to release risk messages to the public through case studies involving formal or alternative media. In addition, we should discuss the ethical and professional implications of such decisions. It is particularly important to teach stories of "heroes of the profession" as "models of moral rectitude and sound ethical judgment," for such cases can demonstrate to students both the difficulty, consequences, and benefits of making ethical decisions and the things they should take into consideration in their own encounters with difficult ethical problems (Dragga 175).

To problematize the use of formulaic solutions in teaching the value of alternative media in communicating health risks, I focus on two challenging issues: the blurry line between the private and public identities of the professional communicators and the limited amount of knowledge that professional communicators can obtain from their institutional positions. Alternative media provide a forum where professional communicators may speak as insiders in risk assessment processes rather than from the institutional sites they occupy. In other words, these sites offer the opportunity to speak as conscientious citizens rather than as authorized spokespersons of governments, industries, or businesses. The decision to speak without authorization blurs the boundary between work and life, public and private, professional and individual, and may usher professional communicators into strange and uncomfortable situations. Of course, to speak is not a straightforward decision, as insiders may only have access to the partial information available in their own local settings. Therefore, they can only speak about the limited knowledge they learn about the risk from their own institutional positions, which may damage the credibility and rhetorical impact of their messages.

Finally, to better prepare students for complicated and difficult communicative situations, we must move beyond the teaching of individual genres in professional communication and scientific writing classrooms. Instead, we must introduce students to the concepts of rhetorical networks, design good cases to help them to examine existing rhetorical networks about existing events, and explore strategies and heuristic tools to map and analyze rhetorical networks about those events. After developing knowledge about rhetorical networks, students can acquire a better understanding of events and explore possible points of contention and points of entry for ethical intervention and civic action.

Rhetoric of Global Epidemics and Their Risks

Emerging epidemics, such as SARS and H1N1 flu, vividly demonstrate not only global interdependence but also intersections of politics, economic development, and public health. When put together, these chapters paint a larger picture about the way rhetoric functions in global epidemics. As a historical study, this project cannot offer predictive or prescriptive rules for rhetorical intervention in future epidemics. It does, however, provide important insight about possible issues that may arise and pitfalls to avoid in the transcultural communication about global epidemics as well as available communicative channels to intervene in the negotiation about such problems. It also highlights possible strategies to avoid unproductive finger-pointing and to better facilitate transcultural collaboration in global epidemics.

Incorporating Ulrich Beck's theory of world risk society into the study of the rhetoric of global epidemics, I highlight the contingency and contention surrounding transnational policies to contain emerging epidemics. Focusing on circulation-related risks, global risk politics attempts to supervise transnational flows of people (and animal products in H1N1 flu) to prevent novel viruses from crossing national borders. Such efforts, however, are often undermined by the constant exchange of people and goods via transcontinental traffic. National authorities, in contrast, often rely more on territorial risk control measures through intensive patrol of national borders and inbound flights. Local communities invent their own tactics, which may employ various combinations of circulation-centric, territorial, or disciplinary (through the creation of completely controlled space, such as isolation wards or quarantine camps) approaches to risk reduction (Bingham and Hinchliff).

My analysis of transcultural participatory risk negotiations reveals the emergence of global and regional publics and their potential to participate in subpolitics to produce alternative lines of action (Beck). "Ad hoc individual participation" may help to forge new linkages to change the "rules and boundaries of the political" and to "shap[e] society from below" (Beck 38–40). My project offers a long list of such heroic individual endeavors, with some of them exerting far-reaching rhetorical influences, that is, Dr. Jiang Yanyong, Dr. Zhong Nanshan, founders of sosick.org, and a Mr. Sheng from Columbia University. Other influentials remained nameless, yet the impacts of their endeavors helped to produce much-needed changes. Such people include anonymous medical-care workers in Guangdong who talked about the mysterious pneumonia despite repeated censorship orders as well as students who participated in local and online deliberations to invent tactics that reduced the risk of both SARS and H1N1 flu. The successes achieved by these individuals are especially remarkable given their status as the "lowest rungs of the ladder of social recognition," a label that tends to discount or silence their lay knowledge as illegitimate.

Lisa Keränen invents the term *biocriticism* to call for "a sustained and rigorous analysis of the artifacts, texts, discursive formations, visual representations, and material practices positioned at the nexus of disease and culture" ("Addressing" 225). Employing the proposed framework of biocriticism, Lisa Keränen argues that public and scientific considerations of bioterrorism-induced risks yield political ramifications including "a powerful interlacing of our public health system and the military industrial complex" ("Bio(in) Security" 228). Numerous publications examine patient activism employed by people living with HIV/AIDS to influence governmental and medical policies, to gain greater access to clinical trials, and to better participate in communication and management of their conditions, which again investigate the interface between disease and culture (Epstein, *Impure Science*, "Construction"; Erni; Scott, *Risky Rhetoric*). My project builds on these studies and sheds new light on possible ways to examine the relationships among emerging epidemics, risks, rhetoric, and deliberation in world risk societies. In addition, it makes distinct contributions to the rhetoric of global epidemics by providing theoretical and methodological tools for in-depth examination of transnational power dynamics among a wide range of cultural, institutional, and grassroots players.

Medicalized globalization is often intricately connected with economic globalization and the accompanying environmental and economic plights it brings to the developing countries. Nick Bingham and Steve Hinchliff's study of Egypt's poultry culling during its avian flu outbreak clearly shows local political economy and household poultry raising as "non-market practices related to U.S. surpluses, military provisioning, cartels, and political power that produced the new food situation in Egypt" (185). Similarly, avian flu outbreaks were more likely to originate in Southern China because of poverty exacerbated by "global modernity" than because of what was seen as the "primitive practices" of "human being living in close proximity with their animals" (Wald 5). Therefore, health emergency measures neglecting the "social realities of the contexts in which they are applied" not only encounter constant local resistance but also find their effectiveness greatly undermined (Lakoff and Collier 20). Meanwhile, questions have been raised about the connections between avian flu and mass-produced, overcrowded, and antibiotic-reliant poultry factories, while the existing theory of wild birds as the origin of avian flu has been challenged (Sargent and Gale, "Bird Flu Trail"; Engdahl; Lean). Similar speculations have been made about the swine flu's infamous birth in the US pig farms (Branswell; Lucas). In addition, the sharing of global research breakthroughs and newly developed vaccines has become a sensitive topic. As a Malaysian newspaper pointed out in mid-May 2009, with most transnational pharmaceutical companies located in developed countries, newly developed vaccines and stockpiled drugs will be used "first to meet the needs of those countries," a practice that in turn will "victimize developing countries" ("Japan's Radically Increased H1N1 Flu Cases").

Given the impacts of globalization, cultures, and rhetoric on transcultural negotiation about global epidemics, it must be acknowledged that no universally applicable truth, coping strategy, treatment, or cure exists to enable individual cultures to contain a global epidemic. As a *Lancet* editorial points out, "history has shown that developing countries are disproportionately affected by an influenza pandemic" because of their lack of adequate public health infrastructure, funding, and expertise ("Swine Influenza" 1495). This observation is confirmed by Mexico's mysteriously high mortality rate at the beginning of the H1N1 flu outbreak. It also suggests that what works for high-income countries may not be transferable to middle-income and low-income countries. Accordingly, each country should base its policies on its unique cultural and economic conditions while learning from successes achieved and lessons illustrated by other countries and regions.

My analysis of the SARS narratives employed by the United States, mainland China, Canada, Hong Kong, and Singapore reveals that individual countries and regions took very different control approaches, which were shaped by individual historical, cultural, political, economic, and material conditions. The United States carried out its work in a scientifically driven and well-coordinated manner. It achieved great success in combating SARS for two reasons: its sophisticated public health infrastructure and emergency-response system, which were greatly improved after the 2001 anthrax scare, and the absence of any serious clusters of cases within its borders. With much-smaller and geographically confined outbreaks, Canada's anti-SARS battle was fought both in the public health arena and through international public-relations campaigns, with political lobbying playing a role as prominent as that of public health intervention and contact tracing. China enlisted individuals and communities at all levels through its mass-prevention and mass-control approach to fight an all-out battle against SARS. Despite the extreme difficulty surrounding contact tracing in worse-affected areas, such as Beijing and Guangzhou, China eradicated SARS after launching a people's war that mobilized patriotism as a rallying force for the entire nation. Singapore took a top-down approach, exerting rigorous contact tracing and encouraging the full cooperation of all citizens both through repeated emphasis of individual responsibilities and by implementing "a zero tolerance policy for breaking quarantine" (Ding and Pitts; Greenfeld 250). In contrast, Hong Kong's work was driven by governmental leadership and citizen intervention. Sosick.org's diligent efforts to map out all locations with recently found SARS patients pushed the government to issue more-transparent risk information after repeatedly rejecting public outcries.

The risk narratives surrounding the 2009 H1N1 flu pandemic tell a different story. With epicenters in North America exporting viruses to other parts of the world, Asian countries tried in vain to argue for travel advisories and border screening to reduce travel-related risks. WHO and top scientists in the United States employed economic rationality and cited the lack of utility of border screening in the SARS epidemic to justify their decisions. Contradictory claims surrounding border control resulted in a credibility crisis among epistemic communities, complaints of putting political considerations above public health, and the chaotic use of border-screening measures in many Asian countries. Official low-risk assurance from WHO and the US CDC did little to alleviate global and regional panic about the quickly spreading flu. Three factors helped to erode the credibility of expert claims: the lack of stockpiled Tamiflu in many developing countries, scientific ambiguity surrounding the health utility of border measures, and the ability of the flu virus to mutate into a much more lethal form, a precedent demonstrated by the 1918 Spanish flu. An editorial in *Scientific American* points out the limited utility of scientific research in emerging and raging epidemics:

> Molecular understanding of a virus can be frustratingly impotent. Researchers deciphered the genetic code of the SARS coronavirus within days. Yet turning that knowledge into weapons against the disease is a much slower, harder task. Developing a SARS vaccine might take at least a year. For now, control of SARS depends largely on the blunt, Dark Ages instrument of quarantine. ("Three Lessons")

Future pandemics will witness similar impotence of scientific research because of huge time delays between the cracking of a virus's genetic code and the research and development of vaccines and drugs. Without vaccines or treatments, the world may again resort to measures such as quarantine, sterilization, mass mobilization, and border control, as it did during SARS.

One key lesson taught by SARS is that global public health is everyone's business, and one missed case may quickly trigger a global outbreak. When SARS started to wane in early June, public health officials all over the world were put on alert again by a second outbreak in Toronto in late May 2003, weeks after the most recent new case had been reported. Moreover, several valuable insights can be gained from anti-SARS work in China and other parts of Asia, including possible strategies to deal with future pandemics in the absence of vaccines, treatments, or cures. To start with, mainland China,

Hong Kong, Singapore, Vietnam, and, in late May, Taiwan, took top-down risk control measures while also encouraging mass mobilization to combat SARS. Their successes in eradicating SARS were driven by strong governmental leadership, rigorous accountability systems, well-coordinated institutional responses, heroic narratives, transparent risk communication practices, and participatory prevention and control networks. John H. Powers and Xiao Xiaosui's edited collection emphasizes the importance of building heroic narratives and mobilizing national ideologies of patriotism, which helped to boost local morale and to win public support in local anti-SARS campaigns. My analysis of China's people's war against SARS demonstrates that in order to have informed publics, there is the essential need to educate concerned citizens, interest groups, and local communities about prevention and control measures. Moreover, for mass prevention and mass control, authorities must offer emotional and valuative support, channels for active participation, and mechanisms to keep everyone committed to the epidemic-control work. In other words, the public needs not only participation in risk reduction work but, more important, participation in risk decision-making processes.

The people's war against SARS in China witnessed the emergence of ad hoc civic infrastructure to "complement and enhance government's capacities and responsibilities" (Schoch-Spana, Franco, Nuzzo, and Usenza 11). Civic infrastructure at all levels served most of the functions listed in Monica Schoch-Spana, Crystal Franco, Jennifer B. Nuzzo, and Christiana Usenza's study on community engagement in catastrophic health events: to transmit educational risk information to dispersed and diverse populations, to energize social trust between authorities and communities, to utilize local knowledge to improve the feasibility and acceptability of risk management plans, and to provide self-organized and innovative solutions in unforeseen circumstances (11–12). With poor public health infrastructure, rural areas resorted to mass mobilization to identify all possible sources of infection (potential carriers and infectors) and to sever transmission channels to avoid importing SARS cases to the region. Rural families with members working in epicenters were mobilized, and parents and stay-at-home wives were recruited to dissuade sons and husbands from returning home. In addition, collaborative agricultural teams were organized to relieve migrant workers of the practical need to return home for physically demanding planting and harvesting work. In city districts, residents were rallied to protect local buildings and communities against SARS. Neighborhood committees converted all citizens into vigilant, amateur epidemiologists who were on constant lookout for SARS symptoms both in others and in themselves. With citizens well-informed and actively participating in SARS control work, communities at all levels constructed strong defenses against local transmission.

As the proverb goes, all roads lead to Rome. The goal of rhetorical study of global epidemics is not achieving consensus, which may require imposing master narratives and hegemonic knowledge amid uncertainty, ambiguity, and fear. Rather, the rhetoric of global epidemics endorses what Jean-François Lyotard calls a "listening game," or the respect for dissensus and differences and the willingness to live with ambiguity, resisting the temptation to impose one's own ideas upon other cultures with vastly different material conditions.

Domestically in China, SARS "exposed serious deficiencies in China's public health system, which [had] been weakened by insufficient funding, decentralization, and privatization over the nearly three decades of market-oriented reform" and "highlighted the devastating impacts of health-related non-traditional security threats" (Kaufman 4). As a direct result of SARS, "previous arguments about the negative downward spiral between infectious disease, economic growth, social and political stability, and national security suddenly gained currency in academic and policy circles" (Y. Zhang, "Politics" 97). In November 2003, health security began to play a prominent role in national policies, and for the first time, HIV/AIDS was listed as one of the six nontraditional security threats, along with extreme poverty and environmental security (Huang, "China" 86).

In addition, institutions at all levels started to collaborate with local communities to adopt flexible risk measures to contain and eradicate SARS. This newly acquired interest in listening also produced positive changes in China's AIDS prevention and treatment policy, which now "endorses many best practices and is promoted by the senior leadership and praised by international observers" (Kaufman 4). Despite its "newfound political will to tackle AIDS through public service provision," the government began to "realize that it lacks the full capacity to accomplish its goal and needs help from both civil society and the private sector" (Kaufman 5). With official endorsement, nongovernmental organizations proliferated to better engage hard-to-reach populations, such as gay men, to provide outreach and education (Kaufman 6).

Internationally, with China and WHO developing their own case definitions of and diagnostic criteria for SARS, Western media and WHO repeatedly questioned the credibility of China's definition and its role in downplaying the magnitude of local outbreaks. China's clinical case definition of SARS, developed in Guangdong as early as mid-February, served as the foundation for MOH's further definitional revisions and updates. Whereas the CDC and the WHO relied on the two categories of suspect and probable cases in their epidemiological surveillance, the MOH resorted to a more detailed and meticulously divided scale of cases in its attempt to contain SARS on the primary battlefield of infectious-disease hospitals.

This vast disparity in case definitions demonstrates the context-dependent and locally determined nature of medical knowledge about emerging epidemics, which is developed in response to local exigencies and material conditions. Both the US CDC's proactive approach and the MOH's reactive approach achieved great success in their national anti-SARS campaigns, attesting to the equal efficacy of coexisting yet highly different models in the battles against global epidemics. Compared with attempts to impose "universally applicable" standardized medical knowledge on individual countries, the use of locally invented and adapted case definitions may work more effectively to contain local epidemics.

The rhetoric of global epidemics also advocates a "sharing game," which requires a commitment to share the latest findings and lessons learned about epidemics. It took Guangdong medical experts months to learn about the importance of rigorous disinfection and isolation practices and the absolute need to set up designated hospitals and fever clinics to avoid cross-infection. These important lessons were not shared with the neighboring harbor city of Hong Kong. One consequence was that in late March, Hong Kong's Department of Health still ordered suspected SARS cases to report once a day to designated hospitals, "therefore guaranteeing that several hundred fever patients would be traveling on crowded mass transit daily" (Greenfeld 249). In future pandemics, mechanisms of real-time exchange and sharing of clinical and scientific data can help all countries and regions to effectively combat such pandemics and to contain them on a country-by-country basis.

Fortunately, Hong Kong and Mainland China started to build sharing mechanism at all levels after the SARS crisis. "Post-SARS exchange[s] of infectious disease intelligence" were institutionally guaranteed because of both "a Tripartite Agreement with Guangdong Province and Macao" and "a Memorandum of Understanding signed with the China's MOH" (Tsang 84). Moreover, Hong Kong and Mainland China collaborated in other areas, such as outbreak investigations, "exchange programs for epidemiology and laboratory staff," and "annual joint contingency exercises on avian influenza" (Tsang 85). This close collaboration will definitely help both parties to better cope with future epidemics through transparent risk communication and resource sharing.

The widespread use of hate speech, vicious rumors, and racial discrimination against Chinatowns and Asian communities during SARS resulted in unnecessary panic and alienation as well as sharp economic losses. These practices also brought huge burdens of public health and public-relations work as well as reduced tax incomes for several cities while also demonizing immigrants and ethnic communities. These practices inserted theories of social contagion and transgression into epidemics and pathologized certain groups and communities based on skin color, ethnic and cultural background, or country of origin.

To combat "systemic racism" in epidemics (Leung), governmental agencies, mass media, and ethnic communities must collaborate closely both to combat public misconceptions and to release transparent information in a timely manner to reduce rumormongering. In addition, affected communities can benefit from aggressive media campaigns and from government-academy-community partnerships to actively participate in both risk communication and risk decision-making processes. One admirable example of community activism is the forty-five-page, community-based report on the impact of SARS released by the Chinese Canadian National Council (CCNC), briefly discussed in chapter 4. The report employs both media analysis and individual testimonies from "members of the Chinese and Southeast Asian Canadian communities including workers, small business employers and staff from community agencies" to provide detailed documentation of the mental, psychological, and emotional impact of the social crisis caused by SARS. This powerful academia-industry-community partnership enabled the CCNC to pool resources and to launch a strong argument for systemic reform based on the collective testimony it compiled. The quality research done for the report certainly boosts its credibility and effectiveness as an advocacy statement.

Internationally, the "sharing game" requires the confidence that through close collaboration, each culture can and will determine a solution that is locally situated, empirically tested, and culturally appropriate in its own anti-epidemic campaign. Claiming that "an authoritarian impulse channeled into public health could show positive results," Karl Taro Greenfeld describes how Singapore reacted to SARS "with its usual heavy hand," home quarantining nearly one thousand citizens, with "their front doors monitored by video camera" (249). Hong Kong, "with its greater civil liberties and laissez-faire tradition," improved its institutional coordination and worked out its own unique mix of anti-SARS measures by determining "what [was] legal and what would be viewed as a violation of civil rights" at the early stage of the epidemic (Greenfeld 249). In contrast, Japan was little influenced by SARS despite its proximity to epicenters. Good personal and environmental hygiene contributed to Japan's escape from SARS. Such practices include a prohibition on spitting and an emphasis on frequent hand washing and disinfection, voluntary mask wearing when cold or flu symptoms appear, complicated water-processing systems, and well-defined recycling practices of household garbage ("Why Japan Escaped SARS"). Japan's strong public health and hygiene systems helped to greatly slow the transmission of SARS and gave the country precious time to learn about best practices from other nations and regions. These three different anti-SARS approaches provide useful models of coping strategies for future pandemics.

In sum, pandemics are the worst time for scapegoating and division. Because countries must increasingly rely on one another to combat global epidemics, governments must rally all forces and call for mass support and participation to combat epidemics. Instead of causing internal divide through scapegoating, it works better to mobilize shared national values, such as patriotism and heroism, as well as to engage in international collaboration.

After all, we are all in this together. Aren't we?

Appendix

Notes

Works Cited

Index

Appendix: Additional Notes on Methodology and Sources

It is my belief that thick description of research methods should not be a convention and privilege of ethnography but one that would strengthen any study with methodological challenges.

When discussing my studies about the transcultural communication about SARS, people have repeatedly asked me the following questions: How did you conduct the study? How did you gather and analyze your data? How did you deal with the complicated issues surrounding global communication? To answer these questions, I follow Mary Lay's lead in writing in detail about my methodology and sources, which may offer future researchers of transcultural/intercultural professional communication some insight into possible approaches to data collection, data analysis, and theoretical revision.

Data Collection Processes about a Global Epidemic

I came to this project through encounters with the Foucauldian theory of biopower, intercultural professional communication theories, and research methodologies. Deeply intrigued by the immense and far-reaching impact of SARS in April 2003, I started to collect whatever data I could find related to SARS at the beginning of the epidemic, knowing that I might use the data for a large research project later on. The data-collection processes have been ongoing until the final revision and completion of this book. Throughout the nine years from 2003 to 2012, I examined a wide range of sources, including independent overseas Chinese websites; mainstream media; public health documents, press releases, and publications; regional media in Hong Kong and Guangdong Province; scientific publications in English and Chinese; archival research of classified official documents, such as directives and circulars; informal personal interviews with residents in Beijing and Guangdong to obtain narratives of first-person experiences; graphics, such as photos and cartoons about SARS or statistic representation of SARS cases; Internet bulletin board system (BBS) posts about personal experiences with SARS; humorous or alarming text messages regarding SARS; and interviews with health officials and medical experts at national and regional levels in China.

Critical Contextualized Methodology and Data Analysis

The data-collection process seems lengthy, painstaking, and time-consuming, but it becomes much less complicated and challenging when compared with the task of data analysis. As a researcher with experiences in empirical research, linguistic and discourse analysis, and rhetorical studies, I use critical reflection, or praxis as advocated by Patricia Sullivan and James Porter, in my research projects by writing notes and journals about my ongoing struggle with the need to fairly represent all cultural players when conducting historical transcultural studies. Constantly overwhelmed by the vast amount of data about the three key players from different sources, I experienced great difficulty in initiating and writing up my first case study about the media construction of SARS. Traditional content analysis methods or rhetorical methods did not work well when transferred to studying the interaction and competition among discourses from three cultures/institutions. I often felt at a loss as to where to start, how to choose and pursue worthy lines of inquiry, and how to justify my data selection and data-analysis criteria and procedures. This state of paralytic confusion and loss lasted for over half a year, during which I continued to accumulate newly published or discovered materials about SARS while considering the possible use of existing methods or methodologies. My reading of methodological discussions and studies in intercultural communication or intercultural professional communication offered little help to overcome my paralyzed-by-data syndrome. It was during this period that I drafted another long case study examining the Guangdong Province's regional media discourse about SARS, without realizing that I actually had two separate studies (regional media and alternative media).

At the end of my first year working on the project, I began to question seriously the feasibility of transferring any monocultural methodology to a cross-cultural context. I also wondered whether methodological invention or contribution would be a result of my yearlong struggle with the study of the intercultural professional communication about SARS. In my teaching, I also grew increasingly dissatisfied with the limited explanatory power and pedagogical implications of intercultural communication theories and the limited theoretical basis for intercultural professional communication.

I started to think seriously about the struggles I had experienced in the project, the ways I came up with solutions, and possible approaches to theorize and present a more systematic way to cope with intercultural professional communication studies in other situations and for pedagogical use. That was how the critical contextualized methodology started to emerge. The articulation and application of the critical contextualized methodology (CCM) to case studies streamlined the organization of various parts and sped up the inventing, writing, and revising processes. As demonstrated by the four historical cases, the CCM is a highly flexible and dynamic tool that can be adapted for different types of projects.

The CCM's emphasis on contexts and interaction also helped me to better address challenges posed by the complicated layers of power, institutions, and key players. A shift of focus from institutions to interaction among key players enabled me to move beyond institutions to examine individuals who tactically employed alternative media and guerrilla media to fight against institutional censorship and to influence the risk communication practices, as demonstrated in chapter 3 (see Ding, "Rhetorics of Alternative Media," for more details).

New Challenges and Theory of Transcultural Communication

Research methodologies and theoretical frameworks are inseparable and, for me, were constantly evolving and developing. Although the critical contextualized methodology helped to streamline my research and data-analysis processes, I somehow felt restrained by the intercultural communication framework and the focus on nation-states as cultural players. Such a focus failed to account for the fluid population of immigrants and travelers. It also neglected the influence of global networks and the Internet, which I came across repeatedly in my reading about the global spread of SARS and the risk communication about SARS across institutional and national boundaries. I was fortunate to have Blake Scott as one of the reviewers of both my *Technical Communication Quarterly* article and my book manuscript, for he introduced me to the theories of world risk society and transcultural rhetorics and gently pushed me to think more in-depth about transcultural risk communication. I started to reformulate the theoretical framework of intercultural professional communication in a transcultural context, which helped me to cope with restraints and limitations imposed by the focus of intercultural professional communication on nation-states.

Possible Methods for Transcultural Rhetorical Studies

Methodological questions accompany theoretical revision. Once I opened the research project to transcultural communication about SARS, more challenges arose. How can one analyze transcultural communication practices adequately since such a study would include more complicated layers of key players, power relations, and interaction? After incorporating small parts of transcultural rhetorical studies in chapters 3 and 4, I started a full-scale transcultural study of the global risk conflicts about SARS in chapter 5, which posed more questions about research methods. Listed below are some of my findings.

To adequately analyze such transnational rhetorical networks of risk conflicts, one has to move beyond the usual analytical tools offered by the immediate rhetorical situations, discourse communities, or Aristotelian concepts and has to examine the cross-cultural, postproduction, multi-institutional, and transnational trajectories of related discourses. In addition, the encounters, contradictions, transformations, and negotiations among various actors exert indelible impacts on the way the transnational rhetorical networks operate and function. Therefore, transnational rhetorical study requires the mapping of a wide range of national, institutional, and cultural key players. It also involves analyzing their interacting power dynamics before investigating the way rhetoric operates to mediate transnational knowledge production and legitimation processes and to help resolve transnational risk conflicts. For instance, my study of the transnational risk conflict surrounding the Toronto travel advisory examines not only discourse employed by the health authorities of WHO and Health Canada but also those employed by Canadian federal government, opposing party leaders, Canadian media, and the general public. In addition, the Centers for Disease Control and Prevention (CDC) of the United States participated in the transnational risk conflicts surrounding travel in Toronto by issuing a downgraded travel alert that directly contradicted WHO's travel advisory. Therefore, one has to examine the CDC's telebriefing and reports about rationales for its travel alert as well as the media coverage about the CDC's travel advice in the United States and Canada.

Finally, with the ongoing H1N1 flu outbreak threatening to become another pandemic, I find it necessary to examine the connection between my theorization about transcultural communication about SARS and the communication practices surrounding the H1N1 flu. Such analysis would produce insight not only about transcultural rhetorical networks surrounding global epidemics but also about possible ways to build a rhetoric about global epidemics. Therefore, when appropriate, transcultural rhetorical studies should examine interconnected events in different historical periods in addition to crossing cultural, institutional, and professional boundaries.

To sum up, researchers should be open to theoretical and methodological challenges and, when possible, undertake the difficult tasks of theoretical and methodological revisions and inventions. Such efforts can help us to better address new questions and to produce findings transferrable to other research contexts.

For those readers who hope to learn more about how I applied the critical contextualized methodology in the four chapters (from chapters 2 to 5), I describe in great detail the research and thinking processes as well as the use of various heuristic tools offered by the methodology below.

Chapter 2 and the Use of Critical Contextualized Methodology and Enthymemic Analysis

Chapter 2 focuses on the official risk communication about SARS in the Guangdong Province from November 2002, when the first case of SARS took place in Foshan, Guangdong, to March 2003, when the regional media in Guangdong stopped investigating about SARS risks because of repeated orders of censorship. It examines the rhetorical contestations about the actual scope of and risks posed by the emerging atypical pneumonia in mainstream and commercial regional media, governmental discourses, and expert discourses. In what follows I explain my use of the critical contextualized methodology and transnational rhetorics to guide the analytical processes (see "Chapter 5 and the Use of Critical Contextualized Methodology and Transcultural Theory" for data-collection procedures).

Chapter 2 uses critical contextualized methodology to help identify tipping points, time-space axes, and key players during the official risk communication processes before March in Guangdong. I started with the identification of tipping points for this chapter, which include the two rounds of panic buying on February 8 and 10, 2003, the first and only official press conference on February 11, the heated media discussions in mid-February, and the abrupt change to media silence starting in early March. Then I moved on to the time-space–axes analysis. The spatial mapping focused on the locations in the Guangdong Province that witnessed panic buying and outbreaks of atypical pneumonia in hospitals. On the time axis, I mapped the earliest reports about atypical pneumonia cases, official and unofficial risk assessment and risk communication efforts, and patterns of media silence and underreporting from November 2002 to March 2003.

The next step was the identification of key players in the event. I started by identifying key media players, which included both mainstream media and commercial media in the region. After collecting news reports, commentaries, and retrospective reviews from the regional newspapers, I compiled all of them into one corpus and looked for types of risk communicators recorded in the media. Very quickly in my repeated readings of news reports, it became apparent that governmental institutions played a dominant role in defining the risk situations in the region. Another major force was medical experts, who were often reported and cited as the authoritative voice claiming that the local outbreaks were under control. It seemed that both key players helped to define the official risk messages delivered by the media. However, as I went on reading critical commentaries and retrospective reviews about the development of the local outbreaks, I realized that another parallel layer of classified risk communication took place among governmental institutions, medicine, and the regional media that produced radically different risk message. This classified risk communication process employed inside notifications, administrative orders of censorship, and disciplinary measures of critique and personnel removal to force the two institutions of medicine and media into silence about the actual SARS situations in the region.

To investigate the two parallel risk communication processes through the use of publicly released and classified governmental discourses, I employed the analytical tools of interaction analysis and power-knowledge analysis. The former investigates the way governmental institutions, media, and medicine interacted, negotiated, competed, and collaborated intentionally or unintentionally to shape the risk messages circulated in the region, that is, both those released to the public and those circulated via classified governmental discourses. The latter examines the power dynamics among power apparatuses, the regional media, and medicine, the types of knowledge claims each of them created, and the way such claims got legitimated, discounted, or silenced in their rhetorical contestations. Finally, context analysis was performed throughout the study because of the intricate connections among political structures, forces of mediascapes and financescapes in the region, communication practices, and economic interests. The risk communication practices only started to make sense once I took into consideration the complicated contextual factors that shaped the two simultaneously ongoing yet highly contradictory risk communication approaches.

As I focused on the risk information contained in both governmental and media discourses, I found it necessary to analyze the rhetorical messages and persuasive approaches in both types of discourses. Because of the complicated types of risk messages delivered by various key players to different audiences, it is important to really focus on the ways such messages helped to persuade the public that the local outbreak was indeed under control despite the quickly spreading epidemic. I experimented with various rhetorical theories and found enthymemic analysis the most appropriate tool to analyze the way covert and partial censorship helped to calm down the public. My enthymemic analysis helped to highlight the way governmental institutions and regional media exploited the successes in controlling rumormongering, panic buying, and overpricing to create the false impression that SARS was indeed under control.

Chapter 3 and the Use of Critical Contextualized Methodology and Transcultural Theory

Chapter 3 focuses on the tactical extra-institutional risk communication that occurred about SARS during the official silence and censorship before April 2003. It examines the rhetorical contestations about health risks posed by the emerging atypical pneumonia in the cultural sites of regional, national, and transnational mediascapes and ideoscapes.

In this chapter, I used critical contextualized methodology to help first to identify key players, time-space axes, and tipping points during such tactical risk communication processes. I started by defining key players as the individuals or groups who sent out risk messages about the spreading atypical pneumonia outbreak to the larger community. I could not pinpoint the key players, however, before first examining the time-space axes to determine the temporal-spatial dimension of my study and then the tipping points to look for key players that helped to bring drastic changes in the risk communication processes about the emerging local outbreaks. The two places I examined were the Guangdong Province before March and Beijing before mid-April, when both places witnessed not only little official coverage of the emerging local outbreaks but also a flood of risk messages from alternative media, ranging from the so-called inside news to wild rumors about city closure. The tipping points included the two rounds of panic shopping on February 8 and February 10, the official press conference held on February 11 by Guangdong health authorities to dispel rumors about local atypical pneumonia outbreaks, and the open letter released by Dr. Jiang Yanyong to communicate to the global community the actual scope of the SARS outbreak in Beijing. After performing the time-space–axes and the tipping-point analyses, I gathered reports from mainstream, commercial, and alternative media about local outbreaks in Guangdong and Beijing and analyzed the reports to find risk communicators who sent risk messages out to the wider community amid official denial and selective media censorship (see chapter 3 for more detail). It was only after repeated recursive readings and analyses that I identified anonymous professionals, whistle-blowers, and greedy merchants as the three key players in the extra-institutional risk communication processes. Finally, I employed the heuristic tools of power-knowledge, interaction analysis, and context to examine how the extra-institutional players competed with governmental authorities and mainstream media in delivering contesting risk messages and how the media policies and media structures in China helped to shape such interactions.

Chapter 4 and the Use of Critical Contextualized Methodology, Corpus-Assisted Discourse Analysis, and Transcultural Rhetorics

Chapter 4 reviews the features of comparative rhetoric as a field dealing with intercultural rhetorics and discourses. With its focus on nation-states, comparative rhetoric usually examines classical literary, philosophical, and rhetorical works and figures to understand the features of the cultural rhetorics of individual nation-states. Therefore, speaking of methodology and approaches, comparative rhetoric takes a more historical approach and focuses on classical works and figures within national boundaries to identify rhetorical terms and frameworks unique to individual nation-states.

Despite its rapid growth as a subfield of rhetorical and intercultural studies, comparative rhetoric is limited by its methodological focus on nation-states. Therefore, it cannot address the challenges posed by the constantly ongoing transnational rhetorical flows, interactions, and negotiations among countries, international governances, and transnational groups surrounding global events. To go beyond the existing nation-state focus in comparative rhetorical analysis and to analyze various competing rhetorics surrounding the global epidemic of SARS, I looked at different cultural, institutional, and rhetorical sites to examine narratives surrounding the outbreak of SARS, to highlight their contextual settings and the impacts of such settings on the employed rhetorics, and to interrogate the complicated cultural, economic, political, and ideological forces motivating rhetorical transformations in transcultural SARS narratives.

To achieve all the goals mentioned above, I applied the critical contextualized methodology to study the transcultural SARS discourses employed by WHO, the United States, and China. I identified four key players in this comparative rhetorical study: WHO, leading national media in the United States and China, and regional media (including transcultural ethnic Chinese media) in the United States. As China was the origin and epicenter of SARS, my investigation here focused on how the American media and WHO constructed the SARS epidemic in China and interpreted the SARS-China relations from the beginning of the epidemic to the removal of Beijing from the WHO's travel advisories in late June 2003. In other words, this study examines the rhetorical interactions about SARS in global mediascapes and ideoscapes as well as contesting transnational forces in operation in the global cultural economy surrounding SARS.

Some of the tipping points that I focused on include WHO's early visits to China, its releases of important travel advisories, China's eradication of SARS, and WHO's withdrawal of travel advisory for Beijing in June. I also included two key transformational moments in China's anti-SARS campaign: April 20, when China broke its silence for the first time and officially apologized for its underreporting of SARS cases; and May 1, when the new Xiaotangshan Hospital was constructed and put to use, which greatly reduced the stress on the overloaded hospitals in Beijing and helped to end the increasing trend of the number of new SARS cases in Beijing. Focusing on these important transformational moments enabled the in-depth analysis of contending media negotiations about the implications of these changes and their interpretation of motivations driving such changes.

Here I also adopted Arjun Appadurai's theory on an adjective approach to culture that emphasizes the "dimensionality" rather than "substantiality" of culture (13) and the "context-sensitive, contrast-centered" approach (12) to the study of cultures. The heuristic tool of context analysis, a key component of the critical contextualized methodology, examines the "situated and embodied differences" that "express or set the ground for the mobilization" of cultural values and identities (13). In addition, power-knowledge analysis and interaction analysis yield new insight about the way global and national key players worked with one another to participate in the transnational risk management of SARS.

To explore how the Communist Party of China interacted with WHO during the SARS outbreak, I employ corpus-assisted discourse analysis to examine SARS coverage in *People's Daily* because of the method's capacity to generate descriptive statistical data for the analysis of trends and changes. Combining both descriptive statistics and contextual analysis, this method provides additional insights that nicely complement rhetorical findings discussed earlier about the WHO-China interaction.

Chapter 5 and the Use of Critical Contextualized Methodology and Transcultural Theory

Chapter 5 investigates the transcultural risk management of SARS and the H1N1flu through the use of travel advices. It investigates the way global risk management discourses operated in mediascapes, ideoscapes, and financescapes. I started by defining the key players: the countries, international governances, institutions, communal groups, and individuals who helped to shape international, national, and regional risk management approaches that either restricted international and domestic travel or supervised the movement of transnational or translocal travelers. When mapping the time-space axes, I decided to cover the two periods from early February to late June in 2003 and from late April to late May in 2009, which witnessed sustained and active transnational negotiations about best approaches to managing the risks posed by SARS and the H1N1 flu. My spatial mapping highlighted the United States, Canada, mainland China, and Hong Kong as countries and regions that were seriously influenced by both epidemics. They negotiated with one another about best ways to employ travel advices to contain the epidemics and to prevent the export of viruses to other parts in the world. The tipping points for SARS include WHO's April 2 travel advisory for Guangdong and Hong Kong, its April 23 travel advisory for Beijing and Toronto, and its decision to remove Toronto from its travel advisory on April 30. The tipping points for the H1N1 flu pandemic include China's first few confirmed case traveling from North America in early May and the release of a bottom-up travel advice calling for self-restraint and responsible action by canceling or postponing trips back to China.

After performing the time-space–axes and tipping-point analyses, I identified WHO, the CDC of the United States, Health Canada, and the Ministry of Health (MOH) of China as the institutional key players. I also identified two individual key players: a Hong Kong health minister speaking as an institutional authority and an overseas Chinese student issuing online statements of grassroots travel advice advocating voluntary travel restraint. The power-knowledge and interaction analyses examine how various transnational and institutional players legitimated their definitions of risks posed by transnational travelers and their use or rejection of travel advices by mobilizing political, economic, cultural, and scientific forces. Finally, contextual analysis investigates the political, economic, cultural, and material contexts that helped to shape risk responses from various cultural and communal players.

Notes

Introduction: Transcultural Flows, Communication, and Rhetorics during a Global Epidemic

1. *Panic buying* refers to the act of a large number of people rushing to purchase large amounts of limited and often special types of products because of the fear of health, environmental, or manufacturing crises, a possible huge price increase, or potential shortage of those goods. For instance, panic buying of vinegar, antiviral drugs, rice, cooking oil, and water took place in Guangdong and Beijing when people learned about the atypical pneumonia amid official silence. While some existing research labels such acts as irrational and unreasonable responses to crises, I argue that emotions and values should function as integral parts of decision-making processes of risk communication and risk management instead of being condemned as interfering noises that should be excluded from such processes.

2. I use the two terms *transcultural communication* and *transcultural rhetorics* interchangeably in the rest of the book because I consider them closely interconnected and intricately related.

3. Appadurai defines *ethnoscape* as the landscape of persons who constitute the shifting world in which we live: "tourists, immigrants, refugees, exiles, guest workers, and other moving groups and individuals constitute an essential feature of the world and appear to affect the politics of (and between) nations" (33). Ethnoscapes are driven by "increasingly complex relationships among money flows, political possibilities, and the availability of both un- and highly-skilled labor" (34).

Technoscape refers to the "global configuration of technologies and the fact that technologies, both high and low, both mechanical and informational, now move at high speeds across various kinds of previously impervious boundaries" (Appadurai 34).

Financescape refers to the global movement of capital, which "is a more mysterious, rapid, and difficult landscape to follow than ever before, as current markets, national stock exchanges, and commodity speculations move megamonies through national turnstiles at blinding speed, with vast, absolute implications for small differences in percentage points and time units" (Appadurai 34).

4. Here and throughout the rest of the book, the terms *biopolitics* and *biopower* are used in the Foucauldian sense. Foucault defines biopower as technologies on the body at two levels: "the regulatory technology of life" at the population level and "the disciplinary technology of the body" at the individual level (*Society* 249). The regulatory technology employs biological and statistic tools to exert bioregulation by the state, as reflected in "a whole series of mechanisms," such as health-insurance systems, child care, pension systems, epidemic prevention, and rule of hygiene to promote the longevity and productivity of the population (*Society* 251). Managing life, growth, health, and the care of the population, biopower brings "life and its mechanisms into the realm of explicit calculations and made knowledge/power an agent of the transformation of human life" (Foucault, *History of Sexuality* 143). Medicine, in turn, becomes a political intervention technique that links the scientific knowledge of biological processes related to the population and disciplinary processes related to individuals.

For Foucault, biopolitics and its associated technologies, as the counterpart of disciplinary technologies, manage the population as a scientific and political problem for the state through the use of mechanisms, such as forecasts, statistical estimates, and overall measures. It "derive[s] its knowledge from, and define[s] its power's field of intervention in terms of the birth rate, the mortality rate, various biological disabilities, and the effects of the environment" (*Society* 245). In addition to managing the "universal" phenomena of populations and health, it also intervenes in the "accidental" events of epidemics (*Society* 245).

5. *Extreme case sampling method* is a type of purposeful sampling, a method often used to select participants in qualitative studies. Purposeful sampling attempts to select information-rich case for study and allows arguments about "the validity of in-depth qualitative findings" (588). Patricia Goubil-Gambrell states: "Extreme case sampling focuses are subjects who are unusual or special in some ways. The logic is that 'lessons must be learned about unusual conditions or extreme outcomes' that are relevant to typical cases" (588). She offers the study of both novice writers and experienced writers as an example of extreme case sampling.

6. Throughout the book, the two terms *health risk communication* and *risk communication* are used interchangeably because they share many similarities in terms of communication channels, approaches, and potential pitfalls. As a subgenre of risk communication, health risk communication about global epidemics has received relatively little attention, and this book contributes to the existing understanding about how emergency health risk communication operates in a global setting.

1. Critical Contextualized Methodology for Transcultural Communication Study

1. Here the term *intercultural professional communication* is used in reviewing existing literature; I shift to the new term *transcultural professional communication* when discussing my own theoretical and methodological frameworks. The purpose is to achieve consistency in references and to avoid confusion caused by the shift between the two theoretical frameworks. A lot of the health risk communication practices I examined go beyond the professional arenas: they were no long controlled by journalists, governmental spokespersons, experts, or public health officials. Instead, concerned citizens and affected communities intervened in the emergency communication processes to make their voices heard and their interests considered in risk decision-making processes. Therefore, I use the term *transcultural communication* throughout the book to refer to this wide variety of communication practices. The question whether they were authorized or unauthorized, official or grassroots, institutional or extra-institutional, verified or unverified, is no longer relevant in the study of emergency health risk communication about global epidemics. It is more useful to focus on all existing communication practices, media, and technologies in such global risk events and on their impacts on the global risk management processes.

2. Similarly, in her discussion of feminist and multicultural critique of objectivity and epistemological agency, Donna J. Haraway advocates "limited location and situated knowledge," for "positioning is the key practice grounding knowledge organized around the imagery of [permanently embodied] vision" ("Situated Knowledge" 190–95). The metaphor of vision requires the researcher's acknowledgment of his/her situatedness in specific cultural, disciplinary, and historical contexts as well as accompanying beliefs and values, which, according to Haraway, is the precondition for "credible witnessing" (*Modest Witness* 33).

3. Given the complicated nature of rhetorical situations and global events, we may not easily identify a clear-cut beginning or ending point of such events. If this is the case, it may help to divide the event under study into distinct developmental stages before employing the time-space axes to map out their temporal-spatial dimensions.

4. The pentagon core of the critical contextualized methodology shares nothing in common with Kenneth Burke's pentad except the fact that it consists of five dimensions or components as the core of the methodology. The critical contextualized methodology is driven by different research questions and aims to answer questions very different from that of Burke's pentad.

2. Risk Communication about an Emerging
Epidemic in Guangdong, China

1. *Partial disclosure* refers to the practice of offering excessive amount of information about the nonessential, more controllable, and less alarming aspects of the emerging risk, for instance, tips about the prevention of new epidemics and reports of the impacts of such epidemics on the daily life of local communities. It strategically selects what to cover in risk communication processes and remains silent about the essential aspects of the risk, for instance, the actual nature and scope of the risk, its extent and geographical areas of influence, and the damage it has brought and will continue to bring.

2. This book stresses the distinction between the actual epidemic of SARS and its side effects, that is, inflation, rumor dissemination, mass panic, and panic buying. The Guangdong media used the enthymeme that the control of side effects, such as inflation and panic buying, meant that the actual epidemic of SARS was also brought under control by interchanging the actual development of the epidemic with its more visible side effects.

3. In China, two different phrases were commonly used to refer separately to atypical pneumonia (fei dian) and SARS (sa si), although the former was more popular because of its wide use in the Chinese media before the WHO's definition in March. To remain faithful to the original Chinese texts, I use the exact word as the original texts in my citations and translations but stick to SARS in my discussion of the SARS outbreak.

4. Ban lan gen, a very popular herbal medicine in China, is usually used to combat flu and the hepatitis B virus.

5. The two mainstream regional newspapers examined for this study are *Guangzhou Daily* and *South Press*. Commercialized regional newspapers discussed here include *Yangcheng Evening, New Press*, and *Southern Cosmopolitan*. All those newspapers are based in Guangzhou. Guangdong has three major newspaper corporations, Yangcheng Evening Co., Guangzhou Daily Co., and Nanfang Daily Co. *Guangzhou Daily* is owned and operated by the Municipal Communist Party of China (CPC) of Guangzhou; *South Press* is owned and operated by the Provincial CPC, and *Yangcheng Evening* is an independent provincial newspaper. *New Press* is jointly owned and operated by Yangcheng Evening Co. and Hong Kong Qiaoxing Co.

To examine the news reports, reviews, and commentaries published by the regional media, I used four different databases in addition to online search to collect news reports and commentaries about SARS published between November 2002 to March 2003 from the mainstream and commercialized regional newspapers, namely, the Database of Chinese Media and the three databases of publication operated by the South Press Group, the Guangzhou Daily Group, and the Yangcheng

Evening Group. To ensure the location of all related reports, I used a variety of Chinese keywords in the search, that is, flu, pneumonia, unknown pneumonia, mysterious pneumonia, and mysterious disease. I also went through the unsorted corpus of publication within each Group database dating from February 1 to March 30 to search for reports and commentaries discussing the SARS event without using any terms related to pneumonia. Altogether, 603 reports, reviews, and commentaries on SARS were published from February 11 to February 20 by newspapers owned and operated by the three corporations.

6. This commentary was widely reprinted in various regional newspapers and websites and won the top award of excellent commentaries during the SARS outbreak in the Guangdong Province.

7. It took me over two years of research in mainstream and nonmainstream media as well as the official websites of Ministry of Health and CDC before I came across a link that redirected me to the Guangdong CDC web pages with SARS documents. My examination of the portal page indicated nothing about the existence of those files.

8. The regulations are expansion of the 1988 State Secret Law. See "Regulations on State Secrets in Public Health Work, Their Level of Secrecy and Details."

9. The 1989 Law on the Prevention and Control of Epidemics provided clear definitions of class A, class B, and class C epidemics, which all comprised existing contagious diseases, such as cholera, plague, and anthrax. The law stipulated that health-care workers and epidemiologists who found cases of the three classes of epidemics must report such cases to local health stations. Epidemiological stations that observed local outbreaks of contagious disease included in the three classes or came across outbreaks of AIDS and anthrax must report such outbreaks to local health departments, which then must report to local governments, upper-level health bureaus, and the Ministry of Health.

3. Rhetorics of Alternative Media, Censorship, and SARS

1. China was forced to collaborate with WHO to improve its disease surveillance and reporting mechanism after WHO issued a travel alert on April 2 recommending postponing nonessential travel to the Guangdong Province. An increasing number of reports about SARS appeared in Chinese media in early April. On April 20, the Chinese government offered an official apology about the undercalculation of SARS cases and fired both the minister of health and the mayor of Beijing because of their incompetence in dealing with the SARS outbreak in Beijing.

2. Heterogeneous in content, forms, and functions, *gossip* refers to "the exchange of information about absent third-parties," usually from social networks outside the immediate family (Foster 81). It may serve an important form of social

communication that serves to bind people together (Dunbar) or a way of inquiry and cultural learning (Baumeister, Zhang, and Vohs).

I adopt Tamotsu Shibutani's theory of rumor, namely, rumor as "a recurrent form of communication through which men caught together in an ambiguous situation [and collective tension] attempt to construct a meaningful interpretation of it by pulling their intellectual resources together" (17). As a collective trans-action of unauthenticated yet plausible news and cooperative improvisation of interpretations, rumor diffuses through informal communication, particularly oral interchanges. It is a form of collective problem solving taking place when "the demand for news in the public exceeds the supply made available through institutional channels" (Shibutani 57–63). Shibutani also points out that rumors follow lines of acquaintances and travel fast.

3. *Ming Pao* is a leading newspaper founded in 1959 in Hong Kong. It focuses on local news in Hong Kong and devotes some attention to news from mainland China and around the world. It enjoys high credibility in the region, and many of its news reports have won awards for their high quality.

4. Besides the four major databases as mentioned in chapter 2, I did online searches to collect news reports, commentaries, and personal narratives about the SARS outbreak. Again I used various keywords to refer to SARS at the early stage of the outbreak to find reports and commentaries about SARS in overseas Chinese websites and Hong Kong news media. Major Chinese commercial websites offering text-messaging services were searched regularly to collect short messages about SARS. However, because of the Internet censorship, most text messages available in those websites were either preventive tips or humor or satire about SARS.

Because of the transient and dynamic features of guerrilla media, such as mobile-phone text messaging, phone calls, and word of mouth, the data-collection processes of messages delivered via guerrilla media are challenging and time consuming. The fact that China imposed censorship on both the Internet and print media during the SARS outbreak further complicates the research processes. Whereas the overseas Chinese websites reported witness narratives about panic buying and alarming text messages, those reported in regional media in Guang-dong are far more scattered, buried in success stories about anti-SARS campaign in Guangdong, and thus harder to find. One interesting thing is that the Guangdong media enjoyed a ten-day period of selective censorship before being forbidden to talk about SARS, during which they reported anything related to the local SARS outbreak from November 2002 to February 11, 2003, but the actual number of SARS cases or the SARS development in the region. Commercialized newspapers played an active role in reviewing events that helped produce mass panic buying, many of which were related to rumors circulated in text messages. Mainstream media also analyzed the "harmful effect" of the public's unselective reception of false alarms and rumors in commentaries and retrospective reports, which also helped to preserve widely circulated text messages as examples of "irresponsible and alarming rumors" ("Disease under Control"). Ironically, news reports and commentaries aiming to promote the official narrative of "SARS is under control" are put to a different use for this study: they preserve the historical traces of text messages addressing the risks of SARS and serve as historical evidences of guerrilla media's role in participatory risk communication.

The data analysis process has been highly recursive. Whenever I obtained new insights from newly found reports, commentaries, narratives, or text messages, I used them to reanalyze existing data and to reevaluate their function in producing the panic buying and in informing the public of the emerging epidemic of SARS. I started with identifying and collecting personal narratives that differed from or contradicted official reports. Sources reporting about those narratives differed in credibility and authority. Some overseas Chinese websites published reports about word of mouth, for instance, "some professionals told a story about SARS, but their names are not revealed to protect their privacy," or "here is an insider story from a friend who works in a hospital specialized in infectious disease." Most news reports from Hong Kong or American media also used pseudonyms or witnesses' last names either out of the intention to protect their interviewees' privacy or because of the interviewees' refusal to reveal their real identities. Given the huge personal risks one would have when breaking the censorship, such use of anonymous narratives helped to protect those who actually sent out risk messages. Then I also found several personal narratives in which the narrators did reveal their actual identities for various reasons, so I categorized personal narratives into two types, one as being told by anonymous professionals and the other as being told by whistle-blowers and examined their rhetorical features.

My analysis of the rest of the data shows that they were all anonymous mobile-phone text messages. Most of those messages were widely circulated and helped to produce the two waves of mass panic buying throughout the Guangdong Province. Because of their huge social impact, it was impossible to leave them out. I examined them in-depth, analyzed their content, format, and impact, and finally coded them as a third category of means of risk communication.

4. Constructing SARS: The United States, China, and WHO

1. A *synecdoche* is a figure of comparison in which a part or quality of a thing is used to stand for the whole thing or vice versa.

2. Zhang Wenkang, a native of Shanghai, had served as a military physician before Jiang Zemin appointed him as the Minister of Health. As a strong ally of Jiang during the power transition in early 2003, Zhang covered up the spread of SARS before April and contributed to its quick spread to different regions in

China. In his book *China Syndrome: The True Story of the 21st Century's First Great Epidemic*, Karl Greenfeld analyzes the role Zhang played in the SARS underreporting amid the power change:

> Zhang Wenkang had inadvertently become a pawn in the power struggle between factions supporting the new president and party secretary, Hu Jintao, and the former party secretary and current central military commander, Jiang Zemin. The paralysis in terms of responding to SARS was in part due to bureaucratic uncertainty as to who was actually running the country. (340)

3. Here, I use Ken-ichi Hashimoto and Ken Tabata's definition of public health infrastructure: "Public health infrastructure is defined as the public capital that enhances the health status of individuals and improves their survival probability and labor productivity. Therefore, public health infrastructure can be interpreted as sewerage and drainage systems, waste disposal, clean water supply, and basic health care." (549). As the basic architecture of public health systems, they may be developed, owned, and operated by local or central governments or sometimes private or state-run enterprises.

4. Corpus-assisted discourse analysis (CADS) draws on techniques commonly used in corpus linguistics, that is, word frequency, keyword collocation, and concordances, to find recurring discursive patterns and lexical features, using quantitative and qualitative techniques. As a multimethod tool, CADS corpora allow qualitative and descriptive analyses that cannot only define, categorize, and count discursive features but also connect to contextual significance through the creation of concordances, or passages containing certain keywords (Aston; Flowerdew).

5. Transnational Risk Management of SARS and H1N1 Flu via Travel Advisories

1. The WHO used the term *travel advisory* to refer to nonspecific travel warning and travel advice to refer to recommendation of postponing nonessential travel to specific places, whereas the CDC uses a travel advisory to recommend that nonessential travel be deferred and uses travel alerts that instead of advising against travel, inform "travelers of a health concern and provides advice about specific precautions" ("SARS Travel Alert Reinstated"). The CDC travel alerts and advisories were disseminated through media advisories, press briefings, e-mail notifications, and US State Department advisories.

Works Cited

Abbate, Gay. "Virus's Link to China May Fuel Racism, Leaders Say." *Globe and Mail* Apr. 1, 2003: A8. Print.

"About 10,000 Students Studying Abroad Isolate Themselves at Home after Returning to Jingsu for the Summer Break." *Contemporary Express*, June 14, 2009. Web. Jan. 10, 2010. <http://news.163.com/09/0614/15/5BPFV86H0001124J.html>.

"Accountability of Officials in Panic Buying in Guangzhou." *New Press* [Guangzhou] Feb. 18, 2003: 5. Print.

Ali, Harris S. "Stigmatized Ethnicity, Public Health, and Globalization." *Canadian Ethics Studies* 40.3 (2008): 43–64. Print.

Alphonso, Caroline. "Illness Spawns Some Shunning of Asians." *Globe and Mail* Apr. 3, 2003: NA9. Print.

Alphonso, Caroline, and Geoffrey York. "Canadian Health Officials Rapped by WHO." *Globe and Mail* June 13, 2003: A1. Print.

Alred, Gerald J. "Teaching in Germany and the Rhetoric of Culture." *Journal of Business and Technical Communication* 11.3 (1997): 353–79. Print.

Altman, Lawrence. "The SARS Enigma: Drop in Cases Encourages the WHO, But Fears and Questions Remain." *New York Times* June 8, 2003: A18. Print.

———. "W.H.O. Expresses Optimism China Can Control SARS." *New York Times* May 13, 2003: A14. Print.

Altman, Lawrence, and Keith Bradsher. "China Bars W.H.O. Experts from Origin Site of Illness." *New York Times* Mar. 26, 2003: A7. Print.

Ammara, Fethi, and Franck Portaneri. "Arabization of Graphical User Interface." *International User Interface*. Ed. Elisa M. del Galdo and Jakob Nielsen. New York: Wiley, 1996. 127–50. Print.

"Analysis of Reasons Leading to Panic about Atypical Pneumonia in Guangzhou." *New Press* [Guangzhou] Feb. 14, 2003: 9. Print.

Andrews, Deborah C. "Teaching International Technical Communication." *Technical Communication Quarterly* 7.3 (1998): 329–39. Print.

"Angels in White Devoted to Treatment of Atypical Pneumonia Patients." *Guangzhou Daily* Feb. 18, 2003: 12. Print.

"Announcements from Health Bureau: Atypical Pneumonia under Control." *New Press* [Guangzhou] Feb. 12, 2003: 2. Print.

Appadurai, Arjun. *Modernity at Large: Cultural Dimensions of Globalization.* Minneapolis: U of Minnesota P, 1996. Print.

Applegate, John S. "The Precautionary Preference: An American Perspective on the Precautionary Principle." *Human and Ecological Risk Assessment: An International Journal* 6.3 (2000): 413–33.

"April 30 News Press by Beijing SARS Control and Prevention Working Group." *Guangzhou Daily* Apr. 30, 2003. Web. Aug. 20, 2003. <http://gzdaily.dayoo.com/gb/content/2003-04/30/content_1051160.htm>.

Artuso, Antonella. "Chinese Take Heat; Asians Cite Racial Slurs, Shunning." *Toronto Sun* Apr. 4, 2003: 5. Print.

Aston, Guy. "Small and Large Corpora in Language Learning." *Practical Applications in Language Corpora.* Ed. Barbara Lewandowska-Tomaszczyk and Patrick James Melia. Lodz, Poland: Lodz UP, 1997. 51–62. Print.

Atkinson, Dwight. "Contrasting Rhetorics/Contrasting Cultures: Why Contrastive Rhetoric Needs a Better Conceptualization of Culture." *Journal of English for Academic Purposes* 3.4 (2004): 277–89.

Atton, Chris. *Alternative Media.* London: Sage, 2002. Print.

"Attracting Foreign Investment China's Long-standing Policy." *People's Daily*, Dec. 3, 2004. Web. June 5, 2005. <http://english.people.com.cn/200412/03/eng20041203_166074.html>.

August, Oliver. "Fear Spreads in China over Mysterious Lung Virus." *Times* [London] Feb. 12, 2003: 20. Print.

———. "New Leaders Struggle to Restore Credibility." *Times* [London] Apr. 21, 2003. Web. June 5, 2005. <http://www.thetimes.co.uk/tto/news/world/article1987128.ece>.

Bak, Per. *How Nature Works: The Science of Self-Organized Criticality.* New York: Springer-Verlag, 1996. Print.

"Bao Manman: Who Is He? The First H1N1 Flu Case in China Bao Xueyang." *bbs.0596.net*, May 15, 2009. Web. Oct. 2, 2009. <http://bbs.0596.net/thread-18864-1-1.html>.

Barnes, David. *The Making of a Social Disease: Tuberculosis in Nineteenth-Century France.* Berkeley: U of California P, 1995. Print.

Barry, Dan. "Anthrax Pranks? You've Got to Be Kidding." *New York Times* Nov. 4, 2001: 4.2. Print.

———. "Determined Volunteers Camped Out to Pitch in." *New York Times* Sept. 23, 2001: B1. Print.

Baumeister, Roy, Liqing Zhang, and Kathleen Vohs. "Gossip as Cultural Learning." *Review of General Psychology* 8.2 (2004): 111–21. Print.

Beck, Ulrich. *World Risk Society.* Malden, MA: Polity, 1999. Print.

Beech, Hannah. "How Bad Is It?" *Time*, May 5, 2003. Web. Sept. 16, 2009. <http://content.time.com/time/world/article/0,8599,2047288,00.html>.

"Behind Beijing's Sustained Decrease of SARS Cases: Gradual Understanding and Control of Sources of Infection." *Xinhua,* May 13, 2003. Web. Sept. 29, 2009. <http://www.sina.com.cn>.

"Beijing Air Travel Hotel Mass Quarantined Travelers Because of the Stay of Mainland's First H1N1 Flu Case." *Jinghua Time* May 12, 2009: 12. Print.

"Beijing Farmers Say 'No' to SARS." *People's Daily* May 1, 2003. Web. Oct. 13, 2005. <http://english.peopledaily.com.cn/200305/01/eng20030501_116129.shtml>.

"Beijing Health Bureau Suggesting Returning Overseas Chinese Avoiding Taking Buses If They Develop Swine Flu Symptoms." *Jinghua Times* May 23, 2009: 7. Print.

"Beijing Municipal Guideline for the Strengthening of SARS Control Work in the Communities." *Beijing Morning* Apr. 29, 2003: 2. Print.

"Beijing's Rigorous Examination of Anti-SARS Work in Construction Sites." *Xinhua,* May 11, 2003. Web. June 5, 2011. <http://www.hebei.gov.cn/syscolumn /lshm/fzfd/fzfdxxzb/index.htm>.

Bell, D. M., and World Health Organization Working Group on Prevention of International and Community Transmission of SARS. "Public Health Interventions and SARS Spread." *Emerging Infectious Disease* 10.11 (2004). *CDC.gov.* Web. Sept. 29, 2009. <http://www.cdc.gov/ncidod/EID/vo110no11 /04-0729.htm>.

Benitez, Mary Ann, and Stella Lee. "Legal Snag Delays SARS List; as Infections Are Confirmed at Yet Another Kowloon Bay Estate, a Plan to Name All Infected Blocks Has Run into Problems'" *South China Morning Post* [Hong Kong] Apr. 11, 2003: 1. Print.

"Between a Virus and a Hard Place." *Nature* 459.9 (2009): 9. Print.

Bi, Ke. "'The Biggest Political Task for Physicians Is to Prevent and Treat Disease Well': The Anti-SARS Warrior Zhong Nanshan." *South Cosmopolitan* [Guangzhou] May 21, 2003: 1. Print.

Bingham, Nick, and Steve Hinchliff. "Mapping the Multiplicities of Biosecurity." *Biosecurity Interventions: Global Health and Security in Question.* Ed. Andrew Lakoff and Stephen Collier. New York: Columbia UP, 2008. 173–93. Print.

Bitzer, Lloyd F. "The Rhetorical Situation," *Philosophy & Rhetoric* 1.1 (1968): 1–14. Print.

Blackwell, Tom. "WHO Drops Toronto from SARS List: 'We Are Delighted'; Finnish Man Did Not Contract Disease Visiting the City." *National Post* May 15, 2003: A2. Print.

Blatchford, Christie. "Beware SARS Symptom: Curdled Sense of Humour." *National Post* Apr. 4, 2003: A1. Print.

Bloom, Barry. "Lessons from SARS." *Science* 300 (2003): 701. Print.

Bowdon, M., and Blake Scott. *Service-Learning in Technical and Professional Communication.* New York: Longman, 2003. Print.

Bradsher, Keith. "Flu's Possible Return Worries Hong Kong." *New York Times* Feb. 22, 2003: A1. Print.

———. "Relapse by SARS Patients Probably Not from Syndrome." *New York Times* May 5, 2003: A5. Print.

Brandt, Allan. *No Magic Bullet: A Social History of Venereal Disease in the United States since 1880.* New York: Oxford UP, 1987. Print.

Branigan, Tania. "How China's Internet Generation Broke the Silence." *Guardian*, Mar. 24, 2010. Web. May 3, 2011. <http://www.guardian.co.uk/world/2010/mar/24/china-internet-generation-censorship>.

Branswell, Helen. "Flu Factories." *Scientific America* 30.4 (2011): 46–51. Print.

Britt, Elizabeth. "The Rhetorical Work of Institutions." Scott, Longo, and Wills 133–50.

Brookes, Tim, and Omar A. Khan. *Behind the Mask: How the World Survived SARS, the First Epidemic of the 21st Century.* Washington, DC: Amer. Public Health Assn., 2005. Print.

Brookey, Robert Alan. *Reinventing the Male Homosexual: The Rhetoric and Power of the Gay Gene.* Bloomington: Indiana UP, 2002. Print.

Brown, DeNeen L. "Canada to Screen for Fevers at Airports." *Washington Post* Apr. 29, 2003: A18. Print.

Burke, Kenneth. *Permanence and Change: An Anatomy of Purpose.* 3rd ed. Berkeley: U of California P, 1984. Print.

Burress, Charles, and Sabin Russell. "Cal Bans Students from Areas Hit by SARS / Hundreds from Asia Will Miss Summer Classes." *San Francisco Chronicle* May 6, 2003. Web. Aug. 7, 2004.<http://www.sfgate.com/health/article/Cal-bans-students-from-areas-hit-by-SARS-2618496.php>.

Cai, Yichen. "SARS Prevention in the Countryside: Beware of 'Black Buses' on the Highway as Blind Zones of Anti-SARS Work." *Xinhuanet*, May 13, 2003. Sept. 29, 2009. <http://news.xinhuanet.com/newscenter/2003-05/13/content_868182.htm>.

Cai, Zhiqiang. "Reasons for and Solutions of Solidified Social Class Structure." *Study Time* June 27, 2011: 12. Print.

"Call for Action: Let Bao Manman Face His Real Identity, We Should Stop an Irresponsible Person from Enjoying Heroic Treatment." *Third Media,* May 13, 2009. Web. Oct. 12, 2009. <http://ido.3mt.com.cn/Article/200905/show1476952c12p1.html>.

"Call for Media Groups to Pool Their Resources." *New Straits Times–Management Times* Aug. 7, 2003: 5. Print.

Canagarajah, A. Suresh. *A Geopolitics of Academic Writing.* Pittsburgh: U of Pittsburgh P, 2002. Print.

Castells, Manuel, Mireia Fernandez-Ardevol, Jack Linchuan Qiu, and Araba Sey. *Mobile Communication and Society: A Global Perspective.* Cambridge, MA: MIT P, 2007. Print.

"CDC Cautions on SARS Overreaction." *New York Times* May 15, 2003: A18. Print.

Centers for Disease Control and Prevention. "CDC Briefing on Public Health Investigation of Human Cases of H1N1 Flu (Swine Flu)." *CDC.gov*, Apr. 30, 2009. Web. Jan. 6, 2010. <http://www.cdc.gov/media/transcripts/2009/t090430.htm>.

———. "CDC's Response to Reports of SARS." *CDC.gov*, Apr. 24, 2003. Web. Jan. 6, 2010. <http://www.cdc.gov/media/transcripts/t030424.htm>.

———. "Interim Travel Alert: Toronto, Ontario, Canada." *CDC.gov*, Apr. 23, 2003. Web. June 12, 2003. <http://www.cdc.gov/ncidod/sars>.

———. "Outbreaks of SARS—United States." *Morbidity and Mortality Weekly Report* May 2, 2003: 357–60. Print.

Chang, Iris. "Fear of SARS, Fear of Strangers." *New York Times* May 21, 2003: A31. Print.

Chao, Loretta. "SARS Fears Grip Chinatown: After Rumors of Illness, Vendors Struggle." *Washington Square News*, Apr. 9, 2003. Web. Sept. 8, 2003. <http://media.www.nyunews.com/media/storage/paper869/news/2003/04/09/UndefinedSection/Sars-Fears.Grip.Chinatown-2396640.shtml>.

Chen, Guangteng, Cuilin Wang, and Gongwei Duan. "Calm Response to Settle the Crisis—Historical Records of Guangdong's Battle against Atypical Pneumonia." *Southern Daily* [Guangzhou]. Feb. 20, 2003: 1. Print.

Chen, Jian. "Hot Topic: Unknown Pneumonia in Zhongshan." *New Press* [Guangzhou] Feb. 3, 2003: 2. Print.

Chen, Margret. "Concern over Flu Pandemic Justified: Address to Sixty-Second World Health Assembly Geneva, Switzerland." *World Health Organization*, May 18, 2009. Web. May 20, 2009. <http://www.who.int/dg/speeches/2009/62nd_assembly_address_20090518/en/index.html>.

———. "Statement Made at the Secretary-General's Briefing to the United Nations General Assembly on the H1N1 Influenza Situation." *World Health Organization*, May 4, 2009. Web. May 6, 2009. <http://www.who.int/entity/dg/speeches/2009/influenza_a_h1n1_situation_20090504/en/index.htm>.

Chen, Stephen. "Italian Quarantined at Tibetan Border Town." *South China Morning Post* [Hong Kong] May 20, 2009: 5. Print.

———. "Mainland Net Users Vent Anger at Apologetic Overseas Chinese." *South China Morning Post* [Hong Kong] May 19, 2009: 4. Print.

Chen, Weiming. "SARS May Be Bioterrorist Weapon Created to Attack China." *Chinese Youth* [Beijing] Oct. 8, 2003: 9. Print.

Chen, Young. *Chinese San Francisco 1850–1943: A Trans-Pacific Community.* Stanford: Stanford UP, 2000. Print.

Chen, Zhihua, and Yunyong Jia. "One-Hundred-Day Record of Atypical Pneumonia: A Baby Named 'Saddam Deng Atypical Pneumonia.'" *Southern Cosmopolitan* [Guangzhou] May 22, 2003: 3. Print.

"China Creates SARS Task Force, Special Fund." *People's Daily* Apr. 24, 2003: 5. Print.

"China Holds Press Conference on SARS." *People's Daily* Apr. 21, 2003: 3. Print.

"China Planning Mechanism for Public Health Emergencies." *People's Daily* Apr. 15, 2003: 3. Print.

"China Safe despite SARS Epidemic: FM Spokesman." *People's Daily* Apr. 1, 2003: 8. Print.

"China's Efforts Lead to Decreasing SARS Cases." *People's Daily* Apr. 3, 2003: 1. Print.

"China Sets Up Health Emergency Systems." *People's Daily* Apr. 10, 2003: 2. Print.

"China Sheds More Funds for SARS Prevention in Rural Areas." *People's Daily* May 11, 2003: 2. Print.

Chinese Canadian National Council. *Yellow Peril Revisited: Impact of SARS on the Chinese and Southeast Asian Canadian Communities.* June 2004. Web. May 21, 2009. <http://www.ccnc.ca/sars/SARSReport.pdf>.

"Chinese Leaders Mobilize Cities to Combat SARS." *People's Daily* May 2, 2003: 4. Print.

"Chinese Media Urged to Boost Morale of the Nation." *People's Daily,* Apr. 26, 2003. Web. Oct. 13, 2005. <http://english.peopledaily.com.cn/200304/26/eng20030426_115833.shtml>.

"Chinese New Leadership Wins Trust: Commentary." *People's Daily,* June 30, 2003. Web. Oct. 13, 2005. <http://english.peopledaily.com.cn/200306/27/eng20030627_118955.shtml>.

"Chinese President on SARS Control, Economic Development." *People's Daily* May 14, 2003: 02. Print.

Christiansen, Flemming. *Chinatown, Europe: An Exploration of Overseas Chinese Identity in the 1990s.* New York: Routledge, 2003. Print.

"Chronology of China's Fight against SARS since April 20." *People's Daily* May 1, 2003: 4. Print.

Chu, L. L. "Continuity and Change in China's Media Reform." *Journal of Communication* 44.3 (1994): 4–21. Print.

Cohn, Martin Regg. "WHO Rebukes Canada for SARS Lobby." *Toronto Star* June 17, 2003: A01. Print.

Confucius. *Analects of Confucius.* Trans. Lai Bo and Xia Yuhe. Beijing: Sinolingua, 1994. Print.

Connor, Ulla. "Intercultural Rhetoric Research: Beyond Texts." *Journal of English for Academic Purposes* 3.4 (2004): 291–304. Print.

"Contain." Def. 2. *Oxford Dictionary.* Web. Aug. 6, 2006. <http://www.oxforddictionaries.com/us>.

"Control." Def. 1. *Oxford Dictionary.* Web. Aug. 6, 2006. <http://www.oxforddictionaries.com/us>.

Coogan, D. "Service Learning and Social Change: The Case for Materialist Rhetoric." *College Composition and Communication* 57 (2006): 667–93. Print.

Couldry, Nick, and James Curran. "The Paradox of Media Power." Couldry and Curran, 3–15.

———, eds. *Contesting Media Power: Alternative Media in a Networked World.* Lanham, MD: Rowman and Littlefield, 2003. Print.

"Croak a Cola." *Snopes.com,* May 6, 2005. Web. Mar. 9, 2006. <http://www.snopes.com/rumors/poisoncoke.asp>.

Crosby, Alfred W. *America's Forgotten Pandemic: The Influenza of 1918.* Cambridge: Cambridge UP, 2003. Print.

de Certeau, Michel. *The Practice of Everyday Life.* Berkeley: U of California P, 1984. Print.

Denby, David. "Call the Doctor: Contagion." *New Yorker,* Sept. 19, 2011. Web. May 12, 2012. <http://www.newyorker.com/arts/critics/cinema/2011/09/19/110919crci_cinema_denby>.

Deng, Lihong. "Recommended Chinese Traditional Medicine Recipe by Head of Health Bureau of Shenzhen." *Guangzhou Daily* Feb. 13, 2003: 12. Print.

Derfel, Aaron. "Global Response Faulted; Swine Flu. ICAO Seeks Harmonization." *Gazette* [Montreal] May 21, 2009: A3. Print.

de Souza, Rebecca. "The Construction of HIV/AIDS in Indian Newspapers: A Frame Analysis." *Health Communication* 21.3 (2007): 257–66. Print.

"Developing Countries Ill-Prepared for Swine Flu Outbreak." *Money Times,* Apr. 29, 2009. Web. June 20, 2009. <http://www.themoneytimes.com/20090429/developing-countries-ill-prepared-swine-flu-outbreak-id-1065860.html>.

Devoss, Dànielle, Julia Jasken, and Dawn Hayden. "Teaching Intracultural and Intercultural Communication: A Critique and Suggested Method." *Journal of Business and Technical Communication* 16.1 (2002): 69–94. Print.

"Diagnosing SARS in China." *New York Times* May 19, 2003. Print.

"Dial 12358 to Report Illegal Inflation." *Guangzhou Daily* Feb. 11, 2003: 10. Print.

DiMassa, Cara Mia. "UC Berkeley Modifies SARS Ban to Allow More Students." *Los Angeles Times* May 11, 2003: 21. Print.

Ding, Huiling. "Confucius' Virtue-Centered Rhetoric: A Case Study of the Analects with Mixed Research Methods." *Rhetoric Review* 26.2 (2007): 142–59. Print.

———. "Rhetorics of Alternative Media in an Emerging Epidemic: SARS, Censorship, and Participatory Risk Communication." *Technical Communication Quarterly* 18.4 (2009): 327–50. Print.

Ding, Huiling, and E. Pitts. "Singapore's Quarantine Rhetoric and Human Rights in Emergency Health Risks." *Rhetoric, Professional Communication, and Globalization* 4. 1 (2013): 55–77. Print.

Ding, Huiling, and Jingwen Zhang. "Social Media and Participatory Risk Communication during the H1N1 Flu Epidemic: A Comparative Study of the United States and China." *China Media Research* 6.4 (2010): 80–91. Print.

"Disease under Control: No Need to Panic." *Guangzhou Daily* Feb. 12, 2003: 2. Print.

"Dismissing Rumors, a Large Number of College Graduates from All Over the Country Went to Job Fairs in Guangzhou." *Guangzhou Daily* Feb. 18, 2003: 8. Print.

Donnelly, Christl A., Matthew C. Fisher, Christophe Fraser, Azra C. Ghani, Steven Riley, Neil M. Ferguson, and Roy M. Anderson. "Epidemiological and Genetic Analysis of Severe Acute Respiratory Syndrome." *Lancet Infectious Disease* 4.11 (2004): 672–83. Print.

Dragga, Sam. "A Question of Ethics: Lessons from Technical Communicators on the Job." *Technical Communication Quarterly* 6.2 (1997): 161–78. Print.

"Drug Firm in Trouble: Making Profit by Disseminating Rumors?" *International Finance* Feb. 18, 2003: A1. Print.

Duffin, Jacalyn, and Arthur Sweetman, eds. *SARS in Context: Memory, History, Policy.* Montreal: McGill-Queen's UP, 2006. Print.

Dunbar, Robin. *Grooming, Gossip, and the Evolution of Language.* Cambridge, MA: Harvard UP, 1998. Print.

Eckholm, Erik. "As Cases Mount, Chinese Officials Try to Calm a Panicky Public." *New York Times* May 1, 2003: A10. Print.

——. "With Virus at Gate, the Drawbridge Is Up." *New York Times* Apr. 28, 2003: A14. Print.

"Economic Impact of SARS, The." *CBC News Online. cbc.ca*, July 8, 2003. Web. Dec. 12, 2006. <http://www.cbc.ca/news/background/sars/economicimpact.html>.

Edbauer, Jenny. "Unframing Models of Pubic Distribution: From Rhetorical Situation to Rhetorical Ecologies." *Rhetoric Society Quarterly* 35.4 (2005): 5–25. Print.

"Editorial Calls for Workers to Support Battles against SARS." *People's Daily* May 1, 2003: 2. Print.

Eichelberger, Laura. "SARS and New York's Chinatown: The Politics of Risk and Blame During an Epidemic of Fear." *Social Science & Medicine* 65.6 (2007): 1071–310. Print.

"806 SARS Cases Found in China: WHO Official." *People's Daily Online*, Mar. 28, 2003. Web. Oct. 13, 2005. <http://english.people.com.cn/200303/28/eng20030328_114162.shtml>.

Eisenman, Joshua. "A Shift in China's Leadership Style?" *Straits Times* [Singapore] May 8, 2003: 13. Print.

Emery, Theo. "SARS Fear Roils Chinatown Neighborhoods in Boston, New York, and San Francisco." *Fox News*, Apr. 8, 2003. Web. June 8, 2005. <http://www.foxnews.com/story/2003/04/08/sars-fear-roils-chinatown-neighborhoods/>.

Engdahl, F. William. "Bird Flu and Chicken Factory Farms: Profit Bonanza for US Agribusiness." *Global Research*, Nov. 27, 2005. Web. Jan. 23, 2006. <http://www.globalresearch.ca/bird-flu-and-chicken-factory-farms-profit-bonanza-for-us-agribusiness/1333>.

"Entire History of Atypical Pneumonia Event, The: The First Case in Guangzhou Was a Peddler." *New Press* [Guangzhou] Feb. 13, 2003: 9. Print.

Epstein, Steven. "The Construction of Lay Expertise: AIDS Activism and the Forging of Credibility in the Reform of Clinical Trials." *Science, Technology, and Human Values* 20.4 (1995): 408–37. Print.

———. *Impure Science: AIDS, Activism, and the Politics of Knowledge.* Berkeley: U of California P, 1996. Print.

Erni, John Nguyet. *Unstable Frontiers: Technomedicine and the Cultural Politics of "Curing" AIDS.* Minneapolis: U of Minnesota P, 1994. Print.

"Events in Atypical Pneumonia Outbreak." *Asian Weekly* [Hong Kong] June 3, 2003: 15. Print.

"Exit Screening Should Be Part of Swine Flu Fight." *South China Morning Post* [Hong Kong] May 18, 2009: 10. Print.

"Experience of a Recovered Doctor." *Guangzhou Daily* Feb. 12, 2003: 15. Print.

"Expert Reminded: It Is Safe to Go Out." *Guangzhou Daily* Feb. 13, 2003: 10. Print.

"Experts Denounced Rumors: Panic Absolutely Unnecessary." *South Cosmopolitan* [Guangzhou] Feb. 11, 2003: 5. Print.

"Experts Predict That New SARS Cases Will Be Further Decreasing in Guangdong This Month." *Shaanxi Daily* Apr. 8, 2003. Print.

"Experts: The Cause of Atypical Pneumonia May Be Virus." *Sohu.com*, Feb. 14, 2003. Web. Jan. 20, 2004. <http://health.sohu.com/36/75/harticle17297536.shtml>.

"Extremely Despise and Doubt Bao's Motivation and Reasoning." *Tianya.cn*, May 16, 2003. Web. Aug. 12, 2009. <http://www.tianya.cn/publicforum/Content/funinfo/1/1460948.shtml>.

Fagan, Amy. "WHO Seeks Perspective in SARS-Related Actions; Outbreaks Now Severe Only in China." *Washington Times* May 17, 2003: A04. Print.

"Failing Connection between Cell Phone and Home Phone Last Night." *Yangchen Evening* [Guangzhou] Feb. 11, 2003: 5. Print.

Fairclough, Norman. *Media Discourse.* New York: St. Martin's, 1995. Print.

Fang, Ye. "Chendu Started Emergency Mechanism to Prevent and Control H1N1 Flu with Four Measures." *Sichuan Daily* May 10, 2009: 1. Print.

Farmer, Paul. *AIDS and Accusation: Haiti and the Geography of Blame.* Berkeley: University of California Press, 1992.

Fidler, David. *SARS, Governance, and the Globalization of Disease.* New York: Palgrave, 2006. Print.

Finlay, Christopher. "The Toronto Syndrome: SARS, Risk Communication and the Flow of Information." *Times 2007 Annual Conference Proceedings* 1–21. Web. Jan 20, 2008. <http://www.inter-disciplinary.net/transform/Finlay-Sars.pdf>.

"First Imported Atypical Pneumonia Patient in North China Talked about Experiences for the First Time." *Chinese Youth* [Beijing] May 22, 2003: 6. Print.

Fleck, Fiona. "How SARS Changed the World in Less Than Six Months." *Bulletin of the World Health Organization* 81.8 (2003). Web. <http://www.ncbi.nlm.nih.gov/pmc/articles/PMC2572529/pdf/14576896.pdf>.

Fletcher, H. "Human Flesh Search Engines: Chinese Vigilantes That Hunt Victims on the Web." *Times Online*, June 25, 2008. Web. Jan. 16, 2011. <http://technology.timesonline.co.uk/tol/news/tech_and_web/article4213681.ece>.

Flowerdew, Lynne. "The Argument for Using English Specialized Corpora to Understand Academic and Professional Language." *Discourse in the Professions: Perspectives from Corpus Linguistics.* Ed. U. Connor and R. Upton. Amsterdam: John Benjamins, 2004. 11–36. Print.

Foster, Eric. "Research on Gossip: Taxonomy, Methods, and Future Directions." *Review of General Psychology* 8.2 (2004): 78–99. Print.

Foucault, Michel. *The Archeology of Knowledge.* Trans. A. M. Sheridan Smith. New York: Harper, 1976. Print.

———. *The Birth of the Clinic: An Archeology of Medical Perception.* Trans. A. M. Sheridan Smith. New York: Vintage, 1975. Print.

———. *Discipline and Punish: The Birth of the Prison.* Trans. Alan Sheridan. New York: Pantheon, 1977. Print.

———. *The History of Sexuality.* Trans. Robert Hurley. New York: Random, 1990. Print.

———. *Society Must Be Defended: Lectures at the College de France, 1975–76.* Trans. D. Macey. New York: Picador, 2003. Print.

Frieden, Thomas R. "Latest Update on SARS in New York." New York City Department of Health and Mental Hygiene. May 14, 2003. Web. Dec. 3, 2005. <http://www.nyc.gov/html/doh/downloads/pdf/public/press03/pr051-0514.pdf>.

Fukuoka, Waka, and Jan H. Spyridakis. "Japanese Readers' Comprehension of and Preferences for Inductively Versus Deductively Organized Text." *IEEE Transactions on Professional Communication* 43.4 (2000): 355–68. Print.

Fukuoka, Waka, Y. Kojima, and Jan Spyridakis. "Illustrations in User Manuals: Preference and Effectiveness with Japanese and American Readers." *Technical Communication* 46 (1998): 167–76. Print.

Gao, Feng. "117 Officials Punished Because of Slack Anti-SARS Performance in Shanxi." *Xinhua*, May 14, 2003. Web. Jan. 20, 2008. <http://www.sina.com.cn>.

Gao, Liping, and Yongxia Wang. "Liuliang, Shanxi: Ten Thousand Civilian Soldiers Mobilized to Prevent SARS' Entry into the Countryside." *Xinhua*, May 12, 2003. Web. Jan. 20, 2008. <http://www.sina.com.cn>.

Gertz, Bill. "VOA Radio Broadcasts to China Signing Off, While Beijing Boosts Propaganda: Critics Point Out Sino-Cast Expansion." *Washington Times* Feb. 15, 2011. Web. Oct. 18, 2011. <http://www.washingtontimes.com/news/2011/feb/15/obama-admin-to-cancel-voice-of-america-china-broad/?page=all>.

Gladwell, Malcolm. *The Tipping Point: How Little Things Can Make a Big Difference*. New York: Back Bay, 2000. Print.

Glanz, James, and John Markoff. "U.S. Gives Web Tools to Dissidents; Internet Detour Provides Ways to Evade Censors in Repressive Countries." *International Herald Tribune* [New York] June 13, 2011: 1. Print.

Glass, Thomas A., and Monica Schoch-Spana. "Bioterrorism and the People: How to Vaccinate a City against Panic." *Clinical Infectious Diseases* 34. 2 (2002): 217–23. Print.

Goossen, Tam, Cynthia Pay, and Avvy Go. "Healing the Scars in Post-SARS Toronto." *Toronto Star* May 19, 2003: A15. Print.

"Gossip and Rumor More Dangerous Than Epidemics: Investigation of the Development of Rumors." *Southern Cosmopolitan* [Guangzhou] Feb. 12, 2003: 7. Print.

Gostin, L., R. Bayer, and A. Fairchild. "Ethical and Legal Challenges Posed by Severe Acute Respiratory Syndrome: Implications for the Control of Severe Infectious Disease Threats." *JAMA* 290.24 (2003): 3229–37. Print.

Goubil-Gambrell, Patricia. "A Practitioner's Guide to Research Methods." *Technical Communication* 39.4 (1992): 582–91. Print.

Grabill, Jeffrey T. "The Study of Writing in the Social Factory: Methodology and Rhetorical Agency." Scott, Longo, and Wills 151–70.

Grabill, Jeffrey T., and Michele Simmons. "Toward a Critical Rhetoric of Risk Communication: Producing Citizens and the Role of Technical Communicators." *Technical Communication Quarterly* 7.4 (1998): 415–41. Print.

Grady, Denise. "W.H.O. Alert Says a Global Spread of Flu Is Likely." *New York Times* Apr. 30, 2009: A1. Print.

Granatstein, Rob. "T. O. Fights Back; Billions of Dollars Are at Stake at Key WHO Meeting." *Toronto Sun* Apr. 29, 2003: 4. Print.

Greenfeld, Karl Taro. *China Syndrome: The True Story of the 21st Century's First Great Epidemic*. New York: HarperCollins, 2006. Print.

Grewal, Inderpal. *Transnational America: Feminisms, Diasporas, Neoliberalisms*. Durham: Duke UP, 2005. Print.

Grigsby, Darcy Grimaldo. "Rumor, Contagion, and Colonization in Gros's Plague-Stricken of Jaffa (1804)." *Representations* 51 (1995): 1–46. Print.

Guangdong Health Bureau. "On the Control and Prevention of Unexplained Pneumonia." Feb. 3, 2003. Web. June 6, 2005. <http://www.xdyy.net/ap/file/1.htm>.

"Guangdong Media's Reflection of Pneumonia: Interview of Lei Yulan." *Yangchen Evening* Feb. 21, 2003: 3. Print.

Gudykunst, William B., Carmen M. Lee, Tsukasa Nishida, and Naoto Ogawa. "Theorizing about Intercultural Communication: An Introduction." *Theorizing about Intercultural Communication*. Thousand Oaks, CA: Sage, 2005. 3–32. Print.

"Guizhou's Zhenning County Mobilized Civilian Soldiers to Facilitate Spring Planting and SARS Prevention." *People's Daily*, May 11, 2003. Web. Feb. 19, 2005. <http://www.people.com.cn/>.

Hai, Wen, Zhong Zhao, Jian Wang, and Zhen-Gang Hou. "The Short-Term Impact of SARS on the Chinese Economy." *Asian Economic Papers* 3.1 (2004): 57–61. Print.

Hall, Edward T. *Beyond Culture*. New York: Anchor, 1976. Print.

Han, Junjie, and Zhixian Pan. "Henan: Government Will Help Migrant Workers' Families with Wheat Harvesting and Fall Planting." *Chinese Youth* [Beijing] Apr. 28, 2003. Print.

Haraway, Donna J. *Modest_Witness@Second_Millennium.FemaleMan_Meets_OncoMouse: Feminism and Technoscience*. New York: Routledge, 1997. Print.

———. "Situated Knowledges: The Science Question in Feminism and the Privilege of Partial Perspective." *Feminist Studies* 14.3 (1988): 575–99. Print.

Harrison, Bridget. "Chinatown's Business Leaders Yesterday Wooed Tourists with Assurances." *New York Post* Apr. 29, 2003: 8. Print.

Hashimoto, Ken-ichi, and Ken Tabata. "Health Infrastructure, Demographic Transition and Growth." *Review of Development Economics* 9.4 (2005): 549–62. Print.

Health Canada. *Learning from SARS: Renewal of Public Health in Canada*. Ottawa, Canada: Health Canada, 2003. Print.

"Hebei Province Chief Ji Yunshi: Hebei's Anti-SARS Work Forms the Defense Line for Beijing." *Xinhuanet*, May 2, 2003. Web. Feb. 16, 2006. <http://www.xinhuanet.com>.

He, Jie. "Test in Spring 2003: Memorandum of the Event of Atypical Pneumonia." *Nanfang Daily* [Guangzhou] Feb. 15, 2003: 5. Print.

Henson, Bertha. "Do Your Part, Stop Selfish Behavior; in War on SARS, There Is No Excuse for Anyone in Singapore Not to Know The Part He Has to Play." *Straits Times* [Singapore] May 3, 2003: 3. Print.

He Qiang. "Background of the Earliest Reports about SARS in Guangzhou: CPC's Strategic Manipulation of Mass Media." *MyCND*. Web. Feb. 16, 2006. <http://mycnd.org/modules/wfsection/article.php?articleid=2199>.

———. "Scientific Definition Manipulated, Execution of Law of Infectious Disease Is Challenging for Doctors." *Xin Yu Si*, May 11, 2003. Web. Feb. 16, 2006. <http://www.xys.org>.

Herman, Edward S., and Noam Chomsky. *Manufacturing Consent: The Political Economy of the Mass Media*. New York: Pantheon, 1988. Print.

Hermida, Alfred. "Behind China's Internet Red Firewall." *BBC*, Sept. 3, 2002. Web. July 7, 2003. <http://news.bbc.co.uk/2/hi/technology/2231101.stm>.

Herndl, Carl G. "Teaching Discourse and Reproducing Culture: A Critique of Research and Pedagogy in Professional and Non-Academic Writing." *College Composition and Communication* 44.3 (1993): 349–63. Print.

Hesford, Wendy, and Eileen E. Schell. "Configurations of Transnationality: Locating Feminist Rhetorics." *College English* 70.5 (2008): 461–70. Print.

"Heyuan Zhongshan Clarifying the Rumor: No Atypical Pneumonia Outbreak." *New Press* [Guangzhou] Feb. 14, 2003: 12. Print.

Hoftstede, Gert Jan. *Culture's Consequences*. 2nd ed. Beverly Hills, CA: Sage, 2001. Print.

Hoge, Warren. "Britain Adopts Emergency Law to Deter Anthrax Hoaxes after Spate of False Reports." *New York Times* Oct. 22, 2001: B6. Print.

Hong, Ling Chang, and Jason Leow. "China's Deadly Numbers Game." *Straits Times* [Singapore] Apr. 20, 2003: 6. Print.

"How Rumors Were Transformed into Panic." *South Cosmopolitan* [Guangzhou] Jan. 20, 2003: 9. Print.

Hsu, Madeline. *Dreaming of Gold and Dreaming of Home: Transnationalism and Migration between the United States and China, 1882–1943*. Stanford: Stanford UP, 2000. Print.

Hsu, Mei-ling. "Reporting an Emerging Epidemic in Taiwan: Journalists' Experience of SARS Reporting." Powers and Xiaosui 182–99.

Huang, Xiaoyan, and Xiaoming Hao. "Party Journalism vs. Market Journalism: The Coverage of SARS by *People's Daily* and *Beijing Youth News*." Powers and Xiaosui 93–107.

Huang, Yanzhong. "China's New Health Diplomacy." *China's Capacity to Manage Infectious Diseases: Global Implications*. Ed. Xiaoqing Lu. Washington, DC: CSIS. 86–92.

———. "The Politics of HIV/AIDS in China." *Asian Perspective* 30.1 (2006): 95–125.

Hua, Yu. "Scientific Prevention Is Key in SARS Control, SARS Prevention Requires Prevention of Superstition." *Guangmin Daily* May 21, 2003: 4. Print.

"Huge Traffic Jam in Guangdong Telephone System: With Only 20% Connection Rate." *Guangzhou Daily* Feb. 12, 2003: 7. Print.

"Humankind Is Able to Conquer SARS: Commentary." *People's Daily*, Apr. 21, 2003. Web. June 12, 2004. <http://english.peopledaily.com.cn/200304/21/eng20030421_115548.shtml>.

Hung, Lee Shiu. "The SARS Epidemic in Hong Kong: What Lessons Have We Learned?" *Journal of the Royal Society of Medicine* 96 (2003): 374–78. Print.

Hunsinger, R. Peter. "Culture and Cultural Identity in Intercultural Technical Communication." *Technical Communication Quarterly* 15.1 (2006): 31–48. Print.

Huo, Lang, Xiaohua Ma, and Duan Yan. "Investigation of the Transnational Chain of the Imported H1N1 Flu Case." *First Finance Daily* [Shanghai] May 12, 2009: 7. Print.

Hu, Shuli, Yi Luo, and Qiyan Li. "Western Invasion of SARS: Epicenter of Shanxi." *Cai Jin* [Beijing] May 3, 2003: 14. Print.

Iezzoni, Lynette. *Influenza 1918: The Worst Epidemic in American History*. New York: TV Books, 1999. Print.

"Impact of SARS on China." *Voice of America*, May 29, 2003. Web. June 16, 2008. <http://www.voanews.com/uspolicy/archive/2003–05/a-2003–05–29–5-1.cfm>.

"Infection Investigation: Beijing Police Hospital and Chaoyang Hospital." *Finance* [Beijing] May 30, 2003: 11. Print.

Institute of International Education. "International Students in the United States." *Institute of International Education*, Nov. 12, 2012. Web. Jan. 3, 2013. <http://www.iie.org/en/Services/Project-Atlas/United-States/International-Students-In-US>.

"Interior Decoration Company Expelled out of Beijing Market after Mismanaged Employees Left Beijing." *Hebei Government*, May 13, 2003. Web. June 5, 2011. <http://www.hebei.gov.cn/syscolumn/lshm/fzfd/fzfdxxzb/index.htm>.

"Investigation: Over 80% Citizens Did Not Believe Rumors." *Guangzhou Daily* Feb. 17, 2003: 9. Print.

"Isolation: Strict Home Quarantine Aims to Halt Virus Spread." *Hong Kong Information Services Department*, Apr. 10, 2003. Web. Nov. 12, 2008. <http://www3.news.gov.hk/isd/ebulletin/en/category/issues/030410/html/030410en07003.htm>.

Jakes, Susan. "Beijing's SARS attack." *Time*, Apr. 8, 2003. Web. June 29, 2004. <http://www.time.com/time/asia/news/printout/0,9788,441615,00.html>.

"Japan's Radically Increased H1N1 Flu Cases Shocked Neighboring Countries, No Consensus Reached on Global Battle against the Flu." *Global Time* [Guangzhou] May 19, 2009: 14. Print.

Jay, Martin. *The Culture of the Self*. Language Laboratory of the University of California at Berkeley, Spring 1983. Audiocassette.

Jiang, Ying. "SARS Scares Drove Americans Away from Chinatown." *Epoch Times*, Apr. 11, 2003. Web. Jan. 23, 2004. <http://www.dajiyuan.com>.

Johnson-Eilola, Johndan. "Relocating the Value of Work: Technical Communication in a Post-industrial Age." *Technical Communication Quarterly* 5 (1996): 245–70. Print.

Johnson, Robert. *User-Centered Technology: A Rhetorical Theory for Computers and Other Mundane Artifacts*. Albany: State U of New York P, 1998. Print.

Jones, J. R. "Reach Out, Touch Somebody, and Die: In *Contagion*, Your Next Kiss (or Cocktail Peanut) Could Be Fatal." *Sun-Times Media*, Sept. 8, 2011. Web. May 12, 2012. <http://www.chicagoreader.com/chicago/contagion-winslet-damon-disaster-movie-soderbergh/Content?oid=4574330>.

Jordans, Frank, and Maria Cheng. "WHO: Swine Flu Vaccine to Take Months to Produce." *Associated Press*, May 19, 2009, Web. Nov. 21, 2009. <http://abclocal.go.com/wpvi/story?section=news/health&id=6820353>.

Kahn, Joseph. "Analysts See Tension in China within the Top Leadership." *New York Times* July 1, 2003: A1. Print.

———. "Beijing Hurries to Build Hospital Complex for Increasing Number of SARS Patients." *New York Times* Apr. 27, 2003: A19. Print.

———. "China Getting a Black Eye for Early Secrecy on SARS." *New York Times* Apr. 13, 2003: A10. Print.

———. "The Contagion Reaches near the Top of the Chinese Communist Hierarchy." *New York Times* Apr. 30, 2003: A11. Print.

———. "Hu Takes Control as Jiang Resigns; President Now Commands the Military; Orderly Power Transfer Is China's First." *New York Times* Sept. 20, 2004: 1. Print.

Kaplan, Robert. "Cultural Thought Patterns in Inter-cultural Education." *Language Learning* 16 (1966): 1–20. Print.

Katz, Steven, and Carolyn Miller. "The Low-Level Radioactive Waste Siting Controversy *in* North Carolina: Toward a Rhetorical Model of Risk Communication." *Green Culture: Environmental Rhetoric in Contemporary America.* Ed. Carl G. Herndl and Stuart Brown. Madison: U of Wisconsin P, 1996. 111–40. Print.

Kaufman, Joan. "Infectious Disease Challenges in China." *China's Capacity to Manage Infectious Diseases: Global Implications.* Ed. Xiaoqing Lu. Washington, DC: CSIS, 2009. 3–16. Print.

Kelso, J. A. Scott. *Dynamic Patterns: The Self-organization of Brain and Behavior.* Cambridge, MA: MIT P, 1995. Print.

Kennedy, George A. *Comparative Rhetoric: An Historical and Cross-cultural Introduction.* New York: Oxford UP, 1998. Print.

Keränen, Lisa. "Addressing the Epidemic of Epidemics: Germs, Security, and a Call for Biocriticism." *Quarterly Journal of Speech* 97.2 (2011): 224–44. Print.

———. "Bio(in)security: Rhetoric, Science, and Citizens in the Age of Bioterrorism—The Case of TOPOFF 3." *Sizing Up Rhetoric.* Ed. David Zarefsky and Elizabeth Benacka. Long Grove, IL: Waveland, 2008. 227–49. Print.

Kienzler, Donna. "Ethics, Critical Thinking, and Professional Communication Pedagogy." *Technical Communication Quarterly* 10 (2001): 319–40. Print.

Kimball, M. A. "Cars, Culture, and Tactical Technical Communication." *Technical Communication Quarterly* 15 (2006): 67–86. Print.

Kim, Min-sun. "Culture-Based Interactive Constraints in Explaining Intercultural Strategic Competence." *Intercultural Communication Competence.* Ed. R. L. Wiseman and J. Koester. Thousand Oaks, CA: Sage, 1993. 132–50. Print.

Kleinman, Arthur, and James Watson, eds. *SARS in China: Prelude to Pandemic.* Stanford: Stanford UP, 2006. Print.

Kolko, Beth, and Carolyn Y. Wei. "Internet Use in Uzbekistan: Developing a Methodology for Tracking Information Technology Implementation Success." *Information Technologies and International Development* 1.2 (2003): 1–19. Print.

Krestas, Shirley A., Lori H. Fisher, and JoAnn T. Hackos. "Future Directions for Continuing Education in Technical Communication." *Technical Communication* 42.4 (1995): 642–45. Print.

Lai, Chloe. "Lifting the Lid on the Spread of SARS." *South China Morning Post* [Hong Kong] Apr. 23, 2003: 6. Print.

———. "Mainland Students Overseas Under Pressure to Stay Put." *South China Morning Post* [Hong Kong] May 21, 2009: 04. Print.

Lakoff, Andrew, and Stephen J. Collier. *Biosecurity Interventions: Global Health and Security in Question.* New York: Columbia UP, 2008. Print.

Lakshmanan, Indira A. R. "China Had Underreported SARS, WHO Investigators Say." *Boston Globe* Apr. 17, 2003: 9. Print.

Lampton, David. *Same Bed, Different Dreams: Managing U.S.-China Relations, 1989–2000.* Berkeley: U of California P, 2001. Print.

Landler, Mark. "A Democracy Stalwart Struggles to Be Heard; Voice of America Works to Spread Its Message in the Age of the Internet." *International Herald Tribune* [Paris] June 9, 2011: 4. Print.

Lan, Feiyun. "Deliberate Downplay of the Crisis to Avoid Panic: Resulting in Huge Panic." *Asian Weekly* [Hong Kong] 2003: 7. Print.

———. "Journalists in Panic with Official Downplay." *Asian Weekly* [Hong Kong] 2003: 11. Print.

Larkin, Marilynn. "Web Serves as Conduit for SARS Information." *Lancet Infectious Diseases* 3.6 (2003): 388–89. Print.

Lean, Geoffrey. "Factory Farms Blamed for Spread of Bird Flu." *Independent*, Feb 26, 2006. Web. May 7, 2007. <http://www.independent.co.uk/environment/factory-farms-blamed-for-spread-of-bird-flu-467770.html>.

Lee, C. C. "Ambiguities and Contradiction: Issues in China's Changing Political Communication." *Gazette* 53 (1994): 7–21. Print.

Lee, Chin-chuan. "Liberalization without Full Democracy: Guerrilla Media and Political Movements in Taiwan." Couldry and Curran, 163–76.

Lee, Ella. "Health Chief to Press U.S. on Screening." *South China Morning Post* [Hong Kong] May 16, 2009: 4. Print.

———. "WHO's Handling of Flu in Sharp Contrast with SARS." *South China Morning Post* [Hong Kong] May 17, 2009: 2. Print.

Lee, Matthew. "Hunan in Panic over Outbreak Rumours." *Standard* [Hong Kong] Feb. 15, 2003: 16. Print.

"Legal Framework for Tackling Public Health Crises Established." *People's Daily* May 13, 2003: 5. Print.

"Legion Disease and Pestis Are Not Causes of Pneumonia." *Guangzhou Daily* Feb. 12, 2003: 14. Print.

Leiss, William, and Douglas Powell. *Mad Cow and Mother's Milk: The Perils of Poor Risk Communication.* 2nd ed. Montreal: McGill-Queen's UP, 2004. Print.

Leung, Carrianne. "The Yellow Peril Revisited: The Impact of SARS on Chinese and Southeast Asian Communities." *Resources for Feminist Research* 33 (2008): 135–49. Print.

Lev, Michael. "SARS Tally Raises, Heads Roll in China." *Chicago Tribune* Apr. 21, 2003. Web. Oct. 10, 2003. <http://articles.chicagotribune.com/2003-04-21/news/0304210090_1_gao-qiang-sars-new-cases>.

Lewin, Tamar. "China Surges Past India as Top Home of Foreign Students." *New York Times* Nov. 15, 2010: A14. Print.

Liang, Keyi. "Text Messages Played a Complicated Role in Rumor-Induced Panic." *New Press* [Guangzhou] Feb. 17, 2003: 7. Print.

Li, Haipeng. "Emergency Construction of 'Noah's Ark.'" *South Weekly* [Guangzhou] July 24, 2003: 6. Print.

Li, Jian. "Canadian Premier Visited Chinatown." *Dajiyuan Epoch Times* [Washington, DC] Apr. 11, 2003: 6. Print.

Lin, Luming. *Wall of People: Chinese People's Fight against SARS*. Beijing: Xuexi, 2003. Print.

Li, Shiyuan. "Guangdong: Where Did True Accurate SARS Data Come From?" *People's Daily* Apr. 12, 2003: 4. Print.

Li, Shu, Jiangping Ye, Sihai Wang, and Si Yang. "Twenty-Four-Hour Massive Investigation." *Tianjin Daily* May 11, 2009: 9. Print.

"List of Buildings with SARS Cases Released." *Government Information Centre*, Apr. 12, 2003. Web. Nov. 12, 2008. <http://www.info.gov.hk/gia/general/200304/12/0412220.htm>.

Liu, Haiming. "Transnational Historiography: Chinese American Studies Reconsidered." *Journal of the History of Ideas* 65.1 (2004): 135–53. Print.

Liu, Jian. "False Text Messages and 'Messaging Harassment' Going Rampant." *ChinaNet*, Mar. 3, 2003. Web. June 30, 2003. <http://www.chinanet.com/200303/03/125.htm>.

Liu, Wangyong. "College Students in Beijing Hotly Debated 'Whether to Go Home or Not,' Avoid Leaving Campus at Will." *Chinese Youth* [Beijing] Apr. 24, 2003: 8. Print.

Liu, Yameng. "To Capture the Essence of Chinese Rhetoric: An Anatomy of a Paradigm in Comparative Rhetoric." *Rhetoric Review* 14.2 (1996): 318–35. Print.

Liu, Yang. "Beijing Bureau of Labor: No Companies Allowed to Dismiss Migrant Workers." *Beijing Daily* Apr. 30, 2003: 3. Print.

Liu, Yue. "'Bao Man-man' and 'Lu Spread-Spread' Became Famous Because of Disease; 'Isolation Journals' Widely Circulated." *Wenweibo* [Shanghai] May 16, 2009. Print.

Lo, Alex. "A Shrinking World Raises the Risk for Global Epidemics." *South China Morning Post* [Hong Kong] Mar. 14, 2003: 4. Print.

Locke, Michelle. "Berkeley: No SARS-Area Students." *Dailyiowanmedia*, May 6, 2003. Web. Sept. 9, 2004. http://www.dailyiowanmedia.com/archives/?p=432865.

Longo, Bernadette. "An Approach for Applying CS Theory to Technical Writing Research." Scott, Longo, and Wills 111–32.

Lou, Yi. "The History of SARS Attacks on North Jiaotong University and Central Finance University." *Finance* May 12, 2003: 12. Print.

"Love Called Not Returning Home, A." *Wenweibo*, May 22, 2009. Web. June 29, 2009. <http://trans.wenweipo.com/gb/paper.wenweipo.com/2009/05/22/ED0905220010.htm>.

Luard, Tim. "China Rethinks Peasant 'Apartheid.'" *BBC News*, Nov. 10, 2005. Web. June 6, 2011. <http://news.bbc.co.uk/2/hi/asia-pacific/4424944.stm>.

Lucas, Caroline. "Swine Flu: Is Intensive Pig Farming to Blame?" *Guardian*, Apr. 28, 2009. Web. Mar. 3, 2010. <http://www.guardian.co.uk/commentisfree/2009/apr/28/swine-flu-intensive-farming-caroline-lucas>.

Lu, Feng. "Danwei: A Special Organizational Mechanism of Society." *Sociology in China* 5 (1993): 43–66. Print.

Lu, Fuming. "Shandong Initiated 'Green-Love Mail Channel' to Dissuade Floating Laborers Working outside the Province from Returning Home." *Xinhuanet*, May 15, 2003. Web. Jan. 23, 2004. <http://www.xinhuanet.com>.

Lu, Jie, and Hua Liu. "Chinese Student Studying in the U.S. Urged Students Studying Abroad to Postpone Their Trip Back to China." *Guangzhou Daily* May 14, 2009: 3. Print.

Lu, Xing. "Construction of Nationalism and Political Legitimacy through Rhetoric of the Anti-SARS Campaign: A Fantasy Theme Analysis." Powers and Xiao 109–24.

———. *Rhetoric in Ancient China, Fifth to Third Century B.C.E.: A Comparison with Classical Greek Rhetoric.* Columbia: U of South Carolina P, 1998. Print.

Lu, Xueyi. *Study of Contemporary Chinese Social Strata.* Beijing: Social Science Academic, 2002. Print.

Lyotard, Jean-François. *The Postmodern Condition: A Report on Knowledge.* Manchester, England: Manchester UP, 1979. Print.

Lyotard, Jean-Francois, and Jean-Loup Thebaud. *Just Gaming.* Minneapolis: U of Minnesota P, 1985. Print.

Macartney, Jane. "China's Web Censors Are Losing the Battle." *Times* [London], Feb. 16, 2006. Web. July 12, 2008. <http://www.thetimes.co.uk/tto/news/world/asia/article2612190.ece>.

Machin, David, and Theo van Leeuwen. *Global Media Discourse: A Critical Introduction.* New York: Routledge, 2006. Print.

MacKinnon, Mark. "Shamed by SARS, China Vows Transparency; Though It Has Yet to Confirm a Single Case, Beijing Swings into Action against Swine Flu in a Dramatic Contrast to 2003's Policy of Denial." *Globe and Mail* Apr. 29, 2009: A13. Print.

Mahon, Michael. *Foucault's Nietzschean Genealogy: Truth, Power, and the Subject.* Albany: State U of New York P, 1992. Print.

"Major Role for Mass Media in Globalization." *Star* [Malaysia] July 29, 2003: 13. Print.

Mao, LuMing. "Studying the Chinese Rhetorical Tradition in the Present: Re-presenting the Native's Point of View." *College English* 69.3 (2007): 216–37. Print.

Mao, LuMing, and Morris Young, eds. *Representations: Doing Asian American Rhetoric*. Logan: Utah State UP, 2008. Print.

Mao Zedong. *On Guerrilla Warfare*. Trans. Samuel B. Griffith. New York: Praeger, 1961. Print.

Marklein, Mary Beth. "Berkeley to Block Students from Nations Hit by SARS." *USA Today* May 6, 2003: 1A. Print.

Martin, Judith N., and Thomas K. Nakayama. *Intercultural Communication in Contexts*. Boston: McGraw-Hill, 2007. Print.

"Mass Panic: People Waited in Line to Purchase Drugs." *Information Times* Jan. 19, 2003: 4. Print.

Matthews, Karen. "SARS Scare Hits New York's Chinatown." *Associated Press Worldstream*, Apr. 15, 2003. *LexisNexis® Academic*. Web. May 3, 2004.

Maylath, Bruce. "Writing Globally: Teaching the Technical Writing Student to Prepare Documents for Translation." *Journal of Business and Technical Communication* 11.3 (1997): 339–53. Print.

McCabe, Aileen. "China Might Reform Punishing Hukou System; Household Registration: Social Harmony at Stake, Professor Says of Rules for 130 Million Migrant Workers." *Gazette* (Montreal) Mar. 2, 2010: A16. Print.

McLaughlin, Kathleen. "Shanghai Beats SARS with Luck, WHO Says." *San Francisco Chronicle*, May 13, 2003. Web. June 3, 2004. <http://www.sfgate.com/health/article/Shanghai-beats-SARS-with-luck-WHO-says-2617146.php#ixzz2KoQ4wuJk>.

McNeil, Donald G. "World Health Organization May Raise Alert Level as Swine Flu Cases Leap in Japan." *New York Times* May 18, 2009: A9. Print.

Mengin, Françoise, ed. *Cyber China: Reshaping National Identities in the Age of Information*. New York: Palgrave, 2004. Print.

Meng, Yan, and Jianying Fang. "How to Evaluate the Contemporary Determinants of International Public Opinions." *Military Correspondent*, Nov. 10, 2010. Web. Sept. 3, 2013. <http://chn.chinamil.com.cn/jsjz/2010-11/12/content_4332551.htm>.

"Migrant Farm Workers Rode Bikes Home from SARS-Affected Areas, Shangdong Heze Took Risk-Reduction Measures at All Levels." *Chinese Youth* [Beijing] May 4, 2003: 11. Print.

Miles, Libby. "Globalizing Professional Writing Curricula: Positioning Students and Re-Positioning Textbooks." *Technical Communication Quarterly* 6.2 (1997): 179–200. Print.

Miller, Carolyn R. "A Humanistic Rationale for Technical Writing." *College English* 40.6 (1979): 610–17. Print.

———. "What's Practical about Technical Writing?" *Technical Writing: Theory and Practice*. Ed. Bertie E. Fearing and W. Keats Sparrow. New York: MLA, 1989. 14–26. Print.

Ministry of Health. "CDC, MOH: Notification on the Distribution of the Prevention and Treatment of Atypical Pneumonia." *Ministry of Health*, 2003. Web. Oct. 3 2004. <http://www.moh.gov.cn>.

"Ministry of Public Security Criticized Practices of Highway Blockades and Stipulated 'Five Forbiddens' to Ensure Smooth Traffic." *China News*, May 6, 2003. Web. July 9, 2006. <http://www.chinanews.com>.

Minnix, Kathleen. "Flu Week: In 1918, World War I and the Spanish Flu Fed Each Other." *Book of Odds*, n.d. Web. Feb. 10, 2013. <http://bookofodds.com/Accidents-Death/Articles/A0225-Flu-Week-In-1918-World-War-I-and-the-Spanish-Flu-Fed-Each-Other>.

"Miracle: The Construction of Xiaotangshan Hospital." *Xinhuanet*, May 4, 2003. Web. July 9, 2006. <http://news.xinhuanet.com/newscenter/2003–05/04/content_857483.htm>.

Miyazaki, Ichisada. *China's Examination Hell: The Civil Service Examinations of Imperial China*. Trans. Conrad Schirokauer. New Haven: Yale University Press. 1976. Print.

Movius, Lisa. "Mrs. Li Is Watching Me." *Salon*, June 19, 2003. Web. July 9, 2006. <http://dir.salon.com/story/mwt/feature/2003/06/19/sars/index.html>.

Moy, Patsy. "Temperature Checks for Air Travellers; All Passengers Leaving Chek Lap Kok Will Be Tested in An Attempt to Ease Overseas Fears on the SARS Outbreak." *South China Morning Post* [Hong Kong] Apr. 12, 2003: 1. Print.

Mu, Fei. "Rapid Action, the Most Effective Option in Spreading Epidemic: Record-Breaking Construction of Hospital in Eight Days." *Asia Weekly* May 5, 2003. 15. Print.

Mu, Fu. "Liu Jianlun and Jiang Yanyong." *Open Magazine* 2003: 32–34. Print.

Murphy, Dean E. "In U.S., Fear Is Spreading Faster Than SARS." *New York Times* Apr. 17, 2003: A4. Print.

Murphy, Dean E., and Karen W. Arenson. "Students in SARS Countries Banned for Berkeley Session." *New York Times* May 6, 2003: A12. Print.

Murphy, Timothy, and Suzanne Poirier. *Writing AIDS: Gay Literature, Language, and Analysis*. New York: Columbia UP, 1993. Print.

"My Chinese Heart." *Xiami*, Feb. 1984. Web. Oct. 15, 2011. <http://www.xiami.com/song/detail/id/2050781>.

"Mystery Pneumonia under Control: FM Spokesman." *People's Daily*, Mar. 19, 2003. Web. Oct. 15, 2005. <http://english.people.com.cn/200303/19/eng20030319_113540>.

"Newest Report on Highly Contagious Epidemic in Guangzhou: With 280 Deaths." *Peace Hall*, Feb. 10, 2003. Web. Aug. 20, 2003. <http://www.peacehall.com/news/gb/china/2003/02/200302102350.shtml>.

"News Press by State Council News Office: Q & A." *Sina*, May 15, 2003. Web. Aug. 21, 2005. <http://www.sina.com>.

Ng, Michael. "Virus Fears Fuel Rise in Oil, Salt, Rice Sales." *Standard* [Hong Kong] Feb. 14, 2003: 12. Print.

Ng, Michael, and Ella Lee. "Epidemic of Fear Spawns Outbreak of Prejudice." *South China Morning Post* [Hong Kong] Apr. 12, 2003: 8. Print.

"Notifications about the Atypical Pneumonia Coverage Sent by Head of the Provincial Propaganda Department in February and March." *Kang Zhongguo,* Apr. 3, 2003. Web. Dec. 12, 2004. <http://www.kanhzhongguo.com/news/gb /articles/3/4/40652.html>.

"November 2002 to May 2003: Major Events in Guangdong's Battle against SARS." *Yangcheng Evening* May 4, 2003: 5. Print.

O'Brien, Chris. "The Human Flesh Search Engine." *Forbes,* Nov. 21, 2008. Web. May 26, 2009. <http://www.forbes.com/2008/11/21/human-flesh-search-tech-identity08-cx_cb_1121obrien.html>.

"Official Denies Bird Flu Rumors." *China Daily* [Beijing] Feb. 22, 2003: 12. Print.

"Official Explains Rise of SARS Cases in Beijing." *People's Daily* [Beijing] Apr. 20, 2003: 4. Print.

"155 Confirmed SARS Cases in Rural Areas, No Large-Scale Outbreak or Spread." *China Central Television,* May 15, 2003.Web. Feb. 2, 2007. <http://www.cctv. com/news/china/20030515/101078.shtml>.

"One Thousand People Waiting in Line to Buy Antiviral Drugs in Guangzhou." *Yangchen Evening* Feb. 11, 2003: 7. Print.

Ong, Aihwa. *Flexible Citizenship: The Cultural Logics of Transnationality.* Durham: Duke UP, 1999. Print.

———. "Graduated Sovereignty in Southeast Asia," *Theory, Culture, and Society* 17.4 (2000): 55–75. Print.

———. "Urban Assemblages: An Ecological Sense of the Knowledge Economy." Mengin, 238–53.

"On the Control and Prevention of Unexplained Pneumonia." Guangdong Provincial Health Bureau. *Modern Hospital,* Feb. 3, 2003. Web. Feb. 19, 2005. <http: //www.xdyy.net/ap/file>.

Ortiz, Fernando. *Cuban Counterpoint: Tobacco and Sugar.* Trans. Harriet de Onís. Durham: Duke UP, 1995. Print.

Ou, J., Q. Li, G. Zeng, Z. Dun, A. Qin, and R. Fontaine. "Efficiency of Quarantine during an Epidemic of Severe Acute Respiratory Syndrome—Beijing, China, 2003." *Morbidity and Mortality Weekly Report* 52.43 (2003): 1037–40. Print.

Owens, Anne Marie, and Isabel Vincent. "WHO Begins SARS Debate Today: Ontario's Medical Officer Says 'I Have the Science' to Get Advisory Overturned." *National Post* Apr. 28, 2003: A1. Print.

Panem, Sandra. "A Drama and Questions." *Science* Feb. 26, 1998: 1039–40. Print.

Pan, Helin. "Interviewing the First Reported SARS Patient." *Information Time* 2003: 12–13. Print.

Parry, Jane. "SARS May Have Peaked in Canada, Hong Kong, and Vietnam." *BMJ* 326 (2003): 947. Print.

Peiris, M. S., T. Lai, L. M. Poon, et al. "Coronavirus as a Possible Cause of Severe Acute Respiratory Syndrome." *Lancet* 361 (2003): 1319–25. Print.

"People's Interests above Everything Else: Interview of Dr. Jiang Yanyong." *Sanlian Life Weekly* [Shanghai] June 11, 2003: 7. Print.

Perelman, Chaim, and Lucie Olbrechts-Tyteca. *The New Rhetoric: A Treatise on Argumentation.* Notre Dame: U of Notre Dame P, 1969. Print.

Pernick, Martin S. "Contagion and Culture." *American Literary History* 14.4 (2002): 858–65. Print.

"Pestis in Guangzhou Causing Mass Panic." *Peace Hall*, Feb. 11, 2003. Web. Aug. 10, 2003. <http://www.peacehall.com/news/gb/china/2003/02/200302111522.shtml>.

Petersen, Alan, and Deborah Lupton. *The New Public Health: Health and Self in the Age of Risk.* Sydney: Allen and Unwin, 1996. Print.

Philips, Heike. "The Data They Didn't Want to Release; 'It Would Be Difficult to Conclude There Is a Need for Such Information.'" *South China Morning Post* [Hong Kong] Apr. 11, 2003: 1. Print.

Pomfret, John. "China Raises Disease's Death Toll: Under Pressure, Officials Admit Spread of Infection to Beijing." *Washington Post* Mar. 27, 2003: A16. Print.

———. "WHO Lifts Warning on Travel to Beijing: China Credits Party for Stopping SARS." *Washington Post* June 25, 2003: A12. Print.

Pomfret, John, and Rick Weiss. "Hong Kong Quarantines Complex to Control Spread of Epidemic." *Washington Post* Mar. 31, 2003: A02. Print.

Poon, L. L. M., Y. Guan, J. M. Nicholls, K. Y. Yuen, and J. S. M. Peiris. "The Aetiology, Origins, and Diagnosis of Severe Acute Respiratory Syndrome." *Lancet* 4 (2004): 663–71. Print.

Porter, James E., Patricia Sullivan, Stuart Blythe, Jeffrey Grabill, and Libby Miles. "Institutional Critique: A Rhetorical Methodology for Change." *College Composition and Communication* 51.4 (2000): 610–42. Print.

Powers, John H., and Xiao Xiaosui, eds. *The Social Construction of SARS: Studies of a Health Communication Crisis.* Amsterdam: Benjamins, 2008. Print.

"Premier: Prevent Rural Epidemic." *China Daily* May 7, 2003: 2. Print.

"President Hu Calls for "People's War" against SARS." *People's Daily* May 2, 2003: 1. Print.

"Press Conference on SARS Prevention and Control Offered by Vice Health Minister Gao Qiang." *Xinhua News Agency*, Apr. 20, 2003. Web. Aug. 26, 2003. <http://news.xinhuanet.com/newscenter/2003-04/21/content_841098.htm>.

Price-Smith, Andrew T. *Contagion and Chaos: Disease, Ecology, and National Security in the Era of Globalization.* Cambridge, MA: MIT P, 2009. Print.

Qiang, Zongren. "Complete History of Attack of Atypical Pneumonia in Guangdong Province." *Bund Pictorial* Feb. 13, 2003: 15. Print.

Quarantelli, Enrico. "Panic Behavior: Some Empirical Observations," *Human Response to Tall Buildings*. Ed. Donald J. Conway. Stroudsburg, PA: Dowden Hutchinson & Ross. 1977. 336–50. Print.

———. "The Sociology of Panic." *International Encyclopedia of the Social and Behavioral Sciences*. Ed. Neil J. Smelser, and Paul B. Baltes. New York: Pergamon, 2001. 11020–30. Print.

Queen, Mary. "Transnational Feminist Rhetorics in a Digital World." *College English* 70.5 (2008): 471–89. Print.

"Questioning Tamiflu." *Southern Cosmopolitan* [Guangzhou] Feb. 16, 2003: A05–7. Print.

"Railroad Strengthened Sterilization." *Southern Daily* [Guangzhou] Feb. 13, 2003: 9. Print.

Rainey, Kenneth T., David Dayton, and Roy K. Turner. "Do Curricula Correspond to Managerial Expectations? Core Competencies for Technical Communicators." *Technical Communication* 52.3 (2005): 323–52. Print.

Ramen, Fred. *SARS (Severe Acute Respiratory Syndrome)*. New York: Rosen, 2004. Print.

"Reflections on SARS." *Lancet Infectious Disease* 4 (Nov. 2004): 651. Print.

"Regulations on State Secrets in Public Health Work, Their Level of Secrecy and Details." *Encyclopedia on the State Secrets Law of the PRC*. Ed. Zhidong Li. Changchun, Jilin: People's Press, 1999. 372–74. Print.

Ren, Yuan. "SARS and Conspiracy Theories across the Strait." *Epoch Times*, May 1, 2003. Web. Feb. 19, 2005. http://www.epochtimes.com/gb/3/5/1/n306805p.htm.

Ren, Zhongping. "Construction of Our New Great Wall: The Great Anti-SARS Spirit." *People's Daily* May 15, 2003: 1. Print.

"Report on the Unexplained Pneumonia in Guangdong." *Guangdong Provincial Health Bureau*, Feb. 3, 2003. Web. Feb. 19, 2005. <http://www.xdyy.net/ap/file /9.htm>.

Rheingold, Howard. *Smart Mobs: The Next Social Revolution*. Cambridge, MA: Perseus, 2002. Print.

Richburg, Keith B. "In China, Chafing under Ancient Permits; Access to City Services Critics Say 'Hukous' Are Outdated and Discriminatory." *Washington Post* Aug. 15, 2010: A08. Print.

Robinson, Susan, and Wendy Newstetter. "Uncertain Science and Certain Deadlines: CDC Responses to the Media during the Anthrax Attacks of 2001." *Journal of Health Communication* 8 (2003): 17–35. Print.

Roeser, Sabine, ed. *Emotions and Risky Technologies*. Dordrecht: Springer, 2010. Print.

Rosenberg, Charles E. *Explaining Epidemics and Other Studies in the History of Medicine*. Cambridge: Cambridge UP, 1992. Print.

Rosenthal, Elisabeth. "SARS Outbreak Fading Away, Officials Say." *New York Times* June 6, 2003: A10. Print.

Rosenwald, Michael S. "Chinatown Fights Fears Restaurants Slump on SARS Worries." *Boston Globe* Apr. 7, 2003: B1. Print.

Ross, Andrew. "Containing Culture in the Cold War." *No Respect: Intellectuals and Popular Culture.* New York: Routledge, 1989. 42–64. Print.

"Rumor Denounced: No Avian Flu b-2 Virus Was Found in Guangzhou." *Southern Cosmopolitan* Feb. 14, 2003: 4. Print.

"Rumor: SARS Infects Restaurant Workers in Asian Neighborhoods. Netlore Archive: Variants of a Widespread Rumor Claim the SARS Epidemic Threatens Local Communities across North America via Infected Workers at Restaurants and Groceries in Chinatowns and Other Asian Neighborhoods." *Urban Legends*, Apr. 1, 2003. Web. Sept. 8, 2008. <http://urbanlegends.about.com/library /bl-sars-restaurants.htm>.

"Rural Economies May Break Invisible Shackles of Hukou." *China Daily* June 7, 2010. Web. Sept. 8, 2010. < http://www.chinadaily.com.cn/beijing/2010-06/07 /content_12389302.htm>.

"Russian Expert: SARS Is a Bioterrorist Weapon, with the United States Being the Most Probable Manufacturer." *Comsenz*, Apr. 19, 2003. Web. June 3, 2004. <http://bbs.taisha.org/archiver/tid-175094.html>.

Saich, Tony. "Is SARS China's Chernobyl or Much Ado about Nothing?" Kleinman and Watson, 105–21.

Salvo, Michael. "Ethics of Engagement: User-centered Design and Rhetorical Methodology." *Technical Communication Quarterly* 10.3 (2001): 273–90. Print.

Sapp, David. A., and Robbin D. Crabtree. "A Laboratory in Citizenship: Service Learning in the Technical Communication Classroom." *Technical Communication Quarterly* 11.4 (2002): 411–31. Print.

Sargent, Carey, and Jason Gale. "Bird Flu Trail Leads Medical Detectives Back to Farms (Update3)." *Bloomberg*, May 30, 2006. Web. June 12, 2007. <http://www .bloomberg.com/apps/news?pid=newsarchive&sid=a334DK66cvUc>.

"SARS and the Beijing Olympics." *Washington Times* May 18, 2003: B02. Print.

"SARS—an Opportunity China Reshuffles Public Health, Disease Prevention System." *People's Daily*, May 3, 2003. Web. Oct. 15, 2003. <http://english.peo-pledaily.com.cn/200305/03/eng20030503_116188.shtml>.

SARS Expert Committee. *SARS in Hong Kong: from Experience to Action. SARS Expert Committee*, July 21, 2003. Web. July 7, 2004. <http://www.sars-expertcom .gov.hk/english/reports/reports.html>.

"SARS Information Offered by China Informative, Complete." *People's Daily* June 14, 2003: 5. Print.

SARS Investigation. Beijing: Chinese Social Science, 2003. Print.

"SARS Travel Alert Reinstated for Toronto!!" *FreeRepublic*, May 23, 2003. Web. Oct. 21, 2004. <http://www.freerepublic.com/focus/f-news/916817/posts>.

"SARS Virus Infects China's Economy." *People's Daily* May 6, 2003: 3. Print.

"SARS World Tour 2003." *Comedian*, Apr. 3, 2003. Web. Dec. 11, 2003. <http://comedian.blogspot.com/2003_03_30_comedian_archive.html>.

Schaeffer, Robert K. *Understanding Globalization: The Social Consequences of Economic, Political, and Environmental Changes*. Lanham, MD: Rowman, 2003. Print.

Schell, R. "Maoism vs. Media in the Marketplace." *Media Studies Journal* 9.3 (1995): 33–42. Print.

Schiller, Bill. "A Tale of Two Outbreaks; Virologist Asks Whether Double Standard Used in Hard Stance on SARS, Leniency on Swine Flu." *Toronto Star* May 21, 2009: A03. Print.

Schnur, Alan. "The Role of the World Health Organization in Combating SARS, Focusing on the Efforts in China." Kleinman and Watson, 31–52.

Schoch-Spana, Monica, Crystal Franco, Jennifer B. Nuzzo, and Christiana Usenza. "Community Engagement: Leadership Tool for Catastrophic Health Events." *Biosecurity and Bioterrorism* 5.1 (2007): 8–25. Web. DOI: 10.1089/bsp.2006.0036.

Schultz, David A. *It's Show Time! Media, Politics, and Popular Culture*. New York: Lang, 2000. Print.

Scott, J. Blake. "Kairos as Indeterminate Risk Management: The Pharmaceutical Industry's Response to Bioterrorism." *Quarterly Journal of Speech* 92.2 (2006): 115–43. Print.

———. "The Practice of Usability: Teaching User Engagement through Service Learning." *Technical Communication Quarterly* 17.4 (2008): 381–412. Print.

———. *Risky Rhetoric: AIDS and the Cultural Practices of HIV Testing*. Carbondale: Southern Illinois UP, 2003. Print.

Scott, J. Blake, Bernadette Longo, and Katherine V. Wills. *Critical Power Tools: Technical Communication and Cultural Studies*. Albany: State U of New York P, 2006. Print.

Scotton, James F., and William A Hachten. *New Media for a New China*. Malden, MA: Wiley-Blackwell, 2010. Print.

Shen, Fangfei, and Qianyu Jiang. "Urgent Notification from Jiangsu's SARS Prevention Directing Center: All Migrant Workers outside the Province Should Stop Returning to Jiangsu." *Contemporary Express* [Nanjing] Apr. 29, 2003: 7. Print.

Shi, Hanbing. "When Southern Weekly Got Murdered by Prostitutes." *Xici*, Mar. 23, 2002. Web. Sept. 25, 2013. <http://www.xici.net/d4680615.htm>.

Shi, Biao, Hua Li, and Lei Zhu. "Six Rumors Leading to Mass Panic Shopping of Rice and Salt in Guangzhou." *New Press* [Guangzhou] Feb. 14, 2003: 7. Print.

Shibutani, Tamotsu. *Improvised News: A Sociological Study of Rumor*. Indianapolis: Bobbs-Merrill, 1966. Print.

"Side Report: Four 'Firsts' in History." *Jingyang Net*, May 4, 2003. Web. Mar. 16, 2011. <http://www.ycwb.com>.

Simmons, Michelle. *Participation and Power: Civic Discourse in Environmental Policy Decisions.* Albany: State U of New York P, 2007. Print.

Sims, Calvin. "In Asian-American Neighborhoods, Fear and Precaution Are Spreading." *New York Times* Apr. 5, 2003: A1, 7. Print.

Singer, Linda. *Erotic Welfare: Sexual Theory and Politics in the Age of Epidemic.* New York: Routledge, 1993. Print.

"Slack Officials Face Crackdown in SARS Crisis." *People's Daily,* May 8, 2003. Web. <http://english.peopledaily.com.cn/200305/08/eng20030508_116390.shtml>.

Slovic, Paul, Melissa L. Finucane, Ellen Peters, and Donald MacGregor. "Risk as Analysis and Risk as Feelings: Some Thoughts about Affect, Reason, Risk, and Rationality." *Risk Analysis* 24.2 (2004): 311–22. Print.

Song, Hua. "Economies of Asian Countries Most Vulnerable to Swine Flu." *Global Times* [Beijing] May 5, 2009: 11. Print.

Song, Jaymes. "SARS Fears Taking Toll on Chinatown." *Associated Press World Stream,* Apr. 12, 2003. Web. May 3, 2005. <http://www.highbeam.com/doc/1P1-73229911.html>.

Sontag, Susan. *AIDS and Its Metaphors.* New York: Farrar, 1989. Print.

"SoSick.org Timeline." *SoSick.org,* 2003. Web. May 16, 2008. <http://www.sosick.org/timeline.html#chinese>.

"Speech of Mr. Gao Qiang, Executive Vice Minister, Ministry of Health, People's Republic of China." *World Health Organization,* June17 2003. Web. June 9, 2010. <http://www.who.int/csr/sars/conference/june_2003/materials/presentations/qiang/en/ index.html>.

Spyridakis, J., H. Holmbeck, and S. Shubert. "Measuring the Translatability of Simplified English in Procedural Documents." *IEEE Transactions on Professional Communication* 40 (1997): 4–12. Print.

Starke-Meyerring, Doreen. "Meeting the Challenges of Globalization: A Framework for Global Literacies in Professional Communication Programs." *Journal of Business and Technical Communication* 19.4 (2005): 468–500. Print.

"State Council Press Conference: Minister of Health Zhang Wenkang Announced, 'It Is Safe to Live, Work, or Travel in China.'" *China Embassy,* Apr. 3, 2003. Web. Nov. 19, 2003. <http://www.chinaembassy.nl/chn/zt/fzfdxfy/t136109.htm>.

State Statistical Bureau. *China Statistical Yearbook.* Beijing: China's Statistics, 2001. Print.

"State Treasury Gives Full Support to SARS Fight: Finance Minister." *Enorth,* May 7, 2003. Web. Sept. 6, 2004. <http://english.enorth.com.cn/system/2003/05/08/000557003.shtml>.

Stein, Rob. "Incident at Elevator Felt Round World; Chinese Doctor Is Identified as Start of Health Emergency." *Washington Post* Mar. 23, 2003: A11. Print.

———. "Plumbing Suspected in SARS Spread / Outbreak at Hong Kong Apartment Complex Traced to Resident's Brother." *Washington Post* Apr. 18, 2003: A16. Print.

Sternberg, Steve, and Mary Beth Marklein. "College Seeks CDC's Assistance." *USA Today* May 7, 2003: 7D. Print.

"Stories from Recovered Patients." *Guangzhou Daily* Feb. 12, 2003. Print.

"Student Studying in the U.S.A. Issued a Statement Urging Overseas Students to Postpone Traveling Back Home." *Guangzhou Daily* May 14, 2009. Print.

Sullivan, Patricia, and James Porter. *Opening Spaces: Writing Technologies and Critical Research Practices.* Greenwich, CT: Ablex, 1997. Print.

Sum, Ngai-ling. "Informational Capitalism and the Remaking of 'Greater China': Strategies of Siliconization." Mengin 206–35.

Sun, Chuanwei, and Lijuan Guo. "Two Weekly Newspapers in Guangdong Were Temporarily Shut Down Due to Biased Reports." *Lianhe Zaobao* [Singapore] Mar. 16, 2003. Print.

Sun, Huatong. "The Triumph of Users: Achieving Cultural Usability Goals with User Localization." *Technical Communication Quarterly* 15.4 (2006): 457–81. Print.

Surendran, Aparna. "Chinatown Hit by SARS Scare; Business Owners Seek to Allay Fears about the Mystery Illness." *Philadelphia Inquirer* Apr. 9, 2003: A1. Print.

Su, Xueshan. "Atypical Pneumonia in Guangdong: Test for the Government and the Media." *New Press* [Guangzhou] Feb. 14, 2003. Print.

"Swine Influenza: How Much of a Global Threat?" *Lancet* 373.9674 (May 2, 2009): 1495. Print.

Swingler, Steve. "SARS Virus Alert; Chinese Quarter like Ghost Town." *Birmingham Evening Mail* Apr. 17, 2003: 1–2. Print.

"Tackle Western Media: Xinhua." *South China Morning Post* [Hong Kong] Sept. 26, 2003: 1. Print.

Taylor, Chris. "China: SARS and the Politics of Silence. The Chinese Plague." *Age* [Melbourne] May 4, 2003. Print.

Taylor, Mark. *The Moment of Complexity: Emerging Network Culture.* Chicago: U of Chicago P, 2001. Print.

Taylor, Neil. "Net-spread Panic Proves Catchier than a Killer Virus." *South China Morning Post* [Hong Kong] Apr. 8, 2003: 2. Print.

"Ten Questions from Journalists about Atypical Pneumonia in Guangdong and Answers from Related Authorities." *New Press* [Guangdong] Feb. 12, 2007: 9. Print.

"Text of Chancellor Robert Berdahl's May 10 Announcement Modifying Campus SARS Policy for International Summer School Students." *University of Berkeley*, May 10, 2003. Web. Nov. 29, 2003. <http://www.berkeley.edu/news/media/releases/2003/05/10_sars_berdahl.shtml>.

Thatcher, Barry L. "Issues of Validity in Intercultural Professional Communication Research." *Journal of Business and Technical Communication* 15 (2001): 458–89. Print.

Thompson, Allan. "WHO Stands by Travel Alert Despite Appeals from Canada." *Toronto Star* Apr. 25, 2003: A4. Print.

"Thorough Cleaning before School Started." *Southern Daily* [Guangdong] Feb. 14, 2003: 17. Print.

"Three Lessons of SARS." *Scientific American* 289.1 (2003): 8. Print.

Ting-Toomey, Stella. "Toward a Theory of Conflict and Culture." *Communication, Culture and Organizational Processes.* Ed. William B. Gudykunst, Leah P. Stewart, and Stella Ting-Toomey Beverly Hills, CA: Sage, 1985. 71–86. Print.

"Tips from Physician about Infectious Disease." *Guangzhou Daily* Feb. 12, 2003: 13. Print.

"To Return or Not to Return: Concerns about Overseas Students; Chinese Working Together to Combat Swine Flu." *Chinaview News,* May 19, 2009. Web. Oct. 2, 2009. <http://www.chinareviewnews.com>.

Treichler, Paula. "AIDS, Homophobia, and Biomedical Discourse: An Epidemic of Signification." *AIDS: Cultural Analysis/Cultural Activism.* Ed. D. Crimp. Cambridge, MA: MIT P, 1988. 31–70. Print.

———. *How to Have Theory in an Epidemic: Cultural Chronicles of AIDS.* Durham: Duke UP, 1999. Print.

Trifonov, V., H. Khiabanian, and R. Rabadan. "Geographic Dependence, Surveillance, and Origins of the 2009 Influenza A (H1N1) Virus." *New England Journal of Medicine* 361 (2009): 115–19. Print. DOI: 10.1056/NEJMp0904572.

Tsang, Thomas F. "The Experience of Hong Kong." *China's Capacity to Manage Infectious Diseases: Global Implications.* Ed. Xiaoqing Lu. Washington, DC: CSIS, 2010. 83–85. Print.

Tufte, Edward. *Envisioning Information.* Cheshire, CT: Graphics, 1990. Print.

"Twenty Days' Continuous Work." *Southern Daily* [Guangzhou], Feb. 22, 2003: 7. Print.

"Unexplained Pneumonia Suddenly Attacked Zhongshan." *New Press* [Guangzhou], Feb. 11, 2003. Print.

Ungar, Sheldon. "Hot Crises and Media Reassurance: A Comparison of Emerging Diseases and Ebola Zaire." *British Journal of Sociology* 49.1 (1998): 36–56. Print.

———. "Moral Panic versus the Risk Society: The Implications of the Changing Sites of Social Anxiety." *British Journal of Sociology* 52.2 (2001): 271–91. Print.

"Unknown Pneumonia Attacked Zhongshan City." *New Press* [Guangzhou] Jan. 16, 2003: 10. Print.

"Update: Outbreak of Severe Acute Respiratory Syndrome—Worldwide, 2003." *MMWR* 52.12 (2003): 241–48. Print.

van Rijn, Nicolaas. "Britain Warns Its Citizens Not to Travel to Toronto." *Toronto Star* Apr. 24, 2003: A01. Print.

Voice of America. "Number of Foreign Students Rises in US." *Voice of America,*

Nov. 14, 2007. Web. Jan. 8, 2009. <http://learningenglish.voanews.com/con-
tent/a-23-2007-11-14-voa2-83133202/127329.html>.

Waldby, Catherine. *AIDS and the Body Politics: Biomedicine and Sexual Difference.* London: Routledge, 1996. Print.

Wald, Priscilla. *Contagious: Cultures, Carriers, and the Outbreak Narrative.* Durham: Duke UP, 2008. Print.

Waldron, Arthur. "The Chinese Sickness." *Commentary* 2003: 36–43. Print.

Wang, Jiangmin, and Shouming Ji. "Guangdong Reorganized the Media to Keep the Outbreak a Secret: Hong Kong Got Infected." *Asian Weekly* May 2003: 5. Print.

Wang, Junping. "About a Love Called Refraining from Going Home." *People's Daily* May 20, 2009: 7. Print.

Wang, Ling-chi. "UC Berkeley's SARS Student Ban Dangerous, Misguided." *New America Media*, May 6, 2003. Web. Oct. 2, 2009. <http://news.newamericamedia .org/news/view_article.html?article_id=5037ff33f7e9bb4abb3849bb6c66b657>.

Wang, Pang. "Over Six Million Migrant Workers Will Stay in Guangdong during the Spring Festival." *Xinhuanet*, Jan. 13, 2003. Web. Sept. 3, 2006. <http://news. xinhuanet.com/employment/2003-01/13/content_688285.htm>.

Wang, Yanlai. *China's Economic Development and Democratization.* Burlington, VT: Ashgate, 2003. Print.

Wang, Zhu. "Over 55 Million People Used Mobile Text Messages in China." *Xin-huanet*, Oct. 30, 2002. Web. May 4, 2005. <news.xinhuanet.com/china/2002-10 /30/c_132840284.htm>.

Weber, Ian, Tan Howe Yang, and Law Loo Shien. "'Triumph over Adversity': Singa-pore Mobilizes Confusian Values to Combat SARS." Powers and Xiaosui 145–62.

Weiss, Timothy. "Reading Culture: Professional Communication as Translation." *Journal of Business and Technical Communication* 11.3 (1997): 321–39. Print.

Wenger, Dennis E. "Community Response to Disaster: Functional and Structural Alterations." *Disasters: Theory and Research.* Ed. E. L. Quarantelli. Beverly Hills, CA: Sage, 1978. 17–47. Print.

Westfeldt, Amy. "Survey: Chinatown Business Down since 9/11, SARS." *Associated Press State & Local Wire*, Apr. 28, 2003. *LexisNexis® Academic.* Web. Aug. 23, 2004.

"We Worked Together to Conquer Atypical Pneumonia." *Kdnet*, Apr. 20, 2003. Web. June 12, 2004. <http://club.kdnet.net/dispbbs.asp?page=1&boardid=52&id =611883>.

"When Coverage Goes Viral." *Toronto Star* May 9, 2009: IN06. Print.

"WHO: China Takes Appropriate Actions in Preventing H1N1." *People's Daily* May 5, 2009: 9. Print.

"WHO Expert: 'I Trust Our Chinese Counterparts.'" *People's Daily* Apr. 21, 2003: 4. Print.

"WHO Experts: No Big Risk to Stay in Guangzhou." *People's Daily* Apr. 8, 2003: 11. Print.

"WHO Initiates Setting up Surveillance, Response System against SARS." *People's Daily*, May 23, 2003. Web. Oct. 16, 2005. <http://english.peopledaily.com.cn/200305/23/eng20030523_117103.shtml>.

"WHO Prescribes Restraint with Swine-Flu Measures." *Washington Times* May 5, 2009: A01. Print.

"WHO Suggests SARS Observation Network in China." *People's Daily*, Apr. 17, 2003. Web. June 21, 2005. <http://english.peopledaily.com.cn/200304/17/eng20030417_115320.shtml.>

"Why Japan Escaped SARS: No Spitting, Frequent Hand Washing and Show." *Yangchen Evening* [Guangdong] May 5, 2003: 15. Print.

Wilson, Rob, and Wimal Dissanayake, eds. *Global/Local: Cultural Production and the Transnational Imaginary*. Durham: Duke UP, 1996. Print.

Windt, Lynn, and Theodore Hinds. *The Cold War as Rhetoric: The Beginnings, 1945–1950*. New York: Praeger, 1991. Print.

Wong, Margaret. "Cellphone Firm Offers SARS Sites Dial-a-List." *National Post* Apr. 19, 2003: A6. Print.

Wong, Victor. "Racialization of SARS." *Geocities*, 2003. Web. Oct. 7, 2004. <http://www.geocities.com/newsonsars>.

World Health Organization. "Acute Respiratory Syndrome in Hong Kong Special Administrative Region of China/ Viet Nam." *World Health Organization*, Mar. 12, 2003. Web. Oct. 9, 2009. <http://www.who.int/csr/don/2003_03_12/en/>.

———. "No Rationale for Travel Restrictions." *World Health Organization*, May 1, 2009. Web. Oct. 9, 2009. <http://www.who.int/csr/disease/swineflu/guidance/public_health/travel_advice/en/index.html>.

———. "Severe Acute Respiratory Syndrome (SARS)—Multi-Country Outbreak—Update 2." *World Health Organization*, Mar. 17, 2003. Web. Oct. 7, 2004. <http://www.WHO.int/csr/sars/archive/>.

———. "Swine Flu Illness in the United States and Mexico—Update 2." *World Health Organization*, Apr. 25, 2009. Web. May 13, 2010. <http://www.who.int/csr/don/2009_04_26/en/index.html>.

———. "Swine Influenza—Update 3." *World Health Organization*, Apr. 27, 2009. Web. May 13, 2010. <http://www.who.int/csr/don/2009_04_27/en/index.html>.

———. "Update 3—Advice for Travelers." *World Health Organization*, Mar. 18, 2003. Web. Oct. 7, 2004. <http://www.WHO.int/csr/sars/archive/>.

———. "Update 8—Disease Outbreak Reported." *World Health Organization*, Mar. 24, 2003. Web. Oct. 7, 2004. <http://www.WHO.int/csr/sars/archive/>.

———. "Update 9—Updated Travel Advice." *World Health Organization*, Mar. 25, 2003. Web. Oct. 7, 2004. <http://www.WHO.int/csr/sars/archive/>.

——. "Update 10—Data from China, Countries Introduce Stringent Control Measures." *World Health Organization*, Mar. 26, 2003. Web. Oct. 7, 2004. <http://www.WHO.int/csr/sars/archive/>.

——. "Update 11—WHO Recommends New Measures to Prevent Travel-related Spread of SARS." *World Health Organization*, Mar. 27, 2003. Web. Oct. 7, 2004. <http://www.WHO.int/csr/sars/archive/>.

——. "Update 12—SARS Virus Close to Conclusive Identification, New Tests for Rapid Diagnosis Ready Soon." *World Health Organization*, Mar. 27, 2003. Web. Oct. 7, 2004. <http://www.WHO.int/csr/sars/archive/>.

——. "Update 13—China joins WHO Collaborative Network." *World Health Organization*, Mar. 28, 2003. Web. Oct. 7, 2004. <http://www.WHO.int/csr /sars/archive/>.

——. "Update 17—Travel Advice—Hong Kong Special Administrative Region of China, and Guangdong Province, China." *World Health Organization*, Apr. 2, 2003. Web. Oct. 7, 2004. <http://www.WHO.int/csr/sars/archive/>.

——. "Update 18—SARS Outbreak: WHO Investigation Team Moves to China, New Travel Advice Announced [WHO Press Release]." *World Health Organization*, Apr. 2, 2003. Web. Oct. 7, 2004. <http://www.WHO.int/csr/sars /archive/>.

——. "Update 19—China Deepens Its Collaboration to Contain SARS, WHO Revises Its Advice to International Travelers as New Data Come in." *World Health Organization*, Apr. 2, 2003. Web. Oct. 7, 2004. <http://www.WHO.int /csr/sars/archive/>.

——. "Update 25—Interim Report of WHO Team in China, Status of the Main SARS Outbreaks in Different Countries." *World Health Organization*, Apr. 9, 2003. Web. Oct. 7, 2004. <http://www.WHO.int/csr/sars/archive/>.

——. "Update 32—Situation in China and Hong Kong, status of diagnostic tests." *World Health Organization*, Apr. 17, 2003. Web. Oct. 7, 2004. <http://www .WHO.int/csr/sars/archive/>.

——. "Update 37—WHO Extends Its SARS-related Travel Advice to Beijing and Shanxi Province in China and to Toronto Canada." *World Health Organization*, Apr. 23, 2003. Web. Oct. 7, 2004. <http://www.WHO.int/csr/sars/archive/>.

——. "Update 58—First Global Consultation on SARS Epidemiology, Travel Recommendations." *World Health Organization*, May 17, 2003. Web. Oct. 7, 2004. <http://www.WHO.int/csr/sars/archive/>.

——. "Update 72—Situation in China." *World Health Organization*, June 3, 2003. Web. Oct. 7, 2004. <http://www.WHO.int/csr/sars/archive/>.

——. "Update 80—Change in Travel Recommendations for Parts of China, Situation in Toronto." *World Health Organization*, June 13, 2003. Web. Oct. 7, 2004. <http://www.WHO.int/csr/sars/archive/>.

———. "Update 87—World Health Organization Changes Last Remaining Travel Recommendation—for Beijing, China." *World Health Organization*, June 24, 2003. Web. Oct. 7, 2004. <http://www.who.int/csr/don/2003_06_24/en/>.

———. "World Health Organization Issues Emergency Travel Advisory." *World Health Organization*, Mar. 15, 2003. Web. Oct. 7, 2004. <http://www.who.int /whr/2003/en/>.

———. "World Health Report for 2003—Shaping the Future." *World Health Organization*, 2003. Web. Oct. 7, 2004. <http://www.who.int/whr/2003/en/>.

Wu, Ang. "Reflection on Atypical Pneumonia in Guangdong: What Role Should the Government Play?" *Sanlian Weekly* [Shanghai] Feb. 21, 2003: 15. Print.

Wurman, Richard S. *Information Anxiety 2*. Indianapolis: QUE, 2001. Print.

Wu, Xinghua. "Hunan's Stipulation: Anyone Entering or Returning to Hunan Will Be Quarantined." *People*, May 1, 2003. Web. Oct. 7, 2004. <http://www .people.com.cn>.

Xiao, Jie. "SARS Greatly Decreases Chinatown Businesses in Philadelphia." *Dajiyuan EpochTime* [Washington, DC] Apr. 15, 2003: 17. Print.

Xiao, Ping. "Lack of Trust on the Public: Analysis of the Reason Causing Mass Panic in Atypical Pneumonia in Guangzhou." *New Press* [Guangzhou] Feb. 14, 2003: 15. Print.

———. "Reasons Leading to Mass Panic about the Strange Disease in Guangdong: Information Block Being the Culprit." *New Press* [Guangzhou] Feb. 14, 2003: 13. Print.

Xiao, Ping, and Lin Jinjun. "Focus on Atypical Pneumonia in the Guangdong Province." *New Press* [Guangzhou] Feb. 12, 2003: 2. Print.

Yan, Su, Xin Fu, and Pingge Xu. "Vice Governor Visited Medical Workers in the Hospital." *Guangzhou Daily* Feb. 13, 2003. Print.

Yan, Yan, and Helin Pan. "Rumors of Contagious Pneumonia Resulted in Mass Panic: Citizens Waited in Line to Purchase Drugs." *Information Time* [Guangzhou] Jan. 19, 2003: 7. Print.

Yardley, Jim. "A Hundred Cellphones Bloom, and Chinese Take to the Streets." *New York Times* Apr. 25, 2005: A1. Print.

Yeung, Chris, and Mary Ann Benitez. "Outbreak Began in Guangdong, WHO Believes." *South China Morning Post* [Hong Kong] Mar. 22, 2003: 9. Print.

Ying, Leu Siew. "Illness Is Now under Control, Says Province." *South China Morning Post* [Hong Kong] Mar. 22, 2003: 9. Print.

———. "Roche Denies Spreading Guangdong Flu Rumours." *South China Morning Post* [Hong Kong]. Feb. 19, 2003: 1. Print.

Ying, Leu Siew, and Ella Lee. "Panic Grips Guangdong as Mysterious Pneumonia-like Virus Kills 6." *South China Morning Post* [Hong Kong] Feb. 11, 2003: 1. Print.

Young, James G. "My Experience with SARS." *SARS in Context: Memory, History, Policy.* Ed. Jacalyn Duffin and Arthur Sweetman. Montreal: McGill Queens UP, 2006. 19–26. Print.

You, Xiaoye. "The *Way*, Multimodality of Ritual Symbols, and Social Change: Reading Confucius's *Analects* as a Rhetoric." *Rhetoric Society Quarterly* 36.4 (2006): 425–48. Print.

———. *Writing in the Devil's Tongue: A History of English Composition in China.* Carbondale: Southern Illinois UP, 2010. Print.

"Zejiang Province Initiated Strong, Proactive Measures to Prevent Import of SARS." *Metropolitan Express* [Hangzhou] May 1, 2003: 7. Print.

Zeng, Guang. "A Letter to Overseas Chinese Students." *Xinhua*, May 16, 2009. Web. Oct. 7, 2004. <http://www.xinhua.com.cn>.

Zeng, Li, and Chen Shen. "Three Goal in SARS Control in the Countryside: No Mass Spread, No Health Damage, Ensuring Stability." *Chinanews.net*, May 15, 2003. Web. Oct. 7, 2004. <http://www.chinanews.com>.

Zhang, Ed. "Capital Tightening Hukou System to Limit Migrants." *South China Morning Post* [Hong Kong] May 12, 2011: 06. Print.

Zhang, J. "Mass Media in China: Controlled Transformation." *International Communications: A Media Literacy Approach.* Ed. Art Silverblatt and Nikolai Zlobin. Armonk, NY: Sharpe, 2004. 165–69. Print.

Zhang, Yangzhong. "The Politics of HIV/AIDS in China." *Asian Perspective* 30.1 (2006): 95–125. Print.

Zhao, Yuezhi. *Media, Market, and Democracy in China: Between the Party Line and the Bottom Line.* Urbana: U of Illinois P, 1998. Print.

Zhu, Yu. "Minister of Health Zhang Wenkang Announced, 'China Is Safe.'" *Xinghua News Agency* Apr. 3, 2003. Print.

Ziporyn, Terra. *Disease in the Popular American Press: The Case of Diphtheria, Typhoid Fever, and Syphilis, 1870–1920.* New York: Greenwood, 1988. Print.

Index

Italicized page numbers indicate tables and figures.

Huiling Ding is an assistant professor at North Carolina State University, where she teaches technical communication and rhetoric. Her essays have appeared in *Technical Communication Quarterly, Written Communication, Rhetoric Review, Business Communication Quarterly, Journal of Medical Humanities, English for Specific Purposes*, and *China Media Research*. She received the 2008 Editor's Pick New Scholar Award for her article "The Use of Cognitive and Social Apprenticeship to Teach a Disciplinary Genre: Initiation of Graduate Students into NIH Grant Writing."